Health Professionals' Guide to

PHYSICAL MANAGEMENT OF PARKINSON'S DISEASE

Miriam P. Boelen, PT

Human Kinetics

Library of Congress Cataloging-in-Publication Data

Boelen, Miriam P.
   Health professionals' guide to physical management of Parkinson's
disease / Miriam P. Boelen.
         p.   ;   cm.
   Includes bibliographical references and index.
   ISBN-13: 978-0-7360-7492-6 (hard cover)
   ISBN-10: 0-7360-7492-9 (hard cover)
   1. Parkinson's disease--Physical therapy.   2. Parkinson's disease--
Patients--Rehabilitation.   I. Title.
   [DNLM: 1. Parkinson Disease--therapy.   2. Physical Therapy
Modalities.   WL 359 B671h 2009]
   RC382.B57 2009
   616.8'33--dc22

                                                      2009006760

ISBN-10: 0-7360-7492-9 (print)   ISBN-10: 0-7360-8546-7 (Adobe PDF)
ISBN-13: 978-0-7360-7492-6 (print)   ISBN-13: 978-0-7360-8546-5 (Adobe PDF)

The Web addresses cited in this text were current as of January 2009, unless otherwise noted.

Acquisitions Editor: Loarn D. Robertson, PhD; **Developmental Editor:** Elaine H. Mustain; **Managing Editor:** Melissa J. Zavala; **Assistant Editor:** Christine Bryant Cohen; **Copyeditor:** Bob Replinger; **Proofreader:** Pamela Johnson; **Indexer:** Andrea Hepner; **Permission Manager:** Dalene Reeder; **Graphic Designer:** Fred Starbird; **Graphic Artist:** Kathleen Boudreau-Fuoss; **Cover Designer:** Bob Reuther; **Photographer (interior):** Miriam Boelen, unless otherwise noted; **Photo Production Manager:** Jason Allen; **Art Manager:** Kelly Hendren; **Associate Art Manager:** Alan L. Wilborn; **Illustrator:** Keri Evans; **Printer:** Edwards Brothers

Printed in the United States of America   10   9   8   7   6   5   4   3   2   1

The paper in this book is certified under a sustainable forestry program.

Human Kinetics
Web site: www.HumanKinetics.com

United States: Human Kinetics
P.O. Box 5076, Champaign, IL 61825-5076
800-747-4457
e-mail: humank@hkusa.com

Canada: Human Kinetics
475 Devonshire Road Unit 100,
Windsor, ON N8Y 2L5
800-465-7301 (in Canada only)
e-mail: info@hkcanada.com

Europe: Human Kinetics
107 Bradford Road, Stanningley
Leeds LS28 6AT, United Kingdom
+44 (0) 113 255 5665
e-mail: hk@hkeurope.com

Australia: Human Kinetics
57A Price Avenue
Lower Mitcham, South Australia 5062
08 8372 0999
e-mail: info@hkaustralia.com

New Zealand: Human Kinetics
Division of Sports Distributors NZ Ltd.
P.O. Box 300 226 Albany, North Shore City, Auckland
0064 9 448 1207
e-mail: info@humankinetics.co.nz

This book is dedicated to my parents,
Bernard and Mary Boelen,
and all people with Parkinson's disease.

Contents

part I GENERAL ISSUES · · · · · · · · · · · · 1

part II DYSKINESIA · · · · · · · · · · · · · 53

List of Case Examples and Reproducible Items

Abbreviations and Acronyms

ACSM—American College of Sports Medicine

ADLs—activities of daily living

AFO—ankle–foot orthosis

APAs—anticipatory postural adjustments

APDA—American Parkinson Disease Association

BOS—base of support

BP—blood pressure

BPM—beats per minute

CNS—central nervous system

COG—center of gravity

COM—center of mass

COMT—catechol-O-methyltransferase

COP—center of pressure

DBS—deep brain stimulation or stimulator

FOG—freezing of gait

GPi—globus pallidus internus

HEP—home exercise program

L-dopa—levodopa

MAO-B—monoamine oxidase B

MSA—multiple systems atrophy

NPF—National Parkinson Foundation

OH—orthostatic hypotension

OT—occupational therapy or occupational therapist

PD—Parkinson's disease

PT—physical therapy or physical therapist

RAS—rhythmic auditory stimulation

Reps—repetitions

ROM—range of motion

RPE—rating of perceived exertion

S&E ADL Scale—Modified Schwab and England Activities of Daily Living Scale

STN—subthalamic nucleus

TENS—transcutaneous electrical nerve stimulation

POMA—performance-oriented mobility assessment

TUG—timed up and go

UPDRS—Unified Parkinson's Disease Rating Scale

YOPD—young onset Parkinson's disease

Preface

While we await the discovery of a cure for Parkinson's disease (PD), its medical management, which includes pharmacologic and surgical measures, is directed at the control of symptoms. Medical management has its limitations, however, when addressing secondary conditions resulting from rigidity and bradykinesia. Such management does not directly address potential or existing physical impairments such as loss of flexibility, strength, or cardiovascular endurance. Ignoring these aspects of PD can lead to unnecessary functional limitations or substantial disability. Physical interventions, however, can address these issues. Medical and physical interventions can work together to enhance overall quality of life significantly.

Yet in my 30 yr of experience as a physical therapist, the most recent 18 of which have been exclusively in treating patients with PD and similar hypokinetic movement disorders, I have been continually frustrated by the lack of a comprehensive clinical reference for selecting useful physical interventions. Physical therapy curricula provide minimal exposure to the care of people with PD or other movement disorders. Tidbits of information are scattered throughout a number of textbooks on a variety of subjects and are often difficult to obtain. Journal articles present useful research findings, but they often fail to make their way into clinical practice. Over the years I have also stumbled onto effective maneuvers through experience, which I desired to share with the wider caregiver community. This material was begging to be brought together in a single reference that would advance the treatment of patients with PD. This book is the result.

The focus of this text is to fill the existing void by comprehensively addressing the physical component of PD management in a single volume. The book is intended to be a complete yet concise and easy-to-use clinical guide. In addition to exercise, physical interventions covered include compensatory strategies such as visual and auditory cues, attention strategies, and adaptive devices. Although much of the book draws on evidence-based work, a substantial portion of it is based on my clinical experience with patients with PD. This book will be used primarily by physical therapists, although any health care professional who has contact with patients with PD can benefit from its contents.

Part I provides a general understanding of PD and discusses the scope of care provided by therapists, physicians, patients themselves, and their caregivers. Chapter 1 offers an overview of interventions for the physical management of the disease. At the end of this chapter is a case example to illustrate how this book can be used in a clinical setting. Most clinicians will benefit from reading the chapters in part I before they use the rest of the manual.

Because patients with Parkinson's do not all exhibit the same symptoms, the chapters in the remainder of the book are written as independent units to address discrete problem areas. These chapters can be used in any order as the need arises in clinical practice, and a preceding chapter need not be read to understand a subsequent chapter. Typically, the theory or background for each chapter is covered at the beginning of the chapter, and the interventions and practical information follow.

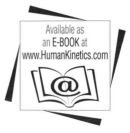

Available as an E-BOOK at www.HumanKinetics.com

Because most readers will not be reading the book from cover to cover but will be looking for answers to specific questions, chapters are extensively cross-referenced. A glossary at the end of the book will help the reader with commonly used terminology. Appendixes provide established PD questionnaires, tests, and norm values. The appendixes also contain patient handouts on compensatory strategies, suggestions for physical therapy goal setting and interventions, and sample evaluation forms that can be used as guides.

Each chapter contains a case example specific to the topic of the chapter. These examples have been simplified to emphasize the area being discussed. The case example in chapter 1 offers additional guidance about how to use this book and how to implement interventions based on problem areas.

Items in appendixes C and D, including informational sheets that can be given to patients, can be reproduced for clinical use. On page ix you will find a listing of these reproducible items as well as a listing of all the case examples.

I hope that you will find this book useful in making your clinical practice more productive and in improving patient outcomes. It is my wish that your patients with Parkinson's disease will be the ultimate beneficiaries of my work. This book was written for them.

Acknowledgments

I would like to thank the following people for their enlightenment, mentorship, support, or guidance.

Louis Boelen

Emma Broussard

Donna Frownfelter

Josephine Gould

Lori Nozaki

Ruth Rice

Mark Rogers

Karen Santelli

Judy Stoecker

Michael Thaut

Hailan Wang

A special thank you to all the people who have allowed their pictures to be printed in this book for the purpose of helping others.

GENERAL ISSUES

This opening part of the book is intended to give you a broad understanding of the umbrella of care required in the management of people with PD. This umbrella encompasses physical management by health professionals such as physical therapists, occupational therapists, speech therapists, and personal trainers. It also includes medical management by physicians, self-management through exercise, and, when self-management is difficult, help provided by the caregiver. This part acquaints you with the symptoms and stages of Parkinson's disease and the benefits of physical management at the various stages. It also guides you in efficient use of this book. Information is provided about medical management, which includes medicinal as well as surgical interventions. The importance of exercise is highlighted, notably its effects on functional abilities and the need for patients to be responsible for self-management. The final chapter in this part discusses caregivers, who are typically closely connected to the patient and often need education to help the patient as well as themselves.

chapter 1

Introduction to Parkinson's Disease and Its Physical Management

Among patients with Parkinson's disease (PD), the rate of progression and severity can vary greatly (Goetz et al., 2000). Some people can have PD for 20 or 30 yr and continue to function independently in the community. For others the disease course is relatively fast and unrelenting. The rate of this clinical progression is directly related to the rate of loss of dopamine-producing cells of the substantia nigra compacta in the midbrain. The cause for this loss is uncertain (idiopathic). The pattern of disease progression has been described by Hoehn and Yahr's staging of PD (Hoehn & Yahr, 1967). Neuroimaging studies have demonstrated a strong correlation with the loss of nigral dopaminergic neurons and the higher stages of Hoehn and Yahr (Goetz et al., 2004). In contrast to idiopathic PD, secondary Parkinsonism is caused by neuropathologies unrelated to the lack of dopamine production. The distinguishing symptoms of secondary Parkinsonism are reviewed in the next section. Regardless of a patient's Hoehn and Yahr stage or whether symptoms are because of secondary Parkinsonism, opportunities for physical and educational intervention are available. These interventions are outlined toward the end of the chapter. Finally, to facilitate efficient use of this book, a sample patient case is illustrated.

Distinguishing Features of Idiopathic Parkinson's Disease and Secondary Parkinsonism

The presentation of symptoms in people with idiopathic Parkinson's disease may exhibit commonalities with secondary Parkinsonism because of basal ganglia involvement. The precipitating underlying pathology, however, results from various causative factors.

Idiopathic Parkinson's Disease

Idiopathic Parkinson's disease (PD, also known as paralysis agitans) is known for its depletion of the neurotransmitter dopamine in the brain. This depletion is due to the death of the dopamine-producing cells in the substantia nigra compacta and is of unknown etiology. Dopamine is responsible for normalization of sequential movements, automaticity of learned movements, and normalization of tone. Symptoms of PD do not become apparent until approximately 80% of the neurons in the substantia nigra compacta are lost (Paulson & Stern, 2004).

The prevalence of PD increases with age. It affects approximately 1% of the population over age 65 and 2% of the population over age 80 (Goldman & Tanner, 1998). Young onset PD occurs in the 21 through 39 age group (Quinn et al., 1987) and accounts for approximately 10% of the population with PD. On rare occasions the onset of PD symptoms may occur before age 21, a circumstance classified as juvenile onset (Sethi, 2003). A preliminary diagnosis of PD requires two of the following three symptoms: bradykinesia (slowness of movement), rigidity, or resting tremor (Dewey, 2000). A more definitive diagnosis depends on the previously mentioned symptoms, a good response to dopamine replacement medications (L-dopa), and the absence of symptoms suggestive of another movement disorder. For example, people with PD do not exhibit initial symptoms of postural instability, orthostatic hypotension, or dementia. These symptoms are suggestive of Parkinson's Plus disorders (Sethi, 2003; Suchowersky et al., 2006). The initial symptoms of suspected PD, however, are typically not treated with L-dopa. Therefore, PD may not be ruled in or out until later in the disease progression, after L-dopa is initiated.

A significant number of people with PD who take L-dopa ultimately develop motor fluctuations and dyskinesias (e.g., choreatic movements). From the standpoint of physical management, therefore, any patient who takes L-dopa medication should be asked whether any mobility variations are related to their medication cycle (see chapter 2, "Medical and Surgical Interventions," pages 11–26). Choreatic movements are not a symptom of PD but a side effect of chronic use of L-dopa in combination with disease progression (Clissold et al., 2006; McColl et al., 2002).

Modified Hoehn and Yahr Staging of PD Progression

In 1967 Dr.'s Hoehn and Yahr published their landmark staging system for PD progression in the journal *Neurology* (Hoehn & Yahr, 1967). The original Hoehn and Yahr system had five full stages. The system was later modified slightly to include half-stages 1.5 and 2.5.

Modified Hoehn and Yahr Stages

- Stage 1 = Unilateral disease
- Stage 1.5 = Unilateral and axial involvement
- Stage 2 = Bilateral disease, balance intact
- Stage 2.5 = Mild bilateral disease with recovery on pull test
- Stage 3 = Mild to moderate bilateral disease; some postural instability; physically independent
- Stage 4 = Severe disability; still able to walk or stand unassisted
- Stage 5 = Wheelchair bound or bedridden unless aided

The modified system remains in general use today for monitoring patients with PD. These stages are listed in "Modified Hoehn and Yahr Stages." For simplicity, only the original full-stage Hoehn and Yahr rating scale will be discussed in this chapter regarding the physical management at each stage.

The Hoehn and Yahr staging system was developed before the use of L-dopa replacement medications, when the symptoms and level of mobility in PD were more predictable. As a result, Hoehn and Yahr stages 2 and 3 were more definitive—postural reflexes were either intact or impaired or absent. Since the advent of L-dopa replacement medications, Hoehn and Yahr stages 2 and 3 have become less static. L-dopa medications give the appearance of improvement in postural reflexes by reducing the symptoms of bradykinesia and rigidity. In addition, L-dopa improves mobility. Patients can therefore move in and out of Hoehn and Yahr stages depending on the effects of the medication (Nieuwboer et al., 2000). For example, during an "on" state, when dopamine levels are optimal, a person can be in Hoehn and Yahr stage 2. The patient then moves to Hoehn and Yahr stage 3 in his or her "off" state, when dopamine levels are suboptimal. The same process applies to Hoehn and Yahr stages 3 and 4.

Secondary Parkinsonism

Patients can present with Parkinsonian symptoms resulting from causes other than the loss of dopamine-producing cells. This circumstance includes a variety of conditions, all known as secondary Parkinsonism. The evaluative and treatment approach would be similar to that used with those who have PD. The causes of secondary Parkinsonism include the following:

• **Medications.** Neuroleptic medications that block dopamine receptors can precipitate Parkinsonian symptoms, but symptoms emerge bilaterally. People with PD initially exhibit unilateral symptoms (Molho & Factor, 2000).

• **Mini CVAs.** Mini CVAs that occur in the basal ganglia area can cause Parkinsonian symptoms. Onset is sudden when compared with PD.

• **Vascular Parkinsonism.** This type of secondary Parkinsonism is due to cerebrovascular disease involving the basal ganglia and subcortical white matter (Sibon et al., 2004). Symptoms primarily affect the lower extremities. Freezing of gait is more predominant than in idiopathic PD. Response to L-dopa is poor. Pyramidal symptoms such as weakness or spasticity may be present (Winikates & Jankovic, 1999).

• **Normal pressure hydrocephalus (NPH).** Patients with this diagnosis exhibit a slow shuffling gait with or without freezing (Giladi, et al., 1997). Unlike in PD, the gait is wide based and the patient will report urinary incontinence. The lateral ventricles of the brain, which are in close proximity to basal ganglia structures, are enlarged. Mild dementia is usually present and can worsen over time (Dewey, 2000). If NPH is suspected, a lumbar puncture is performed and cerebrospinal fluid is withdrawn. If symptoms improve from the spinal tap, the patient is considered an appropriate candidate for the insertion of a ventriculoperitoneal shunt. Symptom resolution is primarily noted in gait (Mori, 2001).

Guidelines for Physical Management

Physical management is necessary to complement the limitations of medical management (pharmacologic and surgical interventions). Various health care disciplines have a specialized focus to minimize musculoskeletal, respiratory, and cardiovascular impairments to optimize function. The ability to take care of oneself, communicate effectively, and optimize transfer and ambulatory abilities is the comprehensive goal.

Multidisciplinary Intervention

These guidelines are directed toward physical therapists. Multidisciplinary intervention, however, is often needed to address the physical management of patients with PD. Occupational and speech therapy in addition to physical therapy and patient education are necessary for optimal outcomes.

- Occupational Therapy (OT)
  - OT can facilitate improved abilities with activities of daily living (ADLs), which may or may not require the use of adaptive equipment.
  - A home safety evaluation can reduce the risk of falls by offering advice on the reduction of environmental hazards.
  - Recommendations on home modifications regarding environmental barriers can reduce difficulties with mobility for both the patient and the caregiver.
- Speech Therapy
  - People with PD are prone to swallowing problems (dysphasia) (Volonte et al., 2002). In advanced PD, swallowing problems may lead to aspiration pneumonia (Potulska et al., 2002). The speech–language therapist can assess for dysphasia and make recommendations for preventing aspiration.
  - Speech intelligibility has been found to be independent of disease severity or disease duration. Therefore, involvement of speech therapy at any of the Hoehn and Yahr stages may be indicated to improve intelligibility (Miller et al., 2007).
  - The speech–language therapist can intervene for problem areas such as voice loudness, articulation, vocal quality, and intelligibility.
- Patient education. All stages of Hoehn and Yahr should include patient education regarding the following issues:
  - Muscle weakness: Patients often think that PD causes muscle weakness. Patients may say that they feel weak, more so when the medication wears off. Although patients may perceive bradykinesia (slowness of movement) as weakness (Dewey, 2000), actual weakness is primarily the result of muscle disuse or other pathological processes unrelated to PD. Patients are often relieved when they discover that they can improve their strength.
  - Individuality of PD symptoms: A common misconception is that all people who have PD have the same symptoms. This population is diverse in their presentations. For example, not everyone has tremor, freezing, poor posture, or dementia. The rate of progression is also variable.
  - Importance of regular exercise and walking: Exercise and walking can optimize flexibility, strength, and mobility. These abilities are critical for long-term management. In the higher Hoehn and Yahr stages they can also reduce strain on the caregiver.
  - Resources: Patients should be made aware of the availability of supportive and educational resources through Parkinson's disease organizations (see chapter 4, page 48).

- Benefits of various allied health disciplines: The patient should be informed of the availability and benefits of physical therapy, occupational therapy, and speech therapy to improve self-management (see appendix D, "Can Therapy Help Me?").

Case Example

Debbie is a 77 yr old woman with a history of PD for 12 yr and now at Hoehn and Yahr stage 3. She is cognitively intact and ambulatory without an assist device. Appropriate resources for obtaining subjective information, objective evaluation procedures, goal setting, and therapeutic interventions are identified in the following sections. The significance of each step is discussed, and cross-references are given to relevant sections of the book.

Subjective Evaluation

Knowing the right questions to ask can bring out problem areas that may not be present at the time of the interview or apparent to the observer. Patients may forget to report problematic activities. Understanding the patient's greatest concerns as well as her or his goals regarding physical management can improve outcomes or in some cases establish realistic expectations. Establishing current exercise habits is critical in guiding long-term maintenance.

- Appendix C contains a sample subjective evaluation form that can be used in guiding questions to ask Debbie. The form includes both mainstream questions and questions specific to the PD population.
- Upon questioning, Debbie reports feeling less steady and losing her balance on occasion with static standing activities. She denies any unsteadiness while walking but believes that she is walking slower. She does not exercise but states that she stays active during the day. No other problem areas were noted.

Objective Evaluation

The objective evaluation helps identify, quantify, and qualify where and why a person is having difficulties so that deficiencies can be targeted through interventions to optimize outcomes. The following measures are taken during Debbie's objective evaluation:

- Appendix C contains a sample objective evaluation form that can be used to help record objective information regarding impairments, dysfunctions, and disabilities.
- Because Debbie reports loss of balance while standing, her postural reflexes are evaluated (see chapter 7, "Postural Instability," pages 80–83).
- Additional balance testing is performed. Appendix B contains established balance tests. The Berg balance test is chosen.
- Chapter 12, "Gait Deviations and Instability," offers procedures for determining gait velocity, which are useful in evaluating all patients with PD, regardless of

(continued)

> subjective reports. Gait velocity is particularly important for Debbie, who thinks that she is walking slower.
> - Appendix B contains gait velocity norms, which are needed for a baseline reference and goal setting.
> - Objective findings: Debbie exhibits impaired postural reflexes, demonstrated by her difficulty in regaining balance when performing the unexpected retropulsive test. Otherwise, the Berg balance score showed that Debbie has good balance. Gait is steady. Gait velocity is 30% below age- and sex-matched norms. She is functionally independent but at risk of falls with static standing activities. Currently, strength and range of motion (ROM) are within functional limits, but she is at risk of musculoskeletal and cardiovascular impairments because of the combined effects of lack of exercise and PD symptoms.

Goals

Goals are based on current subjective and objective problem areas as well as potential areas at risk. Some patients may require only a few goals, and others will have a substantial list. A list of sample goals is provided in appendix C to aid in goal setting. From this list we will pick four goals for Debbie:

- One of the goals is to improve stability with static standing to prevent loss of balance.
- Second, she should be able to perform a stepping strategy in response to a loss of balance to prevent a fall from occurring.
- Third, her gait velocity needs improvement for optimal functional ambulation (see chapter 12, pages 147–149).
- Last, she needs to be independent in a general conditioning, flexibility, and walking program for prevention and maintenance (see chapter 3, pages 27–41).

Therapeutic Interventions

For a quick overview of treatment interventions, refer to "Problem-Oriented Treatment Interventions" in appendix D. For detailed information regarding specific problem areas, including treatment interventions, refer to the applicable chapters. See "Sample Progress Note" in appendix C for suggestions about documenting interventions.

Outcomes

In general, outcomes depend on the following factors: disease severity, comorbidities, cognition, motivation, and adherence to your recommendations. In more severely involved people with PD, the level of care-giving support can also affect outcomes. Each case example in the book has a brief discussion that relates outcomes to the influencing factors. In this case, Debbie is in Hoehn and Yahr stage 3 yet remains at a high level of function and stays active. Cognitively, she is intact. Improvements in her walking can be expected if she adheres to the recommended walking program. Deconditioning can be prevented by consistent participation in an exercise program. Remembering to use compensatory strategies will minimize the risk of falls.

Physical Management at Each Hoehn and Yahr Stage

People in each Hoehn and Yahr stage can benefit from physical interventions, but at each stage the focus becomes progressively more comprehensive and builds on interventions received in previous stages. Adjustments in compensatory strategies are often necessary to optimize movement at various stages, but exercise and activity is important throughout.

- **Stage 1 (unilateral disease).** At this stage the focus is on health promotion (optimizing general strength, flexibility, balance, and endurance) and prevention of potential impairments. Physical therapy interventions can encourage and educate the patient in a lifestyle of conditioning, which can prevent or minimize secondary impairments resulting from PD (see chapter 3, "Exercise and Rehabilitation Considerations," pages 27–41). Asymmetry of gait because of unilateral involvement may interfere with mobility or balance and should be addressed. The patient should be advised in compensatory strategies to improve movement if needed. A compensatory strategy at this stage typically involves paying more attention to movements that lack automaticity or magnitude (attention strategy) (see chapter 13, "Compensatory Strategies for Gait Interventions," pages 160–162).

- **Stage 2 (bilateral involvement without impairment of balance).** Although balance is not impaired at this stage of PD, gait deviations can result in increased unsteadiness and heightened risk of falls. Gait deviations should be addressed to improve steadiness (see part V, "Gait"). Depending on the patient's symptoms, compensatory strategies to prevent falls and control "freezing" should be taught. Besides the attention strategy, compensatory strategies may include a greater scope of sensory cues such as visual or auditory cues. Patients who take L-dopa replacement medications may exhibit motor fluctuations. Differing treatment strategies may be required depending on the medication cycle. Exercises should be performed when dopamine levels are optimal because movement will be less difficult. Multidisciplinary interventions should be promoted as needed.

- **Stage 3 (mild to moderate bilateral involvement; some postural instability but physically independent).** At this stage the main goal is fall prevention, which can be accomplished through conditioning, balance training, use of appropriate ambulatory devices (see chapter 16, pages 187–200), and education in compensatory strategies. The compensatory strategies for balance may include improving stability during static standing by adjusting the position of the feet and learning effective stepping strategies (see chapter 7, pages 85–91) As noted, in stage 2, patients are typically taking L-dopa replacement therapy and usually exhibit motor fluctuations. Caregivers should be educated about how to assist the person with PD. Multidisciplinary interventions should be promoted as needed (occupational therapy or speech therapy).

- **Stages 4 (severe disability but still able to walk or stand unassisted) and 5 (wheelchair bound or bedridden unless aided).** At these stages greater emphasis is placed on educating caregivers and showing them how to assist with bed mobility, transfers, ambulation, and exercises (see chapter 4, "Equipping Caregivers," pages 49–50). Exercises should be directed toward maximizing flexibility for ADLs and mobility. A wheelchair assessment may be necessary to optimize function, maintain comfort, and prevent skin breakdown. Multidisciplinary interventions should be promoted as needed (occupational therapy or speech therapy).

Summary

1. Although idiopathic Parkinson's disease is a progressive neurologic disorder characterized by initial symptoms of rigidity, bradykinesia, or tremor because of the loss of dopamine production in the brain, its rate and severity of progression can vary greatly between individuals.

2. Secondary Parkinsonism manifests with some similar symptoms, which are not due to loss of dopamine production.

3. The Hoehn and Yahr scale provides a way to classify the extent of PD progression.

4. Medical and physical interventions can work together synergistically in people with PD to enhance overall quality of life.

5. Education should be an integral part of therapeutic interventions for people with PD.

6. Multidisciplinary interventions should be considered to optimize self-management.

chapter 2

Medical
and Surgical Interventions

No medication can currently cure Parkinson's disease (PD). Patients who are initially diagnosed with PD may or may not be started on a medication, depending in part on their symptoms. Some drugs are thought to be neuroprotective and are given for that reason. But PD medications do have side effects. Motor fluctuations (a side effect of L-dopa medications) and dyskinesias have been related to cumulative L-dopa dosing in combination with disease progression (Hauser et al., 2006). Dopamine agonists and L-dopa can also lower blood pressure (Bouhaddi et al., 2004; Kujawa et al., 2000). The objectives of PD medications are

- to optimize mobility and
- to minimize the side effects of the medications.

As Parkinson's disease progresses, however, controlling symptoms with medications becomes more difficult. The severity of motor fluctuations and dyskinesias can become disabling. At this point deep brain stimulation (DBS) may be considered to control symptoms. Theoretically, DBS inhibits the hyperactivity of the subthalamic nucleus (STN) or the globus pallidus internus (GPi) through electrical stimulation so that thalamic output can be normalized and thereby improve PD symptoms (Chen et al., 2003). Evidence has supported effective management of PD symptoms with bilateral STN deep brain stimulation (Tir et al., 2007). Anti-PD medications can be substantially reduced when combined with the benefits from the DBS. A study noted continued reductions of anti-PD medications of 47.9% at 3 yr and 39.8% at 5 yr (Piboolnurak et al., 2007). The net result is a reduction in dyskinesias, improved "on" time, and reduced "off" time.

Medications

To facilitate movement and improve mobility, medications work to optimize dopamine levels in the basal ganglia. They do this by replenishing the deficiency of dopamine in the brain, facilitating postsynaptic transmission of the dopaminergic neurons, minimizing enzymatic breakdown of L-dopa or dopamine, or by improving the balance between the neurotransmitters dopamine and acetylcholine. The wide array of medications available for the PD population means that they can be varied in hopes of accomplishing the second objective of medication, namely minimizing the side effects that can result from the combined effects of chronic L-dopa usage and disease progression.

The manipulation of medications is equal parts art and science, a process most effectively managed by a neurologist who specializes in movement disorders. Combinations of medications are typically needed to obtain optimal results, and intermittent adjustments are made depending on disease progression and complications.

Dopaminergic Drugs

Medications are categorized by their neurophysiological affects. For example, the medications that replenish dopamine are called dopamine replacement drugs. The term *L-dopa* is synonymous with any of the dopamine replacement medications. Medications that stimulate the postsynaptic receptors are called dopamine agonists. Medications that interfere with the enzymatic breakdown of dopamine to optimize dopamine levels are called either catechol-O-methyltransferase (COMT) inhibitors or monoamine oxidase B (MAO-B) inhibitors.

Dopamine Replacement Medications

The group of drugs most clinically significant to the rehabilitative professional are the dopamine replacement drugs (L-dopa) because their formulations affect mobility variations more dramatically than any other class of drug does. To date, this group remains the most effective medication in the treatment of PD. You will want to know whether your patient is taking this type of drug. If motor fluctuations are present, mobility problems encountered during both "on" and "off" states should be addressed. "Off" freezing is freezing that occurs while dopamine levels are low. Symptoms that show the greatest improvement in response to this class of drugs are shown in table 2.1. Dopamine depletion may not be responsible for all Parkinsonian symptoms because not all symptoms improve with L-dopa or only minimal improvements may be noted. Table 2.1 also lists symptoms that tend to be resistant to dopamine replacement medications.

Patients can generally take this type of medicine before or after meals. But because L-dopa can cause nausea, those who are subject to this side effect should take it during or just after a meal. Because dietary protein and L-dopa compete for absorption, people with more advanced PD with significant motor fluctuations may need to monitor their dietary protein intake (Hauser & Zesiewicz, 2000).

Carbidopa and benserazide are dopa decarboxylase inhibitors used in combination with L-dopa to block the breakdown of exogenous L-dopa outside the central nervous system, allowing greater concentrations of it to enter the brain. Because of these benefits, dopamine replacement drugs are formulated to have both dopa decarboxylase inhibitors and L-dopa in one pill. The most commonly used dopamine replacement drugs are carbidopa–levodopa (Sinemet) in the United States and benserazide–levodopa (Madopar) outside the United States. The aromatic amino acid dopa decarboxylase is an enzyme that metabolizes L-dopa to dopamine. L-dopa is capable of crossing the blood brain barrier, but dopamine is not. Carbidopa and benserazide do not cross the blood brain barrier and therefore do not interfere with the conversion of L-dopa to dopamine in the brain (Santiago & Factor, 2003). Dopa-decarboxylase inhibitors also help reduce symptoms of nausea and allow lower dosages of levodopa to be administered.

Dopamine Receptor Agonists

Dopamine receptor agonists mimic the action of dopamine and directly stimulate the dopamine receptors. With the exception of apomorphine, these medications may be used

Table 2.1 Dopamine Replacement Medications

Generic name	Brand name	Benefits[1]	Symptoms resistant to this class of drugs[2]	Common side effects*[3]
Carbidopa–levodopa	Sinemet	• Reduced rigidity, reduced tremor reduced bradykinesia • Improved gait • Reduced "off" freezing • Stalevo: reduces motor fluctuations • Parcopa: beneficial for people who have swallowing difficulties	• Postural responses for balance control • "On" freezing • Posture	• Nausea and vomiting • Orthostatic hypotension • Motor fluctuations • Dyskinesias • Confusion • Delusions • Visual hallucinations
Benserazide–levodopa	Madopar			
Carbidopa–levodopa controlled release	Sinemet CR			
Carbidopa–levodopa–entacapone	Stalevo			
Carbidopa–levodopa (orally disintegrating tablet)	Parcopa			

*Side effects related to longer-term use of L-dopa, disease progression, or drug sensitivity.
[1]Brooks et al., 2005; Burleigh et al., 1995; Pavese et al., 2006
[2]Horak et al., 1996; Kompoliti, 2000; Poluha et al., 1998; Shaheda et al., 2005
[3]Not all inclusive; Hauser et al., 2006

as a first treatment option in people with early PD. They can be used with or without L-dopa. Increased "on" time and a reduction of "off" time has been a benefit when taken in conjunction with L-dopa in people who have motor fluctuations (Slawek, 2007). Dopamine agonists have exhibited potential neuroprotective properties. In other words, these drugs may slow the progressive neurodegeneration of dopaminergic neurons (Bonuccelli & Pavese, 2007) (see table 2.2).

Apomorphine can provide a quality of symptomatic benefit that is equivalent to that of levodopa. Apomorphine (Apokyn) is injected subcutaneously and used as needed for severe "off" states. Approximately 10 min are required to relieve the "off" state, and the effect lasts about 90 min. This short-acting drug helps bridge the gap of low dopamine levels until the next dose of carbidopa–levodopa becomes effective.

Pergolide (Permax), a dopamine agonist, has been taken off the market because of the risk of causing heart valve damage (Schade et al., 2007).

Catechol-O-Methyltransferase Inhibitors

Catechol-O-methyltransferase (COMT) is an enzyme that metabolizes levodopa. When carbidopa–levodopa is administered, COMT becomes the primary enzyme to metabolize levodopa to dopamine (Kaakkola, 2000). Inhibiting catechol-O-methyltransferase with the use of COMT inhibitors allows more L-dopa to reach the brain instead of being broken down in the periphery (Jankovic & Stacy, 2007). This class of drugs helps reduce motor fluctuations and prolongs the effect of each levodopa dose. The drug Tasmar can cause liver damage and therefore needs to be monitored (see table 2.3).

Monoamine Oxidase B (MAO-B) Inhibitors

Monoamine oxidase is a major enzyme in the brain that breaks down dopamine. MAO-B inhibitors reduce the breakdown of dopamine at the synaptic cleft, resulting in higher levels

Table 2.2 Dopamine Receptor Agonists

Generic name	Brand name	Mode of administration	Benefits[1]	Side effects[2]
Bromocriptine	Parlodel	Oral tablet	• Improvement of PD symptoms • Reduced "off" time • Increased "on" time • Neuroprotective properties	• Nausea and vomiting • Sleepiness • Hallucinations • Orthostatic hypotension
Pramipexole	Mirapex	Oral tablet		
Ropinerole	Requip	Oral tablet		
Apomorphine	Apokyn	Subcutaneously injected		

[1]Slawek, 2007; Bonuccelli & Pavese, 2007
[2]Stacy, 2003

of dopamine and improvement of PD symptoms (Jankovic & Stacy, 2007). This class of drugs is beneficial when taken alone or with L-dopa (see table 2.3).

Other Drugs

Anticholinergics and amantadine either help to reestablish the balance between the neurotransmitters acetylcholine and dopamine or have been shown to improve PD symptoms, but their mechanism of action is unclear.

• **Anticholinergics.** Anticholinergics can be helpful in reducing resting tremor by improving the balance between acetylcholine and dopamine levels in the striatum. The benefits of this class of drug, however, are varied and modest. Many side effects occur, especially in older people. Side effects include dry mouth, blurred vision, oversedation, urinary retention, confusion, and hallucinations. Because of the risk–benefit ratio, anticholinergics are not often prescribed (Tolosa & Katzenschlager, 2007). Drugs include trihexyphenidyl HCL (Artane) and benztropine mesylate (Cogentin).

• **Amantadine.** Amantadine (Symmetrel), originally intended to be used as an antiviral medication, was accidentally discovered to help symptoms of PD. It is an N-methyl-D-aspartate (NMDA) receptor antagonist. When administered in conjunction with L-dopa it can reduce dyskinesias and improve mobility (Jankovic & Stacy, 2007). One study demonstrated the benefits of amantadine in delaying the onset and severity of dementia in PD (Inzelberg et al., 2006). A possible side effect is edema in the lower extremities.

Challenges of Parkinson's Disease

Although the benefits of anti-Parkinson's medications far exceed the risks, minimizing side effects is a challenge. Observational characteristics and pathogenesis of dopamine levels are discussed in this section. Symptomatic orthostatic hypotension (OH) can be the result of the primary disease process or be exacerbated by anti-Parkinson's medications. Management of OH is needed for fall prevention and is reviewed in this section.

Motor Fluctuations

Motor fluctuations is a term used to identify a change in the ability to move in response to taking L-dopa with or without other anti-Parkinson's medications. Motor fluctuations can be subtle or dramatic and are related to the dopamine levels in the brain.

Table 2.3   Inhibitory Drugs

Catechol-O-methyltransferase (COMT) inhibitors (Kaakkola, 2000)			
Generic name	**Brand name**	**Benefits and considerations**	**Side effects**
Entacapone	Comtan	• Prolongs the effect of L-dopa • Reduces "wearing off" • Reduces motor fluctuations • May allow for reduction of carbidopa–levodopa dosing • Does not increase peak levels of L-dopa • Not effective without carbidopa–levodopa	• Dyskinesias (because of the combined effect with L-dopa)
Tolcapone	Tasmar		• Dyskinesias (because of the combined effect with L-dopa) • Elevated liver enzymes— need regular blood tests to monitor

Monoamine oxidase B (MAO-B) inhibitors			
Generic name	**Brand name**	**Benefits**	**Side effects**

Selegiline (Jankovic & Stacy, 2007; Victor & Waters, 2003)	Eldepryl	• Mild improvements of PD symptoms when used without L-dopa
		• In early PD
		  • delays the need to start L-dopa therapy and
		  • reduces the development of freezing
		• In more advanced PD
		  • reduces motor fluctuations and
		  • allows reduction of L-dopa dosing
			• Side effects most commonly seen when taken with L-dopa
			• Nausea
			• Constipation
			• Diaphoresis
			• Hallucinations
			• Dyskinesias
			• Orthostatic hypotension

Rasagiline (Chen et al., 2007; Oldfield et al., 2007)	Azilect	• Monotherapy—improves symptoms in early PD • Reduces "off" time and improves "on" time with more advanced PD • Five to 10 times more potent than Selegiline • Possible neuroprotective properties	

Low dopamine levels can result in

- worsening of bradykinesia (slowness of movement),
- hypokinesia (reduced amplitude of movement),
- rigidity (increased resistance to passive movement of a limb),
- dystonia (a sustained muscle contraction that produces involuntary twisting and abnormal posturing),

- tremor (rhythmical, involuntary oscillation of a body part), and
- greater balance impairment or a worsening of gait, including increased freezing.

Normal dopamine levels result in normalization of movement. High dopamine levels can result primarily in choreatic dyskinesias. The choreatic type of dyskinesia is a symptom of the L-dopa medication, not PD.

Motor fluctuations may occur with or without choreatic dyskinesias (Hauser et al., 2006). Approximately 50% of people with PD develop motor fluctuations within 3 to 5 yr of starting L-dopa, a proportion that increases to more than 80% after 10 yr (Dodel et al., 2001).

Terminology Related to Motor Fluctuations

Several terms are used in connection with motor fluctuations:

- **"On"**—the general state of improved function when medications are working and dopamine levels are optimal. This term is relative. Some people exhibit "on" states with normal movement and no mobility problems; their "off" states may demonstrate only subtle gait deviations. Other people exhibit dramatic dyskinesias with impaired mobility during their "on" states. When these people are in their "off" states they are no longer dyskinetic but exhibit greater impairments of movement and secondarily potential mobility limitations.

- **"Off"**—Relates to a general state of function that exhibits greater PD symptoms compared with the "on" state. Dopamine levels are less than optimal.

- **Wearing off**—After chronic use of L-dopa in combination with disease progression, a patient will notice that the medication is not lasting as long as it did previously. The patient may start to experience more difficulty with movements 1 h before the next dose. This circumstance is called wearing off—a predictable symptom. The medication may be lasting 3 h instead of 4 h.

- **"On–off"**—The emergence of abrupt and unpredictable symptoms of PD. Unlike wearing off, "on–off" is unrelated to a patient's medication cycle. For example, an hour after taking L-dopa a person could be independent with mobility but suddenly become bradykinetic and unstable. Assistance with ambulation and getting out of a chair may be necessary. Just as abruptly, the person can become independent and regain mobility. "On–off" phenomenon can play emotional havoc and lead to social isolation because the person with PD has no way of knowing when his or her body will be unable to function.

Neurophysiological

Patients, families, and health care professionals who are not familiar with PD often ask, "What causes those wiggly movements?" The theoretical cause for changes in the ability to move and the emergence of choreatic dyskinesias are discussed at the neuronal level. Although the explanation accounts for typical responses to dopamine replacement drugs, it does not account for all responses. For example, why is it that on occasion a person with PD will have no response to a dose of L-dopa when improvements typically occur? Theoretically, dopamine levels should be improved.

- The primary pathology in PD is the loss of cells in the substantia nigra compacta, resulting in reduced dopamine production. Secondarily, a loss of storage occurs in the presynaptic axonal terminals of these cells, which terminate in the striatum. Hence, degeneration occurs in the nigrostriatal axonal projections.

- In the presence of dopamine deficiency, the neuronal postsynaptic membrane becomes hypersensitive to the release of dopamine because of increased receptor formation on the postsynaptic terminal.

- Although L-dopa can increase the levels of dopamine in the striatum of the brain, it cannot increase those levels to normal. But because of the adaptability within the basal ganglia and perhaps the increased postsynaptic sensitivity, these levels can be sufficient to relieve symptoms.

- Dopamine production is a two-step process.
  - Step 1: Amino acid tyrosine is converted to dopa. The first step of endogenous dopamine production (dopamine that the body produces naturally) is rate controlled and tonically released for normalization of movement. As a result, this step places tight reins on the levels of dopamine.

    Amino acid tyrosine + enzyme tyrosine hydroxylase = dopa

  - Step 2: In this step, dopa is converted to dopamine by the aromatic amino acid enzyme decarboxylase so that it can be stored or used for neurotransmission. This step is not rate controlled; it will convert any dopa molecule available regardless of need. This is not a problem when dealing with only endogenous factors. When someone takes L-dopa medications, the brain receives it in the dopa form, and the enzyme decarboxylase eagerly converts it to dopamine regardless of need.

    Dopa + enzyme aromatic amino acid decarboxylase = dopamine

- As dopaminergic cells continue to diminish, the accumulative amount of storage space to hold dopamine for a potential synaptic transmission lessens. When someone is taking L-dopa medications the enzyme decarboxylase indiscriminately converts as much dopa to dopamine as possible. If enough storage is available and the amount of L-dopa is not excessive, normalization of movement should occur. But if insufficient storage is present with relatively too much L-dopa, the excessive dopamine can overflow into the postsynaptic terminals, which are already hypersensitive. The result will be dyskinetic movements (Melamed, 1992).

- An additional contributing factor to motor fluctuations is the inherent inability of the medications to release L-dopa in a smooth, continuous fashion similar to the body's natural mechanisms when no pathology is present. Many strategies can be used to help smooth out the release of dopamine, but peaks and valleys of dopamine levels remain a major hurdle in patient management (van Laar, 2003).

Dyskinesia

Dyskinesia is an umbrella term used to describe involuntary movement disorders, including chorea, tics, tremors, athetosis, myoclonus, and dystonia (Hoff et al., 1999). When referring to PD, the term *dyskinesia* is most commonly associated with choreiform-type movements that are rapidly flowing and unpredictable in direction or magnitude. Dyskinesias are present at rest and with voluntary motions. Dyskinesia is not a symptom of PD but is a side effect of L-dopa in combination with disease progression. Dyskinesias do not occur while a person is sleeping, but they can prevent a person from going to sleep (Ahlskog, 2000). These drug-induced dyskinesias may be described by their presence in the medication cycle:

- Peak dose dyskinesia (most common)
- Biphasic dyskinesia: occurs when the medication starts to take effect and again when the medication is wearing off
- End dose dyskinesia
- Random presentations of dyskinesias (Uitti, 2000)

People with young onset PD (YOPD) are more susceptible to dyskinesias after only a few years of taking L-dopa medication (Jankovic, 2005) than are those with older onset PD, but they have a slower disease progression (Alves et al., 2005; Jankovic, 2001). People with older onset PD disease have the luxury of improved mobility without dyskinesias for about 4 to 7 yr (Dewey, 2000). Onset of dyskinesia varies among people. The Dyskinesia Severity Rating Scale was established to categorize the severity of functional impairment or disability resulting from dyskinesias while performing three activities: walking, putting on a coat, and lifting a cup to the lips for drinking (Goetz et al., 1994). This scale (see the sidebar) has reportedly demonstrated significant inter- and intrarater reliability (Goetz et al., 1994).

Patients are not in a constant dyskinetic state. Dyskinesias occur as part of the motor fluctuation cycle and usually indicate the "on" state of the medication cycle when dopamine levels are high. Patients are typically most mobile at this time. The health care professional cannot affect the occurrence or severity of dyskinesias, but they indicate that the patient has motor fluctuations. These patients will also have periods of increased difficulty with mobility during their "off" states. Accurate identification of mobility or ADL issues related to both "on" and "off" states is advantageous in helping the patient. Clinically observed dyskinesias may range from 0 to 3 on the Dyskinesia Severity Rating Scale. Patients with violent dyskinesias are most likely home bound. Patients with disabling dyskinesias are typically evaluated by a movement disorder neurologist for further medication adjustments or surgical options such as deep brain stimulation. The Dyskinesia Severity Rating Scale can be helpful in giving a more complete picture of the patient's capabilities. Dyskinesias noted during the evaluation could be categorized as mild (1 or 2 on the Dyskinesia Severity Rating Scale), moderate (3 on the Dyskinesia Severity Rating Scale), or severe (4 on the Dyskinesia Severity Rating Scale). The mild, moderate, or severe categorization, although not precise or scientifically calibrated, offers a clinical picture of the patient's potential limitations.

Dyskinesia Severity Rating Scale

0—No dyskinesia. Normal motion.

1—Minimal dyskinesias. No interference with voluntary motion or functional activities.

2—Impairment of voluntary movements, but patient is normally capable of undertaking motor tasks independently.

3—Intense interference with movement control and significant limits on daily activities. May be able to perform activities unassisted but with difficulty, increased time, and effort.

4—Violent dyskinesias. Incompatible with any motor task. Needs assistance with all functional activities.

Dyskinetic movements can vary in location and severity. Observationally, some patients may exhibit greater axial dyskinesias, whereas others have it in one or more of their extremities. Some may exhibit only a mild cervical dyskinesia. The respiratory muscles can also be affected.

Orthostatic Hypotension

Although people can exhibit orthostatic hypotension (OH) for many reasons, autonomic dysfunction is the primary cause of OH in PD (Ahsan Ejaz et al., 2006). Orthostatic hypotension is a fall in systolic BP below 20 mm Hg and diastolic BP below 10 mm Hg from baseline (from lying to standing) within 3 min of being in an upright position (Lahrmann et al., 2006).

Signs and Symptoms

Autonomic hypotension presents with a drop of BP as noted earlier but without a compensatory increase in heart rate (Hilz et al., 2002). This type of hypotension commonly presents with supine hypertension and can cause unsteadiness and falls (Ejaz et al., 2004). The prevalence of symptomatic OH in PD is approximately 20% and has been attributed to autonomic failure in combination with the use of L-dopa (Senard, 2003). Selegeline (Eldepryl) may also contribute to OH (Pursiainen et al., 2007).

Commonly reported symptoms are dizziness, light-headedness, weakness, lethargy, fatigue, paracervical and suboccipital ache (coat hanger ache), and visual disturbances (Mathias & Kimber, 1998; Mathias et al., 1999; Young & Mathias, 2004). Changes from the patient's baseline should be reported to the neurologist or primary physician. Because of the autonomic pathology underlying OH, medical management of orthostatic hypotension is difficult in the presence of supine hypertension (Pathak & Senard, 2006) (figure 2.1).

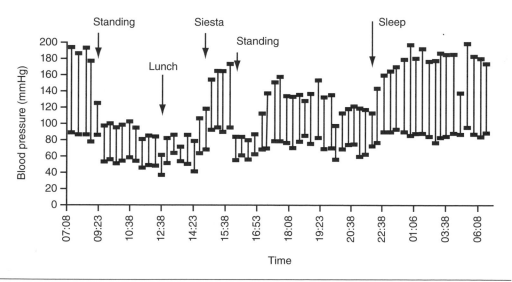

Figure 2.1 Printout of typical 24 h blood pressure monitoring in a patient with Parkinson's disease, orthostatic hypotension, and supine hypertension.

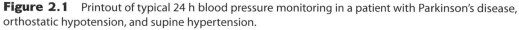

Reprinted, by permission, from A. Pathak and J.M. Senard, 2006, "Blood pressure disorders during Parkinson's disease: Epidemiology, pathology and management," *Expert Review of Neurotherapeutics* 6(8): 1173-1180.

Educational Interventions for OH

Patient education to minimize blood pressure drops should be emphasized. I have found that dehydration is a common contributing factor to OH and have observed improvements in symptoms and systolic blood pressures in patients 10 min after they drank 8 oz (240 ml) of water. Similar responses have been noted in a study in which subjects drank 480 ml and showed improvements in blood pressure after 15 min (Young & Mathias, 2004). In practice, a powerful educational tool (for those who tend to be dehydrated) is to take the patient's blood pressure, have him or her drink 8 to 16 oz (240 to 480 ml) of water, wait 10 to 15 min, and retake the blood pressure. Recommendations such as increasing salt intake or wearing compression hose for daytime use should be cleared by the physician. Patients may be on diet restrictions or have arterial insufficiency, which may result in further complications if wearing compression hose. Patients with symptomatic hypotension should have blood pressure checks in the clinic with position changes and after exercise (Mathias & Kimber, 1998).

See appendix D, "Recommendations for People With Hypotension," for a handout that lists precautions that patients can observe to minimize the effects of hypotension.

Information regarding guidelines for blood pressure monitoring is available through the American Heart Association by calling 800-242-8721 (United States only) or writing the American Heart Association, Public Information, 7272 Greenville Ave., Dallas, Texas 75231-4596. Ask for reprint No. 71-0276 (Pickering et al., 2005).

Deep Brain Stimulation

DBS involves inserting an electrode into the target site. The electrodes are connected by a subcutaneous extension lead wire to a programmable pulse generator (figure 2.2). The pulse generator, similar in size to a cardiac pacemaker, is inserted subcutaneously below the clavicle. About 2 to 4 wk after surgery the neurostimulator is turned on and programmed

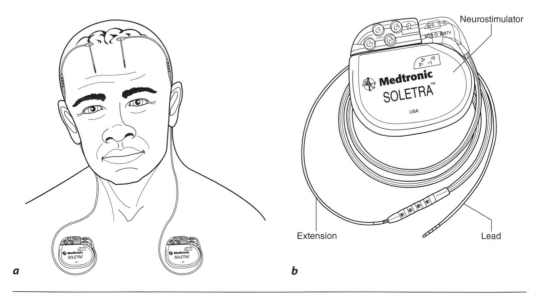

Figure 2.2 *(a)* The location of the implanted DBS; *(b)* a more detailed view of the DBS component.
Reprinted with the permission of Medtronic, Inc. © 2002.

Josh is a 68 yr old male with PD diagnosed 7 yr ago. He is in Hoehn and Yahr stage 2. He lives alone, is ambulatory without an assist device, and drives. Medical history includes hypertension. Josh takes antihypertensive medications. His anti-Parkinson's medications were increased a month ago for relief of PD symptoms.

Subjective Evaluation

Josh reports increased unsteadiness when initially standing up from his bed. When standing for long periods or walking he complains of dizziness (denies room spinning) and paracervical and suboccipital ache (coat hanger ache). Josh admits to not drinking enough fluids during the day. He reports that he has recently started to lose his balance and has fallen a few times in the past month because his knees buckled. He states that although he loves to walk, he has recently started walking only around the house because of feelings of unsteadiness. Josh has not yet told his doctor about these new symptoms.

Objective Evaluation

Because of the patient's complaints, OH is suspect and blood pressure is taken. Supine blood pressure is 110/65, and heart rate is 60. Blood pressure upon initial standing is 90/60, and heart rate is 60. After standing for 3 min the patient becomes symptomatic and unsteady. Blood pressure reading is 75/50, and heart rate is 60. Symptoms resolved after sitting. Minimal strength and flexibility impairments were noted. Postural reflexes are intact (pull test is negative). Berg balance score (see appendix B for Berg balance test) is 29/56, indicating significant instability and the need to use a walker.

Goals

Although the initial apparent goal is to improve balance, Josh's balance is most likely a manifestation of his low blood pressure, which needs to be medically managed first. From the standpoint of physical management, a walker may offer more stability, but it will not prevent a fall if his blood pressure drops too low. Therefore, emphasis will be on education of management or recognition of symptoms to minimize escalation of blood pressure drops. Because he lives alone, the issue of ensuring that Josh has help should be addressed. Josh is becoming less active and is at risk of becoming deconditioned. The initial goals are

- to increase patient awareness regarding physical management of OH-related blood pressure drops for fall prevention,
- to increase awareness and understanding of medical alert systems,
- to be independent with a home exercise program (HEP) that will prevent deconditioning and maintain flexibility, and
- to improve Berg balance score from a new baseline after blood pressure is medically managed.

(continued)

Case Example   *(continued)*

Therapeutic Interventions

Initially, Josh's physician is contacted concerning relatively new onset of symptomatic OH. Josh is given the patient handout "Recommendations for People With Hypotension." Items on this handout are reviewed (see appendix D for a reproducible handout). Although his blood pressure problems may be transient, he is also informed about medical alert systems and given the handout "Medical Alert Systems" (see appendix D for a reproducible handout).

To prevent deconditioning, Josh is instructed in a home exercise program that avoids any standing exercises. Physical therapy is put on hold to allow medication adjustments. Josh's internist reduced his antihypertensive medication, which improved symptoms somewhat. The neurologist started him on midodrine (Proamatine), a medication used for neurogenic OH.

Outcomes

On his next visit the Berg balance score improved to 40/56, indicating a significant improvement in balance capability. The patient was asymptomatic with improved blood pressure readings. Although Josh's blood pressure readings improved, they continued to be erratic with continued periods of instability. He is now deliberately drinking more water. Josh did not follow up with getting a medical alert system because he is reportedly feeling more stable, but he states that he now keeps his cell phone in his pocket. The remaining physical therapy sessions focus on balance training and advancement of his HEP.

(Medtronic). In follow-up visits, the movement disorder neurologist, who is familiar with DBS programming, adjusts the stimulation parameters of the pulse generator and makes anti-PD medication adjustments to optimize mobility and minimize side effects (Moro et al., 2006).

Risks, Benefits, and Candidate Criteria

Before considering surgery, a person must consider the risks and benefits of the procedure itself. If the surgical procedure is considered a viable option, the last matter is establishing the risks and benefits inherent to the person being considered for the procedure.

• **Risks of DBS surgery**. Risks related to the implanted device itself are not high. A study of 204 implants showed complications from the DBS device in 7.6% of the total number of implants. Infections accounted for 6.2% of the total number of implants. Skin erosion and lead wire fractures accounted for 1.4% (Constantoyannis et al., 2005). Risks of the surgery are also low but can be serious. A review of eight studies showed that 905 patients and 1,489 implants exhibited a 6.6% risk of a severe adverse event such as intracranial hemorrhage, seizures, cognitive or behavioral decline, or other neurological deficit, and a 2.5% risk of a permanent neurological deficit (Rezak et al., 2004).

• **Benefits of the DBS surgery**. The procedure is reversible. Additionally, the waveform of the stimulation is adjustable. Initially, and over time as the disease progresses, the stimulation can be shaped to optimize relief of symptoms. Rigidity and bradykinesia are reduced, improving overall mobility. Other benefits include

- improved stride length,
- improved gait velocity,
- improved quality of sleep,
- reduction of dyskinesias,
- reduction of tremors, and
- reduction in anti-PD medications.

• **Criteria for DBS candidates**. For a person with idiopathic PD, the failure of L-dopa to control symptoms is the initial consideration for DBS surgery. These people will have shown a significant decline in mobility resulting from disabling dyskinesias or increased severity of "on" and "off" states. The following criteria are also considered in the screening process:

- Intact cognition: During surgery the person is asked to move the arm or leg in certain directions. If the person is unable to follow these commands, the placement of the stimulator could be suboptimal. Postoperative worsening of dementia is also a greater concern.

- Medical stability: Any comorbidity that may increase the risk of complications or cause the risks to be greater than the benefits is evaluated. For example, patients who have unstable heart disease, active infections, or significant cerebrovascular disease may be considered unstable for surgery (Lang et al., 2006).

- Psychological stability: Neuropsychological testing can establish the patient's preoperative status. Those with neuropsychological impairments are at greater risk of complications in this area postoperatively (Trepanier et al., 2000).

Table 2.4 outlines the benefits and limitations of DBS by neuronal target location.

Physical Therapy for Patients With a DBS

Overall evaluation and treatment approaches to patients with a DBS are similar to those without one as regard to exercise, balance training, and compensatory strategies. Where they differ are the restrictions imposed to preserve the DBS components and secondarily to avoid harm to the patient. Many of the modalities used in physical therapy for musculoskeletal problems are contraindicated for people who have a DBS.

Table 2.4 DBS Benefits and Limitations

DBS target site	Benefits	Limitations
Bilateral subthalamic nucleus (STN) (Salarian et al., 2004; Krack et al., 2003; Davis et al., 2005; Maurer et al., 2003; Chen et al., 2003; Zibetti et al., 2007)	• Improves stride length and secondarily gait velocity • Reduces dyskinesias • Improves "off" freezing • Reduces bradykinesia, rigidity, and tremor • Improves functional mobility • Improves quality of sleep • Allows reduction in anti-PD medications	• Does not improve gait variability (gait rhythmicity), which is an aggravating factor in freezing • Unable to control disease progression • No change in "on" freezing • No change in postural reflexes or trunk righting
Bilateral globus pallidus (GPi) (Group, 2001)	• Benefits similar to STN but not as pronounced	
Thalamus (Alesch et al., 1995)	• Reduces resting tremor and essential tremor	• Does not improve other PD symptoms

Contraindications

Medtronic, the manufacturer of DBS systems, has established guidelines for various modalities or treatments commonly performed by physical therapists. Modalities such as shortwave diathermy, microwave diathermy, or ultrasound anywhere in the body are contraindicated for any patient with an implanted DBS. Energy from any of these modalities can be transferred through the implanted system and cause tissue damage at the location of the implanted electrodes, resulting in severe injury or death (Medtronic, 2005). The only exception is diagnostic ultrasound as in an echocardiogram.

Physical Therapy Guidelines and Precautions

Physical therapists should pay close attention to the following guidelines and precautions for working with patients with a DBS implant:

1. TENS (transcutaneous electrical nerve stimulation): Do not place TENS electrodes so that the TENS current passes over any part of the neurostimulation system. If the patient thinks that the TENS may be interfering with the implanted neurostimulator, the patient should discontinue using TENS until he or she talks with the doctor.

2. Therapeutic magnets (for example, those found in bracelets, back braces, shoe inserts, and mattress pads) can cause the DBS neurostimulator to turn on or off unintentionally. Therefore, patients should be advised not to use therapeutic magnets.

3. The only restriction concerning cervical ROM is that abrupt or high-velocity movements should not be performed because the movement can cause a break in the lead wire.

4. No restrictions exist concerning cervical traction other than patient comfort.

5. Compatibility guidelines have not been established about precautions or contraindications related to interferential current or other electrical modalities. Therefore, these modalities should be avoided (Medtronic, 2005).

Summary

1. Motor fluctuations are unique to people with PD and result primarily from L-dopa medication in combination with the increased difficulty of maintaining constant dopamine levels with disease progression.

2. L-dopa may have little to no effect on posture, postural reflexes, and "on" freezing.

3. L-dopa may relieve symptoms of "off" freezing, bradykinesia, and rigidity and secondarily may improve gait, balance, postural reflex responses (if masked by rigidity and bradykinesia), facial expression, and micrographia (small, cramped writing).

4. Physical management should address mobility problems related to both "on" and "off" states.

5. Autonomic orthostatic hypotension is common in PD.

6. PD medications can exacerbate orthostatic hypotension.

7. Patient education to self-manage hypotensive symptoms is important for fall prevention and safety.

8. Deep brain stimulation of the STN or GPi is effective for improvement of mobility by reducing rigidity, bradykinesia, L-dopa-induced dyskinesias, and motor fluctuations.

9. Symptoms not typically improved from DBS in the STN or GPi are "on" freezing and impaired postural reflexes.

10. Physical therapy evaluation and treatment to improve general functional mobility is similar for people with or without DBS.

11. Every patient with PD should be asked whether she or he has an implanted DBS if modalities or manual therapy is being considered. Follow the contraindications, precautions, and guidelines for patients with DBS.

chapter

3

Exercise and Rehabilitation Considerations

Three main areas of exercise must be considered for rehabilitation—flexibility, strength, and cardiorespiratory endurance. Impairments in any of these categories can lead to disabilities. Flexibility can be restricted by tightness in any of the structures surrounding a joint, by pathology in the joint, or by pain. The terms *flexibility* and *range of motion* (ROM) are used interchangeably in this chapter.

Loss of strength is multifactorial, but from the rehabilitative standpoint it will be addressed in its relationship to inactivity and exercise. Older adults lose cardiorespiratory endurance or stamina primarily because of decreased activity with age *(Physical Activity and Health: A Report of the Surgeon General*, 1996). People with PD go through the same age-related changes in range of motion (ROM), strength, power, and endurance as the general older population does. People with PD, however, have greater risk of secondary musculoskeletal impairments because of their primary disease process. ROM can be affected by decreased amplitude and slowness of movement, rigidity, and proprioceptive impairments. Increased difficulty with movement can lead to a reduction of activities with a secondary loss of strength and endurance.

Medical management of PD may reduce rigidity and bradykinesia but does not directly address physical components such as ROM, strength, and endurance. Physical management is therefore critical in addressing these areas. Optimal patient outcomes require both medical and physical management. To optimize gains, patients should exercise when PD medications are most effective because L-dopa reduces rigidity and bradykinesia (Pavese et al., 2006). No exercise should cause pain, and any that does should be discontinued or modified. When exercises are performed improperly, pain can result. Ensuring proper form may be all that is necessary.

People with PD can also exhibit age-related comorbidities such as osteoporosis, arthritis, or spinal stenosis. Potential areas of impairments appear to be similar in the aging population and in people with PD. Therefore, exercises or community exercise classes that benefit the older population may be additional avenues for conditioning that may be recommended for the PD population.

The focus of this chapter is to offer guidelines and examples of various types of exercises. The goal is to achieve rehabilitation and long-term maintenance through patient education, participation, and adherence. A home exercise program that targets impairments and potential impairments will optimize mobility for the long term and can offer protection against momentary setbacks such as temporary illnesses. The ultimate purpose of exercise is to compress morbidities to the very end of life. In other words, the goal is to help people live a quality life for as long as possible and leave this earth in "optimal condition."

Flexibility

Stretching is a necessary component of a well-rounded exercise routine. Guidelines and practical examples for an effective stretching program are discussed next.

General Considerations

To maximize the effectiveness of flexibility exercises, patients need to be educated about how the three components of stretching can affect their flexibility. First, the patient must achieve the full available range to maintain current flexibility, at least. With the PD population, compensatory strategies are often required. Second, the optimal frequency of stretching must be addressed. Finally, the duration of stretch holding should be determined.

Achieving Maximum ROM

PD symptoms such as bradykinesia and hypokinesia contribute to the underscaling of movement and potential loss of flexibility. Centrally impaired proprioceptive integration can also contribute to hypometric movement (Jacobs & Horak, 2006). To compensate for these neurological impairments, additional cueing strategies can be used to encourage a larger excursion of movement to obtain full range. This approach has been demonstrated in gait by optimizing step length through cuing strategies (Lehman et al., 2005; Suteerawattananon et al., 2004).

Cueing can be helpful in an exercise program as well. Mentally focusing on each exercise (attention strategy) may be sufficient in people with mild PD to accomplish full range. Advising the patient to "think about moving as far as possible, comfortably, with each repetition" can enhance the excursion of movements. People with moderate PD may need additional tactile or visual cues to accomplish optimal flexibility. Sometimes a combination of visual and tactile cues is needed. For example, to optimize trunk rotation, a person can stand with her or his back to the wall. The person is then asked to reach across with the right hand to touch the wall on the left side. Visually, the person follows the hand to get close to the wall. Touching the wall ensures that maximum range has been achieved (figure 3.5c). The type of cueing needed should be assessed on an individual basis. Obtaining full range should be encouraged. Not moving through the available range will not maximize or maintain flexibility.

Frequency

The American College of Sports Medicine (ACSM) guidelines recommend that adults and older adults stretch a minimum of 2 to 3 d per week and ideally 5 to 7 d a week with focus on areas of reduced ROM ("General principles of exercise prescription," 2006). No specific guidelines have been established for people with PD. From my clinical experience, I have observed that people who perform stretching exercises on joints without limitations can maintain their flexibility by performing stretches two to three times a week. Exercises addressing potential areas of tightness should also be performed a few times a week and monitored by the patient or caregiver.

Potential areas of tightness are areas that exhibit rigidity but currently have normal flexibility. If the patient is performing an exercise in proper form but is not maintaining flexibility with the recommended frequency of stretching, the frequency should be increased. Stretching approximately 5 d a week may be necessary for people who are sedentary, have areas with reduced ROM, or have moderate PD. I recommend that people with severe PD stretch daily with assistance to ensure that maximal range is obtained.

Hold Time for Stretches

No strong consensus exists regarding absolute hold time to stretch a muscle. Hold times may depend on the level of tightness, age, and the muscle being stretched. One study compared the gains obtained when stretching tight hamstrings for 15, 30, and 60 s in older people. Improvements were noted in all three categories, but the most significant gain was noted with the 60 s hold (Feland et al., 2001). Another study compared 10 s holds to 30 s holds but kept the total daily stretch time constant; both groups stretched a total of 1 min twice a day. The stretching protocols were found to be equally effective (Cipriani et al., 2003). Another study compared a 5 s hold to a 15 s hold. Total stretch time for each exercise was 45 s (nine repetitions [reps] of the 5 s hold and three reps of the 15 s hold were performed). Passive ROM improved equally in both groups, but the 15 s hold showed greater improvements in active ROM (Roberts & Wilson, 1999).

Most studies evaluating hold durations have been on younger adults and on tight muscle groups. If ROM is being performed for prevention on a joint that exhibits normal flexibility, a shorter hold of 5 s can be sufficient (provided that full range is attained with each repetition). Longer holds are recommended if the intent is to correct ROM. Some patients with arthritic changes may need to perform submaximal gentle active ROM repetitions without a hold to reduce joint stiffness and then proceed to repetitions with a hold. The length of hold may be inversely proportional to the number of repetitions. This approach can help with adherence. For example, if the intended cumulative hold time is 1 min, the following options may be considered: six reps with a 10 s hold, three reps with a 20 s hold, or two reps with a 30 s hold.

Range of Motion Exercises

The final recommendations offered to patients regarding ROM exercises depend on the exercise goal (prevention versus correction), observed effectiveness, tolerance, and potential adherence. The following ROM exercises offer ideas for the more common areas of limitations. People who have PD may also have osteoporosis secondary to being sedentary or to limiting their activities because of fear of falling. Patients with a history of osteoporosis should avoid excessive trunk flexion or axial rotational exercises to minimize the risk of compression fractures. These precautions are noted with the exercises that follow.

Cervical and Shoulder

The following are common areas of limitation in the cervical spine and shoulder. The effects of these limitations are described.

Cervical retraction

A forward head can affect balance and swallowing capabilities. This exercise can be difficult to perform correctly. If the patient sits in a chair with the back against the wall, the wall can serve a tactile cue for head retractions (figure 3.1). For many this exercise can be difficult because of age-related changes in the cervical and thoracic spine. An alternative is

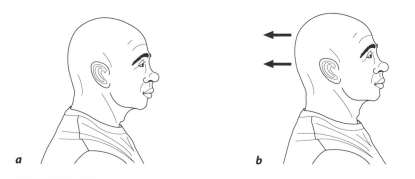

Figure 3.1 *(a)* Beginning position and *(b)* cervical retraction.

to place a pillow between the wall and the head. The patient then tries to squish the pillow while attempting to maintain a neutral spine. The pillow offers tactile feedback. Adding any prop, however, can reduce adherence. This exercise can be performed lying down if sitting is too difficult.

Cervical rotation

This type of motion is important for driving, especially when backing up. Cervical rotation is also needed for walking to have the ability to look left and right. This exercise can also help improve general neck comfort. Cervical rotation should be performed with the cervical spine in the patient's optimal neutral spine position (minimizing a forward head posture) to avoid undue stress to the cervical joints. In other words, the patient should first perform a head retraction and attempt to maintain the retracted position while performing cervical rotation.

Shoulder flexion

This common area of limitation can cause loss of balance backward when reaching up. For example, limited shoulder flexion will restrict the reach of a person trying to reach for a high shelf. A common substitution is to extend and rotate the trunk to reach the object. This position is unstable for someone with postural instability, which can result in a secondary loss of balance backward. Sitting with the back fully supported can help isolate the motion in the shoulder. Folding the hands together (as shown in figure 3.2) can help position the shoulder to avoid rotator cuff irritation. The patient can then focus on excursion rather than arm position. Excessive kyphotic postures will limit shoulder flexion and should not be forced. As with any exercise, the exercise should be performed to comfort. Preexisting shoulder problems may require individualized attention.

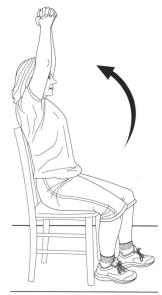

Figure 3.2 Shoulder flexion ROM with hands together and fingers interlaced.

Trunk

Trunk stiffness or tightness is common and often leads to discomfort or pain, which may be partly due to rigidity and bradykinesia. Patients may report improvements in back comfort when they start taking L-dopa medications. Trunk flexibility exercises can help maintain these improvements.

Trunk flexion

Tightness in the low back paravertebrals is common. This tightness can aggravate symptoms from spinal stenosis. Performing forward trunk bending in sitting can frequently offer more immediate relief of symptoms than just sitting. Having the patient lean forward and stretch the low back in a seated position while keeping the hands on the knees can help stretch the back muscles (figure 3.3). The patient can easily perform this exercise as needed for pain control.

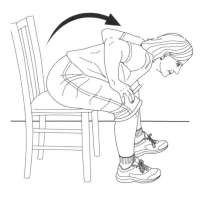

Figure 3.3 Low back stretch. Hands are placed on the knees to protect the spine.

A similar exercise demonstrated in various commercial exercise programs has the person reaching for the floor instead of placing the hands on the knees. Reaching for the floor is not recommended for people diagnosed with osteoporosis or people who have excessive rounding of the thoracic spine (people who are not diagnosed with osteoporosis but are suspect). Axial flexion exercises aggravate compression fractures (Sinaki & Mikkelsen, 1984). Placing the hands on the knees helps prevent excessive trunk flexion, especially in the thoracic spine, but flexion in the thoracic spine should still be monitored.

Trunk extension

Thoracic and lumbar extension are typically limited, and tolerance to these exercises can vary widely. The younger populations have fewer comorbidities that restrict trunk extension and exhibit better tolerance to extension exercises. Trunk extension exercises can range from prone press-ups to a gentler approach of lying supine and performing a longitudinal stretch with reaching arms and legs (figure 3.4). Performing bilateral shoulder flexion in sitting can also facilitate axial extension (figure 3.2). Because extension can aggravate symptoms from spinal stenosis, the patient may need to rely on a gentler approach. The patient's symptoms will be your guide.

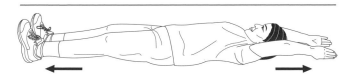

Figure 3.4 Supine postural stretch—a gentler approach to maintaining axial extension.

Trunk rotation

Exercises that improve rotation can be performed supine, sitting, or standing. Modifying the exercise to be functionally meaningful can help significantly with adherence. Golfers usually understand the relevance of this exercise, but both golf and axial rotational exercises that have high-velocity axial rotation components should be avoided in the presence of osteoporosis (Ekin & Sinaki, 1993). See figure 3.5 for variations of rotational exercises. The patient can use tactile cues as in figure 3.5*a* by attempting to touch the elbow to the opposite knee. Patients who have less flexibility may attempt to touch the forearm to the opposite knee. Visual cues can facilitate motion as in figure 3.5*b*, in which the patient attempts to look at a target behind her or him.

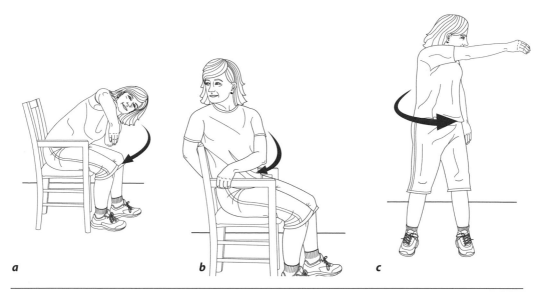

Figure 3.5 Variations on trunk rotation: *(a)* sitting elbow to knee, *(b)* upright sitting, *(c)* standing and reaching high.

Lower Extremity

ROM limitations in the lower extremities can affect balance, gait, ADLs, and transfer abilities.

Hip extension

Although the hip flexors may not always be tight, this area has potential for tightness, especially in someone who becomes more sedentary, exhibits an increased forward-flexed posture (which tends to occur at the hips), or walks with reduced stride length. Tightness of the hip flexors can also contribute to low back strain and aggravate symptoms from spinal stenosis. The ability to perform a hip flexor stretch can vary widely. Using less conventional methods to minimize tightness may be necessary, although they may be less than optimal.

One method of stretching the hip flexors (and the quadriceps) is to lie supine with one leg over the edge of a bed or couch while holding the opposite knee to the chest (figure 3.6*a*). Pulling the knee to the chest prevents arching of the low back. This exercise also helps improve quadriceps flexibility of the ipsilateral lower extremity and improves hip flexion of the contralateral lower extremity. For those who have difficulty pulling the knee toward the chest, the exercise can also be performed in a hook-lying position (figure 3.6*b*). In this position greater attention may be needed to avoid arching the low back. For some people with PD, even the hook-lying stretch is uncomfortable and further modification may be needed. Lying supine with one knee pulled to the chest and performing an isometric of the opposite hip extensors and quadriceps with the leg resting on the bed can improve comfort and reduce difficulties (figure 3.6*c*). In this position only the hip flexors are being stretched.

Active hip extension in standing or when performing a forward lunge may be necessary for those who cannot tolerate the hip flexor stretch in supine. Regardless of stretching position, preventing or minimizing lumbar extension should be integral to this group of exercises to minimize stress to the low back and to isolate the stretch to the hip flexors.

Hip abduction

Tightness of the hip adductors causes limitations in hip abduction. The flexibility of the hip adductors is important with activities such as getting in and out of a car or bathtub and for maintaining hygiene with advanced disease. I have not found a strong correlation between hip adductor tightness and the narrowness of the base of support with standing or ambulating, but over time these habitual movement patterns could result in reduced flexibility. The presence of rigidity and inactivity seems to play a greater role than does a narrow base of support in hip adductor tightness. See figure 3.7 for hip adductor stretch.

Hip flexion

Hip flexion ROM is typically not limited, but when restricted it can interfere with donning and doffing shoes and socks. Lack of forward trunk leaning, which occurs predominantly through hip flexion rather than trunk flexion, can be observed when people get out of a chair. People do not lean forward sufficiently for many reasons, but one common reason is the fear of falling forward. Insufficient forward leaning can reduce the ability to stand up from a chair or sit back down and is often the cause for backward loss of balance. See figures 3.3, 3.6*a*, and 3.6*c* for alternative methods to improve hip flexion ROM.

Quadriceps flexibility

Quadriceps flexibility is necessary to get up from the floor. When in a kneeling position and

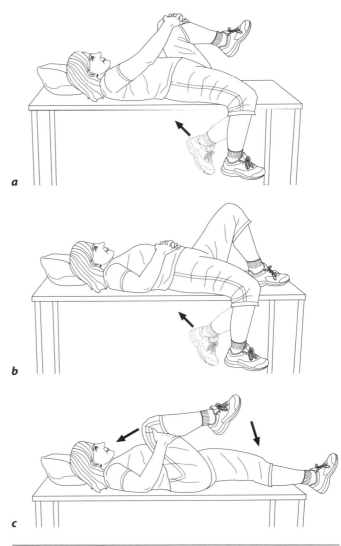

Figure 3.6 Variations on supine hip flexor stretch: *(a)* knee to chest and other leg flat, *(b)* hook-lying hip and quad stretch, *(c)* alternative exercise for those who cannot tolerate the previous two.

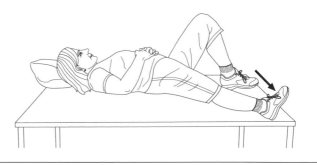

Figure 3.7 Hip adductor stretch.

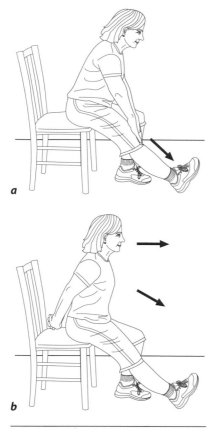

Figure 3.8 Alternatives to stretching the hamstrings: *(a)* effective stretch, *(b)* improved isolation of the hamstrings and greater protection of the spine for those with osteoporosis.

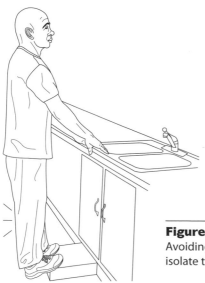

before getting up from the floor, the quads are in the stretched position at both the hip and the knee. Maintaining flexibility can greatly enhance floor transfers. See figure 3.6, *a* and *b* for alternatives to stretch the quadriceps muscles.

Hamstring tightness

Few people are not tight in the hamstrings. Tightness can interfere with bed mobility, especially if the patient is in the habit of long sitting before swinging the legs out of bed. In other words, the patient sits straight up with their legs still in bed instead of rolling to their side while swinging the legs out of bed before sitting up. Performing a hamstring stretch in sitting is often easiest on the patient. To isolate the stretch to the hamstrings, a neutral spine should be encouraged with emphasis on bending at the hips. The patient sits on the edge of the chair with one knee extended and the heel on the ground. The patient slides both hands down the extended leg until he or she feels a stretch while attempting to maintain a neutral spine (figure 3.8*a*). Although this stretch is effective, people with osteoporosis should avoid it. Alternatively, the patient can place both hands behind the low back while leaning forward at the hips to help maintain a neutral spine. This method, safer for people with osteoporosis, strengthens the paraspinals while stretching the hamstrings (figure 3.8*b*). A less complicated approach is active knee extension while seated with the back supported in neutral spine.

Calf tightness
or decreased ankle dorsiflexion

Calf tightness or reduced dorsiflexion is common. Reduced dorsiflexion can be a fall risk. The conventional runner's calf stretch is often too complicated to perform correctly, and it can be uncomfortable for people with spinal stenosis. An alternative method is to stand with the forefeet on the edge of a block of wood or book with the heels resting on the ground. The degree of stretch can be modified by adjusting the forward lean (axis at the ankles) or using a thicker prop (figure 3.9).

Figure 3.9 Static calf stretch. Typically, the gastrocnemius is tight. Avoiding knee flexion and maintaining an upright posture will help isolate this stretch for maximal benefit.

Resistance Training

With increased age comes a loss of muscle mass called sarcopenia, which results in a decline of strength and function. Strength is the ability to exert a force. The cause of sarcopenia seems to be related to a combination of factors such as nutritional changes, inactivity, and changes in the endocrine system, which influences metabolism (Volpi et al., 2004). By the seventh and eighth decade approximately 20% to 40% of maximum voluntary muscle contraction can be lost, which in itself can lead to disability (Doherty, 2003). Much of this loss can result from inactivity. In a questionnaire study, 5,537 community-dwelling people over age 64 were asked about their strengthening-exercise habits. Only 11% performed strengthening exercises two or more times a week and were sufficiently active to prevent deconditioning (Volpi et al., 2004). Muscle weakness is not a symptom of PD but is secondary to inactivity and disuse.

Fortunately, much of the weakness in older adults and in those with PD is reversible. Morphologically, resistance training can increase the cross-sectional area of both type I (slow twitch) and type II (fast twitch) muscle fibers in older people (Dodd et al., 2004). With aging, a relative decline occurs in type II fibers. Neurologically, strength training can increase motor unit recruitment and synchrony of recruitment (Bryant et al., 1998). In one study, institutionalized frail people ranging from 89 to 91 yr old underwent a strengthening program three times a week for 8 wk at an intensity of 80% of one-repetition max. Their strength gains ranged from 143% to 205% (Fiatarone et al., 1990). This finding demonstrates the extent to which older people underuse their muscles.

People with PD have an ability to gain strength similar to that of age-matched controls. Significant improvements occurred in gait velocity, stride length, and posture in people with PD as a result of a strengthening program (Scandalis et al., 2001). People need strength to move. Thus, strengthening is critical to preventing disability and maintaining mobility, balance, cardiovascular health, and bone health. Strength training needs to be a lifetime commitment, especially in older people and those with PD. Training must challenge the muscles to work against greater forces than they are accustomed to, and it needs to be specific concerning speed and muscle groups to optimize functional abilities.

The hip extensors and hip abductors are usually weak in sedentary people. Hip abductor strength is a stabilizing force for lateral balance recovery. In older people the hip abductor muscles are deficient in the fast-twitch muscle fibers that are important to lateral stability and balance recovery (Rogers & Mille, 2003). When a person uses an assist ambulatory device, the hip abductors are at further risk of disuse.

The quadriceps muscle often lacks power strength, which contributes to difficulties when standing up from a chair. Calf muscles also tend to be weak or deconditioned, which may be partly due to reduced push-off during gait and reduced stride length. Exercises for these muscle groups should be addressed preventatively and restoratively. Strength training and power training are two areas of focus in resistance training. Strength training focuses on the amount of resistance. Power training emphasizes speed to develop the fast-twitch muscle fibers. Power training is typically reserved for the lower extremities to improve balance recovery, getting out of a chair, and climbing stairs or curbs.

Training for Strength

As the muscles gain strength, greater resistances can be applied to develop yet greater strength, using the overload principle ("General principles of exercise prescription," 2006).

If their current home exercise program (HEP) becomes easy, patients should be advised how to progress themselves by

- increasing the resistance by changing to a different colored Thera-band, changing the position of the exercise to make it more challenging, or increasing the amount of weight;
- increasing the hold time of an exercise (with controlled breathing); or
- performing the exercise slower.

Sets and Repetitions

Performing three sets of 8 to 12 repetitions of an exercise can require significantly more time than performing one set, and adherence can become more difficult as well. Research supports performance of one set. Performing one set has demonstrated similar results to performing three sets in a study of community-dwelling people between ages 65 and 78. Both groups improved similarly in strength, chair rise, stair climb, and body composition. The group performing three sets showed greater improvement only with the 400 m walk (Galvao & Taaffe, 2005). A study that measured for an increase in thickness of the quadriceps muscle when performing one set of 8 to 12 reps versus three sets found no difference between groups (Starkey et al., 1996). One set of approximately 8 to 12 reps performed two to three times per week (on nonconsecutive days) has been found to be sufficient for strength training (Silverman et al., 2006).

Resistance

The most common method of determining the amount of resistance is based on a percentage of 1RM (one-repetition maximum), the maximum amount of weight that can be lifted only once (because of muscle fatigue) through its full range. Establishing 1RM with older or PD populations, however, involves elevated risk of injury. Thus, determining a safe yet challenging weight for resistance training must be done with special care when working with people with PD, especially with older patients. Here are guidelines to help you do so:

- A safer alternative is to determine 80% to 85% of 1RM by establishing how much weight the patient can lift with good form for a maximum of 7 to 11 reps. According to Lewis and Kellems (2002) 11 reps equate to 80% of 1RM, and 7 reps equate to 85% of 1RM. Determining the percentage of 1RM by the number of repetitions performed should be used as a guide rather than an absolute because the number of repetitions at a given percentage of 1RM can vary between muscle groups and individuals (Silverman et al., 2006).

- The appropriate resistance or intensity can also be determined by the Borg rating of perceived exertion scale (RPE). The level of perceived exertion after performing a set of repetitions should be 12 to 13, or "somewhat hard" ("Exercise testing and prescription for children and elderly people," 2006).

- The patient should be able to perform the established number of repetitions (approximately 7 to 12) in proper form. If this is not possible, the resistance should be lowered so that all repetitions can be performed properly.

- When in doubt, start the patient with a lighter load and progress. But the resistance applied to a muscle must be sufficient to create strength changes.

Strength gains have been noted in older people with intensities as low as 40% of 1RM, but greater gains are noted between 80% and 85% of 1RM. One study of older subjects demonstrated that quadriceps strengthening at 80% of 1RM resulted in significantly greater gains in strength, endurance, and gait velocity than strengthening at 40% of 1RM. The lower-intensity group still showed significant improvements when compared with controls who performed exercises without weights (Seynnes et al., 2004).

Training for Power

The amount of power required for an activity is relative. For example, greater speed and strength will be required to recover from loss of balance and prevent a fall than will be required to stand up from a seated position. Power (high-velocity) strengthening in older people has demonstrated greater functional gains when compared to lower-velocity strength training (Fielding et al., 2002; Miszko et al., 2003) and should therefore be considered part of the exercise program if possible.

Power strength, defined as the ability to exert a force quickly, is deficient in both older people and people with PD. Power depends on strength but is distinct from strength in regard to velocity. Velocity depends on the neuromuscular system to respond quickly. Power is the product of strength and velocity. A deficiency in either strength or velocity affects power output.

Strength training alone can improve power (Slade et al., 2002), but performing higher-velocity exercises at even low resistance can improve power strength. Higher resistance produces even greater gains (de Vos et al., 2005). Specificity of training relative to strength and power is critical for improving power strength. Some people may exhibit good strength but lack the power component. Other people may be deficient in both strength and power, in which case both need to be addressed. To gain power strength, training must incorporate power types of exercises.

The speed at which patients can perform a movement depends on their basic strength and the amount of resistance incurred. For example, Karen, who has relatively weak calves, is asked to perform heel raises quickly but has difficulty going fast because of the resistance of her body weight. But if she uses her arms to assist with this exercise by pushing down on a kitchen counter or other stable waist-high surface, she can perform the exercise quicker. She can reduce the resistance and focus on power strengthening. This exercise works specifically on her power, but she also benefits from strengthening exercises to increase her force production. For strength building she would perform the exercise slowly through her full range both concentrically and eccentrically and adjust her hand pressure for appropriate resistance (the rate of perceived exertion should be "somewhat hard").

The main muscle groups to target for power strengthening are the calves, quadriceps, and hip abductors. One method of assessing lower-extremity power is the chair stand test (see appendix B). Count the number of repetitions of standing up and sitting down in 30 s without upper-extremity support and compare the results with age-matched norms. The results provide a baseline that can be used for goal setting and as a motivator.

From a mechanical and musculoskeletal viewpoint, people with PD tend to have difficulty maintaining lateral stability because of narrow-based gait, reduced trunk righting, reduced trunk flexibility, and reduced hip abductor strength (Dimitrova et al., 2004; Maurer et al., 2003). Addressing any of these deficits may help with balance recovery:

- A sidestepping exercise performed at varying speeds with quick reversals can strengthen this muscle group. A safer alternative is to sidestep a short distance with upper-extremity support on a kitchen counter.

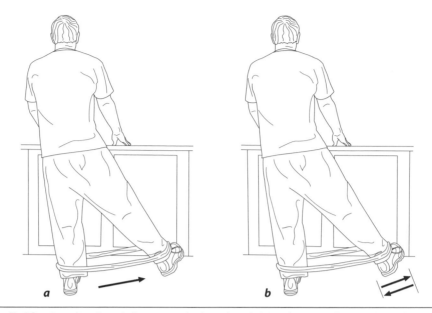

Figure 3.10 Standing hip abduction with Thera-band: *(a)* without oscillation, *(b)* with oscillation.

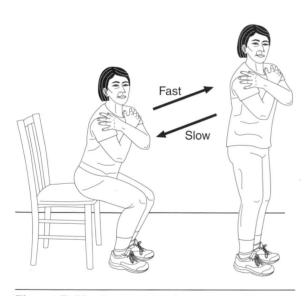

Figure 3.11 Sit to stand with arms crossed. Note that standing is fast, whereas sitting back down should be slow.

• Using a Thera-band around the ankles while abducting the hip in standing position can improve hip abductor strength in both hips at the same time (figure 3.10*a*). To focus more on power, this exercise can be performed with short, quick oscillations at end range (figure 3.10*b*).

• The quadriceps can be strengthened by standing up quickly and sitting down slowly (figure 3.11). For additional suggestions, see chapter 9, "Chair Transfers," pages 115–117. The power of the calf muscles can be enhanced by increasing speed, as reviewed previously in Karen's case. Functionally, more effective stepping strategies in response to loss of balance can result from repeated perturbations sufficient to necessitate a stepping response (see chapter 7, "Postural Instability," pages 86–89 for technique).

Walking at increased speeds with sudden stops (with a staggered stance) can improve control and stability with deceleration. When practicing sudden stops, the patient should wear a gait belt as a precaution for fall prevention.

Cardiorespiratory Endurance

As mentioned earlier, older adults lose cardiorespiratory endurance or stamina primarily because activity decreases with age. This occurrence is common in people with PD as well. Walking is a common and practical mode of exercise to improve endurance. The need to have endurance to perform daily activities is relative and necessary for independence or for minimizing dependence. A goal for one person may be to participate in a 3 km walk. Another person may want to be able to walk with greater independence in the home.

Walking most days of the week for 30 min at moderate intensity is recommended to improve and maintain cardiorespiratory fitness *(Physical activity and health: A report of the surgeon general,* 1996). The same result can be attained by walking for 30 min a day cumulatively for no less than 5 min at a time (Coleman et al., 1999). This alternative allows people who are less conditioned to complete the time needed at tolerable durations. Not all patients are able to walk 30 min daily or for 5 min at a time, but they can work toward this long-range goal to optimize functional abilities.

Although postural changes, bradykinesia, and rigidity can contribute to restrictive pulmonary dysfunction in PD (Sabate et al., 1996), these pulmonary restrictions typically do not interfere with improvements in walking endurance. Improvements in pulmonary function tests have been noted in subjects with PD after the administration of L-dopa, but values remained substantially lower than those of controls (Pal et al., 2007). When initiating a walking program or other types of endurance activities, the clinician should monitor heart rate, blood pressure, and RPE. Older people with PD are more likely to exhibit autonomic dysfunction than other people of comparable age, which can result in hypotension and require closer monitoring. See chapter 2, "Medical and Surgical Interventions," pages 19–22, for further information regarding orthostatic hypotension and see chapter 12, pages 140–149, and chapter 13, pages 156–157, for guidance about a walking program. Gait velocity norms can be found in appendix B.

Lifelong Self-Maintenance

The proportion of fast-twitch muscle fibers in older people is significantly reduced and is susceptible to deconditioning. All gains return to baseline after 4 mo (Fatouros et al., 2005). The effects of exercise start to diminish after 2 wk if a significant reduction in activity occurs. Benefits from exercise can be lost in 2 to 8 mo if exercise is not resumed (Sabate et al., 1996). These findings underscore the need to educate patients from the beginning about engaging in a lifelong conditioning program.

Key Role of Home Exercise Programs

People with PD can improve strength, balance, and gait velocity equally as well by performing a home exercise program (HEP) as they can by performing under the supervision of a physical therapist (Lun et al., 2005). People with PD who perform an HEP have shown significant gains in gait when compared with people with PD who do not perform an HEP (Caglar et al., 2005). The financial saving of guiding the patient initially in an HEP and then having the patient be responsible for self-maintenance can be substantial. After the patient or caregiver demonstrates understanding of an HEP, the therapist can focus on the necessary compensatory strategies, patient education, and specialized treatment interventions.

Patients need to be educated about the cause of deconditioning and its effects on mobility so that they can make educated choices about self-improvement or maintenance by maintaining their HEP. At the very least, they and their caregivers need to be aware that deconditioning results from inactivity. The less active the patient is, the worse the deconditioning will be. Patients and caregivers should also know that 20 to 30 min of daily exercise at moderate intensity is more effective in maintaining mobility than simply being active throughout the day. At the same time, they should realize that if they simply cannot do those 20 to 30 min, they should try to be as active as possible in their ADLs. Any physical activity is better than no activity when attempting to minimize the effects from deconditioning (Brach, 2004).

Adherence to Home Exercise Programs

Motivating patients to exercise can be a challenge. The patient's adherence depends in part on your approach. Patient education, practicality, and the ability to compromise are key factors. Individual exercises that address more than one impairment can help reduce the burden of a maintenance home exercise program. The concept of killing two birds with one stone is almost a necessity and can improve adherence. The time required to perform activities of daily living (ADLs) can more than double for some patients because of the increased difficulty of movement. Minimizing the time doing exercises is important so that patients believe that life is more than just ADLs and exercise. For example, a person with PD presents with a forward-flexed posture, spinal stenosis, and tightness in the hip flexors and quadriceps. The tightness in the hip flexors can potentially affect the person's posture from an orthopedic standpoint and aggravate symptoms from spinal stenosis. Tightness in the quadriceps can interfere with the ability to get up from the floor. One exercise can address tightness in both the hip flexors and the quadriceps (see figure 3.6, *a* and *b*).

Education

Some highly motivated patients do not need to be convinced that they must have an effective HEP. They understand the need to adhere to such a program to maintain a good quality of life. Although many patients want to help themselves, they simply do not understand the effect of exercise on mobility or independence. Again, patients need to be educated in the importance of lifelong conditioning for optimal health and well-being. This concept must be stressed with patients who do not understand until they finally grasp it. Explaining how your previous patients have fared with various levels of exercise adherence can be helpful. For example, patients who adhere to a regular exercise program tend to maintain or improve their strength and flexibility. Others who perform only part of the needed exercise program will improve or at least maintain the areas being addressed but will worsen in neglected areas. Finally, patients who do not exercise typically lose flexibility and strength with secondary worsening of mobility. You can also point out (assuming that it is true in your experience, as it is in mine) that variances from these observations seem to correlate with the patient's overall activity level.

Negotiation

You may need to negotiate with your patient to facilitate adherence to exercise recommendations. Establishing an HEP that is palatable to the patient yet effectively targets the patient's needs requires an open dialogue between you, the patient, and the caregiver. Patients typically avoid exercises that are difficult to get into position to perform. For example, a person who exhibits difficulty with bed mobility and rolling should be directed to perform exercises primarily in the sitting and standing positions.

Logically, then, having the patient involved in the development of the HEP can boost adherence. For example, when patients are asked if they are doing their exercises they sometimes say, "I'm doing the exercises but not all of them." Our job is to explore the patients' reasons for avoiding those exercises.

One reason for exercise avoidance is pain. An exercise that causes pain should be evaluated to determine whether the patient is performing it correctly. Any exercise that is performed correctly but remains painful should be discontinued, and another exercise should be substituted for it to target the original impairment. Time can be another reason for not adhering. If a patient has an extensive HEP, the exercises can be divided up so that the patient performs some on one day and the remainder on the next. This method can reduce daily exercise time yet continue to address necessary or potential impairments. Alternatively, the patients can do all the lying exercises on one day, all the sitting exercises on the next day, and all the standing exercises on the third day. The closer the exercise duplicates a functional activity, the greater the adherence. For example, I have observed that the repeated sit-to-stand exercise exhibits a high level of adherence. Another way of improving adherence is to modify the offending exercise so that it is more suitable or to educate the patient about the functional reason behind a particular exercise.

Case Example: Exercise Programming for YOPD

Lina is 38 yr old and in Hoehn and Yahr stage 1.5 (unilateral disease, axial involvement, balance intact). Other than having young onset PD (YOPD), she is generally healthy.

Subjective Evaluation

Lina's goal is to learn a comprehensive HEP for prevention. She is concerned that PD will make her weak. Currently, she does not exercise but stays active with housework and raising her two children, ages 9 and 12.

Objective Evaluation

Lina exhibits normal general strength. Mild flexibility impairments are noted in the right extremities and trunk rotation. Balance testing demonstrates no deficiencies. Gait deviations exhibit reduced trunk rotation, reduced right arm swing, and reduced stride length on the right.

Goals

The following goals are established:

- Lina needs to demonstrate understanding of HEP (proper form).
- She should demonstrate improved stride length of the right lower extremity during gait.

(continued)

Case Example *(continued)*

Therapeutic Interventions

Lina is educated in the common misconceptions of PD (see chapter 1, "Introduction to Parkinson's Disease and Its Physical Management," page 6) and the benefits of exercise and walking. She is reassured that PD does not cause weakness but that inactivity and lack of exercise can cause deconditioning and loss of flexibility. She is instructed in strengthening exercises that target postural muscles (thoracolumbar extensors and scapular musculature and hip extensors) and conditioning exercises for the lower extremities (hip abductors, quadriceps, and gastrocnemius) that can maintain her ability to balance and perform transfers.

Stretching exercises target the trunk (rotation and extension) and the flexor muscle groups (pectoral muscles, hip flexors, hamstrings, and gastrocnemius). Because Lina is young, she has a greater range of exercise possibilities than is typically possible for older people (with or without PD) who have various comorbidities to contend with and work around. Yoga classes are recommended as an alternative.

Lina is advised to perform exercises daily while undergoing therapy to learn proper technique and expose any exercises that may be incompatible because of pain or difficulties. After her exercise program is solidified, Lina is given further instruction regarding the needed frequency for stretching versus strengthening exercises for long-term maintenance. Suggestions are made about how to progress with strengthening exercises. Gait deviations are addressed with attention strategies. She is advised to walk at least 30 min daily or perform other cardiovascular activity such as biking or swimming. She is advised that the recommended intensity for exercise benefits should be an RPE of "somewhat hard."

Outcomes

Lina quickly learned the needed exercises and was able to improve stride length on the right with attention strategies. She is motivated and therefore will probably prevent the development of potential impairments, a task that is far less difficult than attempting to regain what is already deficient.

Attempting to gain adherence to a home exercise program can be an art. The saying "Something is better than nothing" can encourage a patient to do exactly that. Some of the most difficult patients to motivate are those who are depressed or see the glass as half empty. Some patients will never adhere to recommendations, whether they come from a medical doctor, psychiatrist, or allied health professional. I have found these people to be in the minority. Regardless, patients are ultimately responsible for their health and well-being, and they must live with the consequences of their decisions.

Some patients, of course, are not able to help themselves and must rely on caregivers for their ability to exercise. The burden is then on the caregiver to ensure adherence and optimal mobility. Unfortunately, the caregiver is not always able to handle this burden, in which case alternative resources should be discussed. The next chapter discusses how to assist caregivers in their role.

Summary

1. People with PD and older people have similar musculoskeletal impairments, but people with PD are at greater risk of developing impairments because they have more difficulty with movement.

2. Inactivity plays a major role in muscle weakness and secondary impairment of mobility.

3. When applicable, patients should be advised to exercise when PD medications are most effective to optimize gains because L-dopa reduces rigidity and bradykinesia.

4. Muscle weakness is not a symptom of PD.

5. Stretching for longer hold times is more effective in tight muscles.

6. Strengthening guideline: one set of 8 to 12 repetitions per muscle group with an RPE of "somewhat hard" and performed in proper form is recommended for strength improvements and maintenance.

7. Power strengthening produces greater functional gains than strength training alone.

8. The effects of exercise can start to diminish after 2 wk if a significant reduction in activity occurs. Benefits of exercise can be completely lost in 2 to 8 mo if exercise is not resumed.

9. Patient education that addresses exercise and its importance to mobility and quality of life can improve adherence and prevent deconditioning.

10. Optimizing adherence with an HEP requires an individual approach and open communication with the patient.

4

Equipping Caregivers

The act of caregiving can encompass meeting a variety of needs for the patient including financial, emotional, legal, social, and physical support. The term *caregiver* applies to anyone who gives care to a person who needs it. Typically, care is provided by an informal caregiver, often the significant other, although other family members may share the role. Formal caregivers are hired help.

Caregiving may come more naturally to allied health professionals. Occupational therapists, physical therapists, and nursing professionals have the training to perform transfers safely with proper body mechanics. Occupational therapists learned about adaptive equipment to improve capabilities with activities of daily living (ADLs). People in all three disciplines were instructed in how to help someone walk without putting the patient or health care worker at risk. Most informal caregivers, however, have not received the training necessary to take care of their loved ones optimally and safely. Hired caregivers also have varying levels of knowledge in the physical management of patients. Family members or hired caregivers need to learn how to maneuver the patient safely to prevent injury to themselves or the patient and to reduce potential physical and emotional stress for both. This chapter discusses the limitations of caregivers and ways to improve their physical management of the people they help.

Caregiver Burden and Educational Needs

Studies have shown that the burden of caregiving increases with worsening of mobility (Martinez-Martin et al., 2005; Schrag et al., 2006). Some of the cognitive and physical deficits can weigh more heavily than others. One study demonstrated that the caregiver felt greater burden when the person with PD had problems with hallucinations, depression, confusion, and falls (Schrag et al., 2006). The caregiver's concern with falls is due, in part, to lack of knowledge about how to help and the inability to assist the patient from the floor safely without being injured him- or herself (Davey et al., 2004). Another study reported that the caregiver felt greater burden when the patient had ADL limitations and the caregiver did not know how to handle these problems (Edwards & Scheetz, 2002). In addition, many caregivers are sleep deprived. Sleep disturbances were found in 27% of caregivers in one study, which added further to the burden felt by the caregiver (Happe & Berger, 2002). When the combined effects of sleep deprivation and lack of training in physical management are considered, it is no wonder that caregivers can appear stressed or tired.

Regardless of the level of caregiving needs, education should be an integral part of the health professional's interventions. Education about PD itself, physical management to optimize capabilities, and dispelling any misconceptions can all help with coping (see chapter 1, "Introduction to Parkinson's Disease and Its Physical Management," pages 6–7 regarding PD misconceptions).

Providing information about PD to children of a parent with PD was addressed in one study. Fifty percent of adolescent children and adult children reported not having information about the disease that would have helped them with expectations and coping (Schrag et al., 2004).

Resources for Caregivers

The caregiver and the person with PD can both benefit from various disciplines, services, and resources to address their physical and informational needs. The following suggestions can help the caregiver or the person with PD address commonly encountered problems.

Referrals

Patients or their caregivers can be given the patient handout "Can Therapy Help Me?" (Boelen et al., 2006) to facilitate appropriate referrals for PT, OT, or speech disciplines (see appendix D for a reproducible handout).

Occupational and Speech Therapy

Besides physical therapy, occupational and speech therapy services can facilitate improvements to quality of life for both the person with PD and the caregiver.

Occupational therapy

The caregiver or patient may not be aware of occupational therapy services. Evaluation of the home environment and ADL needs can offer practical insights and solutions to safety hazards and environmental barriers. Gaining knowledge of available equipment may reduce stress of potential future needs and enable greater self-management.

Speech therapy

Intelligibility of speech, a common problem in people with PD, does not appear to be correlated to disease duration and is weakly correlated to disease severity (Miller et al., 2007). The inability to communicate effectively can lead to social isolation as well as frustration when attempting to vocalize even basic needs. People with PD can develop a soft monotone voice and have difficulties with articulation. They tend to have an altered perception of their speech loudness (Sadagopan & Huber, 2007). For example, people with PD perceive their soft voice to be at a normal volume. They perceive speaking at a normal volume as yelling.

Medical management can help improve speech to a limited degree. Strengthening the supporting musculature for speech and respiration, and training to improve articulation and self-perception of loudness require physical intervention. A specialized speech training program called Lee Silverman Voice Treatment (LSVT) has been developed for people with PD to improve volume of speech and intelligibility (Sapir et al., 2007). The caregiver and patient should be aware of such interventions. As with any physical intervention, prevention or optimization sooner rather than later is the better approach.

People with PD can also develop swallowing problems. Aspiration pneumonia may result from swallowing difficulties. Symptoms are coughing or choking during or after eating or drinking. The patient may sound congested and demonstrate a relatively acute physical or mental decline. The speech therapist can assess the patient's swallowing capabilities and make recommendations.

Respite Care

What is respite care? The dictionary definition of the word *respite* is to "offer temporary relief especially from something distressing or trying" or "to give interval of relief from." The caregiver or family member can hire temporary help to relieve family members from their caregiving role so that they can rejuvenate or accomplish duties outside the home. PD organizations may be able to direct families to local respite care agencies. PD organizations or social workers may be able to provide guidance to those with financial limitations so that they can obtain services.

Medical Alert System

Although medical alert systems have gained recognition over the years, many people still do not understand when such a device would be useful or how it works. Included in appendix D is a reproducible handout that explains the medical alert system. Here is what the health care professional needs to know about such systems:

• A patient who cannot get up from the floor even with the assist of the caregiver is advised either to call 911 or to subscribe to a medical alert system.

• Medical alert systems should be recommended for patients who are at high risk for falls and live alone or for people at risk of falls who live with other family members but are alone at times throughout the day or night. The medical alert system is a service. The patient wears either a wristband or a necklace with a push button (see figure 4.1, *a* and *b*). The push-button device is waterproof so that it can be worn in the shower. If the patient falls, he or she pushes the button. The service then calls the patient on a special phone that also acts as an intercom. Some services have only the intercom hookup (see figure 4.2, *a* and *b*). The service then contacts the proper authorities, who will go to the patient's home and provide assistance. Having this system in place relieves stress on the caregiver and family members, and the patient knows that help is available.

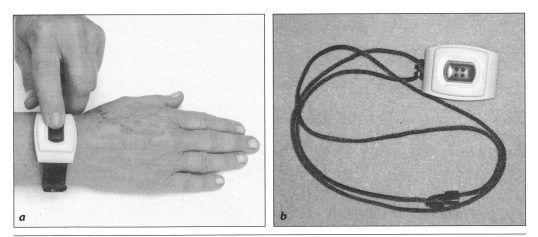

Figure 4.1 Medical alert system push button devices: *(a)* wristband type, *(b)* necklace type.

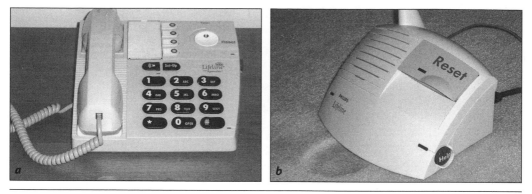

Figure 4.2 *(a)* Medical alert system phone and intercom combination; *(b)* intercom only.

- The following are some of the companies that offer medical alert systems:
  - Lifeline: www.LifelineSystems.com, 800-543-3546
  - Medical Alert: http://medicalalarm.com, 800-588-0200
  - AlertOne: www.Alert-1.com, 800-693-5433
  - Lifefone: www.lifefone.com, 800-882-2280
  - American Red Cross (not available in all states)

Informational Resources

Patients may not be tapped into the resources that they need. Agencies can provide information on PD or direct patients to doctors and facilities who specialize in PD. A great deal of information is available to help the patient, caregiver, and family. The following list describes several helpful resources.

- The information and referral centers of the American Parkinson Disease Association (APDA) (www.apdaparkinson.org) can guide patients and caregivers to sources of help. Information is available about locations and meeting times of support groups and exercise classes in local areas. The APDA has a separate information and referral center for people with young onset PD. The APDA has many free informational publications for patients and caregivers.

- The National Parkinson Foundation (NPF) (www.parkinson.org) has information on centers and physicians worldwide who specialize in movement disorders. The NPF offers free informational publications for patients and caregivers.

- The Parkinson's Disease Society of Great Britain (www.parkinsons.org.uk) offers information on PD for caregivers and health care professionals. Included are Web sites for traveling with special needs:
  - www.access-able.com, "Access-Able Travel Source," is a U.S.-based Web site.
  - www.pwd-online.ca, "Access to Travel—Canada," is a Web site that has general information for people with disabilities including a section on travel.

- The book *Parkinson's Disease: 300 Tips for Making Life Easier* by Shelley Peterman Schwarz (ISBN: 1-888799-65-X) is a helpful and practical guide for the clinician, caregiver, or patient.

Therapist-Provided Training

The physical therapist should take seriously the responsibility to educate their patients' caregivers in the following areas. If the caregiver is not properly trained in these important skills, unnecessary stress, both physical and psychological, can result.

Nighttime Care

People with PD typically do not take L-dopa medication at night because it may cause sleep disturbances or have side effects. Nighttime mobility is therefore more difficult than daytime mobility. Arming patients and caregivers with options to reduce nighttime difficulties may allow more restful nights, which can be critically needed.

- Using a bed assist rail (see chapter 10, "Bed Mobility," pages 122–124) can improve bed mobility at night. If the patient needs assistance to get up at night (sometimes frequently), the caregiver also loses sleep. Using the bed assist rail may enable the patient to get up independently, or at least with less assistance. At best, the caregiver can get the rest needed for adequate functioning during waking hours. At minimum, the caregiver will not need to provide as much assistance during the night. Use of the bed assist rail can also give the patient a greater sense of independence. Patients and caregivers often verbalize great appreciation for this device.

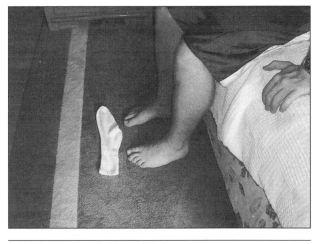

- "Off" freezing occurs when dopamine levels are low. Typically, L-dopa replacement medications are not taken at night, resulting in nighttime "off" freezing that is more responsive to visual cueing than "on" freezing is. Placing a sock on the floor (of a contrasting color) next to the bed can provide a target for the patient to step over on the first step to start walking (see figure 4.3).

- A bedside commode or a urinal can reduce awake time and improve safety. The occupational or physical therapist can offer insights to optimize commode transfers.

Figure 4.3   A visual cue, such as a sock placed in front of the feet, can be helpful for "off" freezing.

- Greater use of night lighting may improve nighttime stability. People with PD tend to rely on vision for balance to compensate for proprioceptive integration deficits (Vaugoyeau et al., 2007).

Dealing With Freezing

The caregiver may need to assist the patient with lateral weight shifting. This process should be reviewed with the caregiver (see chapter 14, "Freezing," pages 169–194, for freezing interventions).

The caregiver may also need to advise the patient how to unfreeze by using various strategies. Issuing a handout on freezing will help reinforce the techniques learned (see appendix D for a reproducible patient handout on freezing strategies).

Floor Transfers

People with PD who are at risk of falls should know how to get up from the floor, and caregivers should know how to help them if needed (see chapter 11, "Floor Transfers," pages 132–135). Most informal caregivers are not knowledgeable in this area and secondarily become hurt when attempting to help (Davey et al., 2004). People with moderately involved PD and their caregivers often voice appreciation and a sense of relief as they learn how to get up from the floor.

An instructional video that reviews floor transfers is *Part Two: Parkinson's Disease & the Art of Moving* by John Argue, www.parkinsonsexercise.com or 510-985-2645. This video also reviews balance exercises and compensatory strategies for freezing and walking.

Recommendations for a gait belt should be made, if necessary to improve transfer abilities. Caregivers do not always know how to use a gait belt and may need instruction in its use.

Ambulation

At times I have seen a caregiver assist a patient with ambulation by simply holding hands. This method is not optimal. Although they may still be holding hands when the patient trips, the patient can fall and hit the ground. Gait training with the caregiver and the patient may be necessary to maximize safety for both. Having the caregiver hold the patient's arm above the elbow offers better leverage for the caregiver to provide balance control. The caregiver may need instruction in compensatory strategies to reinforce optimal gait patterns. See chapter 13, "Compensatory Strategies for Gait Interventions," pages 151–164, and "Attention Strategies," a reproducible patient handout in appendix D, to help teach the caregiver about these compensatory strategies, as well as how to assist with weight shifting.

Home Exercise Program

In the presence of cognitive impairments, the patient may need assistance or guidance with the home exercise program. The therapist should be sensitive to the capabilities of the caregiver and patient. The caregiver should be educated about the importance of exercise for maintaining mobility and secondarily for minimizing the burden on the caregiver.

When you are confident that the caregiver grasps the necessity of regular exercise outside the clinic, the following points may be helpful:

• Exercise classes can make exercising more fun and more social. Getting out of the house can help both the caregiver and the patient. Location and times of exercise classes for people with PD can be obtained from the PD organizations listed earlier.

• A personal trainer for the patient can provide substantial relief for the caregiver. Although the cost may be prohibitive for some people, a trainer is valuable because she or he can take the burden off the caregiver and is usually better equipped than a spouse to motivate a patient.

• If a patient already has a personal trainer, the therapist should avoid duplication of exercises and attempt to complement the current regimen. For a comprehensive approach specific to PD, therapists and trainers should communicate regarding overall deficits, needs, and physical management regarding compensatory strategies. The caregiver or patient can facilitate communications by showing the trainer exercise handouts received in therapy, showing the therapist the log of exercises performed with the trainer, or asking the trainer to attend one of the therapy sessions for instruction on specialized maneuvers.

• Videos strongly motivate some people to exercise. Various exercise videos are available for seniors and for people with PD. Videos should be selected based on the person's capabilities.

Hans has PD and is at Hoehn and Yahr stage 3 (mild to moderate bilateral disease, postural instability, physically independent) during his "on" state. During his "off" state he is at Hoehn and Yahr stage 4 (severe disability, still able to walk or stand unassisted). His wife, Adrienne, is his sole caregiver. She retired early from her job to help take care of him.

Subjective Evaluation

Hans and Adrienne live together in a one-level home that requires only one step to enter the house. Adrienne reports that Hans needs a lot of help in the evening, at night, and in the morning. In the evening when he is ready to go to bed, he needs assistance to get out of a chair and walk to the bedroom. At night he tries to get out of bed to go to the bathroom but is unable to do so. Adrienne's back is now starting to hurt from lifting. In the morning before taking his first dose of L-dopa medication, Hans' gait is narrowly based and he freezes frequently, requiring Adrienne's assistance for ambulation to prevent falls. Hans reports falling a few times a week because of freezing during his "off" state when he attempts to walk without Adrienne's help.

Hans exercises during his "on" state 5 d a week. Both Hans and his wife agree that once his anti-Parkinson's medications start working, he is physically able to function independently. He walks about 20 min daily with Adrienne and does not use an assist device, but he thinks that his strides are shortening. He owns a two-wheeled walker but not a bed assist rail.

Objective Evaluation

During the evaluation Hans is in his "on" state, exhibiting mild dyskinesias in his trunk and extremities. He exhibits normal strength and flexibility. No difficulties are noted with bed mobility or chair transfers. Postural reflexes are impaired, but Hans is able to recover from the pull test without having to be caught, although recovery is marginal. His gait is steady without an assist device. Primary gait deviations are reduced stride length, arm swing, and trunk rotation. No freezing is noted.

Goals

Goals are directed to improving mobility during his "off" state. Achievement of goals will rely on observations during his "on" state to confirm understanding and feedback from Hans and Adrienne when he is in his "off" state. The following were established:

- Hans will be able to get in and out of his bed at night with supervision and minimal assistance by using the bed assist rail.
- Adrienne will demonstrate how to assist Hans with getting out of bed using the bed assist rail with proper body mechanics to minimize back strain.
- Both Adrienne and Hans will demonstrate understanding of proper body mechanics with chair transfers to reduce difficulties in the evening.

(continued)

Case Example *(continued)*

- Hans will demonstrate in therapy how to use his two-wheeled walker properly during turns and linear ambulation during his "on" state.
- Adrienne or Hans will report improved control of freezing and improved stability with walking when using his rolling walker during his "off" state.
- Hans will demonstrate improved stride length with use of rhythmic auditory stimulation during his "on" state.

Therapeutic Interventions

Interventions will require the presence and participation of both Hans and Adrienne. Hans is instructed how to use the bed assist rail and how to position himself to optimize body mechanics when getting out of a chair and to reduce difficulties (Adrienne observes the interventions with Hans so that she can reinforce or advise him, if needed, regarding proper procedure.) Adrienne is instructed how to guide and assist Hans with bed mobility and chair transfers to minimize strain on her back and optimize safety. Hans, in the presence of Adrienne, is instructed how to use the walker. Adrienne is advised how to assist Hans in weight shifting to help control freezing and improve stride length for "off" states. Finally, gait training with rhythmic auditory stimulation is instituted.

Outcomes

Adrienne and Hans report significant improvements in bed mobility. Hans can now pull himself up into a sitting position with the bed rail, although he still needs help with his legs when getting into bed. Adrienne reports that her back is feeling much better. Chair transfers remain difficult but are not as much of a strain. Freezing is significantly reduced with the walker, and Hans now requires only minimal assistance or close supervision for walking when "off." When Hans walks to music he is able to take bigger steps. This type of outcome is not unusual, but achieving it requires both to do their part by consistently performing activities learned in therapy. Following up on the equipment recommendations to reduce difficulties is critical. Other factors affecting outcomes are disease severity, comorbidities, cognition, motivation, health status of the caregiver, and, in some cases, having the financial means to hire a needed caregiver.

Summary

1. Caregivers typically lack the knowledge to take care of a family member, a situation that creates great stress on the caregiver.
2. Physical therapy, occupational therapy, and speech therapy should include caregivers so that the stress on them can be reduced through educational and physical management.
3. Copious amounts of educational materials are available for the caregiver and patient. The health professional should try to connect patients to these resources.

DYSKINESIA

The term *dyskinesia* typically refers to choreatic movements in the Parkinson's disease population and is the side effect of dopaminergic medications. In a broader sense, the term *dyskinesia* refers to other types of abnormal movements. In this part of the book, the types of dyskinetic movements addressed are dystonia and tremors. Both dystonia and tremors tend to be resistant to medical and physical management. The physical management of dystonia therefore focuses on minimizing the effect of existing or potential musculoskeletal, cardiovascular, and respiratory impairments. Camptocormic postures and drop-head postures often necessitate the use of supportive devices to improve ability during activities. The physical management of tremors focuses more on the use of adaptive equipment.

Postural Variations
and Dystonia

Postural deviations vary significantly in the PD population. The Parkinsonian posture is typically associated with a forward inclination of the trunk. Less commonly, some people with PD exhibit an exaggerated forward bent posture (figure 5.1*a*). On the other hand, a person who has had PD for many years may exhibit a normal posture or undergo postural changes that are related to aging rather than PD (figure 5.1*b*). The forward-flexed posture may be one of the contributing factors to gait festination or anterior postural instability. Some people with PD may exhibit a scoliotic posture or a severe forward bent posture that can be caused by dystonia of the abdominal musculature or weakness of the back muscles. Dystonia is a sustained muscle contraction that produces involuntary twisting and abnormal posturing that can become more pronounced with voluntary movements (Tarsey, 2000). Scoliotic trunk deviations can interfere with lateral weight shifting while ambulating, which is already typically reduced in people with PD. In more severe cases, scoliosis can interfere with respiratory capacity.

This chapter focuses on the severe and atypical postural disturbances (camptocormic and drop-head postures) that may or may not have a dystonic component and on ankle and foot dystonia, which is a more common site for dystonia in people with PD and is unrelated to camptocormic and drop-head postures. Evidence of the effectiveness of medical and physical management for all three of these disturbances is limited. The interventions proposed for the physical management of these disturbances are the result of reviewing the medical literature and implementing interventions in an attempt to reduce impairments and ultimately improve function. Knowledge of the benefits and limitations of these measures is helpful in patient education and in determining appropriate interventions. "Axial Dystonia and Exercise" presents general principles of exercise management for those with axial dystonia.

Camptocormic Posture

Camptocormia is defined by marked forward inclination of the trunk (figure 5.1*a*), which worsens while walking, disappears in the supine position, and has little to no response to levodopa (L-dopa) (Djaldetti & Melamed, 2006; Feriha et al., 2004). The forward-flexed trunk angle needs to be greater than 45° to be considered camptocormic (Shaheda et al., 2005). Photographs of camptocormic postures exhibit forward angulation of the trunk occurring with excessive hip flexion (Karbowski, 1999; Shaheda et al., 2005). This type

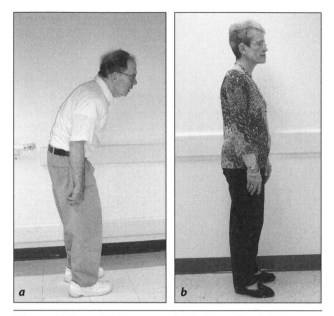

Figure 5.1 *(a)* This person with Parkinson's exhibits a forward-flexed posture that is more exaggerated than the typical Parkinsonian posture. His posture is descriptive of a camptocormic type of posture. *(b)* This person was diagnosed with PD 10 yr ago, yet her posture is normal for her age.

of posture often presents with scoliosis and localized lumbar kyphosis in the absence of excessive thoracic kyphosis.

Camptocormic posturing has been observed in PD, multiple system atrophy disorders, and dystonic disorders (Slawek et al., 2006; Song et al., 2007). Multiple systems atrophy (MSA) is a category of movement disorders that generally responds poorly to L-dopa medication but shares Parkinsonian symptoms. MSA includes the following diagnoses: Shy-Drager syndrome, striatonigral degeneration, and olivopontocerebellar atrophy.

Etiology

Although the cause of camptocormic postures remains unclear, two major theories address their etiology. One suggests that peripheral mechanisms—myopathic changes in the paravertebral musculature—are at the root of these postures (Charpentier et al., 2005; Ozer et al., 2007; Schabitz et al., 2003). Another theory postulates that central nervous system (CNS) mechanisms trigger abdominal dystonia (Bloch et al., 2006; Djaldetti et al., 1999).

Axial Dystonia and Exercise

Follow these general guidelines for prescribing and supervising exercise for those with axial dystonia:

- The primary focus is maintaining strength and flexibility to avoid contractures (Tarsy & Simon, 2006).

- Avoid any exercise position that triggers dystonia. Choose positions that minimize dystonia. Typically, the patient is a good resource regarding triggers and can help to determine optimal positions.

- Dystonic responses will dictate interventions. Modifications of the home exercise program may be necessary to avoid aggravation of symptoms and to optimize intended outcomes.

- Dystonic triggers are specific to the individual. These triggers should be noted and avoided.

My experience supports both theories. Patients with camptocormic postures often report a pulling or tensing sensation in their abdominal muscles and low back fatigue that progresses to low back pain with increased ambulation. Some patients experience back fatigue without dystonia which becomes painful and limits ambulation. I have also observed that dystonia of the abdominal muscles is triggered with walking and in static standing when patients attempt to raise their arms. Ambulation and standing endurance become limited. These patients are at risk of becoming deconditioned.

Management

Although limitations in the management of camptocormic postures persist, maintaining or improving functionality is still possible with physical management. Medical management of camptocormic posture remains a challenge but is still being explored.

Medical Management

The benefits of medical management for camptocormia are limited. A study that looked at the effectiveness of Botox for treating dystonic abdominal muscles showed that improvement occurred in four of the nine patients (Shaheda et al., 2005). A few case studies address the effects of deep brain stimulation (DBS) on camptocormic postures. People with PD who underwent bilateral DBS of the subthalamic nucleus or the globus pallidus internus have shown improvement of this posture (Hellmann et al., 2006; Micheli et al., 2005; Yamada et al., 2006).

Although L-dopa medications can improve other symptoms in people with PD, this medication offers little or no benefit toward camptocormic postures (Shaheda et al., 2005). See table 2.1, Dopamine Replacement Drugs, page 13, for benefits and limitations of L-dopa medications.

Physical Management

The lack of evidence for the physical management of camptocormic posture brings me to share a pattern of interventions that I have developed over the years from working with this population. Although improving strength in the extensor musculature is possible, these gains are insufficient to have any significant effect on posture, walking endurance, and pain. Soft lumbar supports without stays have demonstrated limited benefits with ambulation endurance and comfort. Restrictive and supportive corsets have reportedly been too difficult to don and are impractical or uncomfortable, which has resulted in poor compliance.

I have found that supporting and protecting the spine by using a walker has resulted in optimal functional outcomes. As this benefit became increasingly apparent to me, I began to speak more frankly with patients about the benefits and limitations of physical therapy interventions. Introducing to a patient the idea of using a walker is often an emotional moment. Many have not previously entertained the thought of using a walker, and their balance is typically intact. Here are guidelines that I have found effective for this population:

- Patient education
  - Discuss realistic expectations from therapy interventions, particularly the need to rely on external support to reduce severity of forward bent posture or back strain. Establish the connection between poor posture and pain.

- Review guidance about types of chairs. Soft deep chairs only worsen postural alignment. Chairs should be comfortable yet supportive to optimize posture. For optimal back support, the buttocks need to be as far back in the seat as possible. This position can be accomplished by leaning forward, scooting the buttocks to the back of the seat, and then sitting up straight. Encouraging patients to do this "buttocks check" will reinforce the concept. An exception to this suggestion is the person who exhibits an inflexible lumbar kyphosis, which causes the buttocks to slide forward when attempting to sit up straight.

- Advise your patient on the importance of maintaining the flexibility and strength of the surrounding tissues for optimal bone and joint health, respiratory capacity, and minimization of discomfort or pain. See the section "Adherence With Home Exercise Programs" (chapter 3, "Exercise and Rehabilitation Considerations," pages 40–42) for material on increasing patient adherence.

- Progressive stretching and strengthening program for the postural, respiratory, and proximal musculature (shoulders and hips)
  - Focus should be on a home exercise program for long-term maintenance.
  - Depending on dystonia and standing tolerance, exercises may need to be performed in lying and sitting to minimize triggering of dystonia or back discomfort.
  - See chapter 3 for exercise suggestions to benefit posture.

- Ambulating with a walker. Walking with a walker offers significant improvements in back comfort and ambulation endurance necessary to prevent deconditioning. Although the walker helps maintain current posture, it is not intended to correct posture. Patients often report arm fatigue when using a walker, a problem that seems to be related to the severity of their abdominal dystonia.
  - Adjusting the walker to the proper height can be a challenge, but consideration should be given to the patient's most comfortable or attainable postural position when walking.
  - Typically, patients ask to have the walker handles adjusted on the tall side because they believe that the high position will help them walk more erectly. Having the walker handles higher, however, results in excessive elbow flexion because of the inability to maintain an erect posture when walking. This position creates undue strain on the upper extremities and neck area (figure 5.2a). If the walker handles are too high, some patients tend to extend their elbows fully, causing them to lag farther behind the walker. Both scenarios place greater strain on the patient, and the latter situation can be unsafe because the patient will have difficulty controlling the speed of the walker.
  - Walker handle heights need to be adjusted lower than conventional adjustments to minimize upper-extremity fatigue and allow the patient to ambulate in the new "natural" posture (figure 5.2b).
  - When adjusting for proper walker height (handle height at wrist level with arms relaxed at the side), patients will attempt to stand taller than their "natural" posture. After they start walking, their natural posture will dominate. The handle heights should be adjusted to this more natural posture to avoid excessive elbow flexion and strain. Some patients with a stronger dystonic component may require an even lower handle height so that the elbow is close to full extension to minimize arm fatigue.

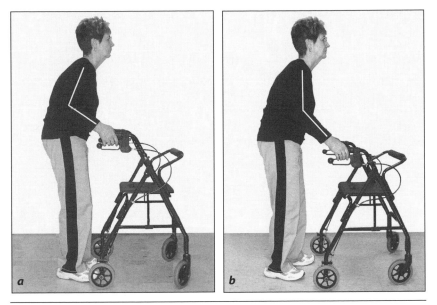

Figure 5.2 *(a)* A higher handle position that does not improve posture and causes greater strain; *(b)* a lower handle height that reduces strain and does not worsen posture.

Case Example: Camptocormic Posture

Jose is 64 yr old and has PD (Hoehr and Yahr stage 2). His physiatrist has recommended therapy for back pain. X rays demonstrate degenerative changes in the lumbar spine.

Subjective Evaluation

Jose reportedly started walking with a cane 6 weeks ago due to recent onset of walking bent over. He states he needs the cane for back support to reduce back discomfort. Prior to this he reportedly exercised regularly. Ambulation is now limited due to back pain which progressively worsens with increased ambulation. He has no back pain when sitting or lying. Back pain escalates to 8/10 when walking. He has become a household ambulator except for running errands. Currently his walking endurance is about 2 minutes. His goal is to be able to walk 15 minutes with less back discomfort.

Objective Evaluation

Jose's posture is camptocormic with right thoracolumbar "C" scoliosis and lumbar kyphosis. He is forward bent and leaning to the left. His lumbar spine exhibits a reversal of the normal lumbar lordosis. Jose's bilateral upper and lower extremities have normal strength. Palpable muscle contraction is noted only in the lumbar paravertebrals.

(continued)

Range of motion: Limitations are noted in bilateral hip extension, bilateral shoulder flexion, lumbar extension (able to reduce lumbar kyphosis to a flat lumbar position but unable to obtain a lordotic posture), and left lateral chest expansion.

Jose's gait shows progressive worsening of camptocormic posture with use of a cane. Ambulation endurance is limited to 100 ft (30 m) because of back fatigue and low back pain 8/10. No balance deficits are noted.

Goals

Short-term goals for Jose are the following:

- He will become independent with a home exercise program to optimize rib cage mobility, respiratory function, and axial and proximal flexibility and strength.
- The patient will demonstrate understanding of proper sitting postures to optimize axial alignment (by minimizing lumbar kyphosis in sitting).

Long-term goals for Jose are the following:

- He will increase ambulation tolerance to 0.25 mi (0.4 km) or 15 min with a walker.
- He will demonstrate proper use of the walker in several ways:
  - Effectively use handbrakes for velocity control, ramps, and curbs and when sitting down or standing up from the walker seat.
  - Stay within close boundaries of the walker to minimize strain and maintain control of walker speed.
  - Perform proper turns with the walker—turning the body with the walker as a unit and keeping the feet within the boundaries of the two rear wheels.
  - Reduce low back pain with ambulation from 8/10 to 3/10 when using a walker.

Therapeutic Interventions

- The patient was educated about outcome expectations, back protection, pain reduction, and the importance of a home exercise and walking program for self-maintenance.
- Jose was instructed in an HEP that emphasized the following:
  - Flexibility exercises that target the spine, hips, rib cage, and shoulders
  - Strengthening exercises performed primarily in lying or in the hands-and-knees position because these positions do not trigger Jose's abdominal dystonia
- Strengthening exercises:
  - Supine: upper-extremity and upper-back strengthening using a Thera-band (progressed with increased resistance); bridging (progressed to single-leg bridging)

(continued)

Case Example   *(continued)*

- Side lying: side plank, hip abduction (progressed with ankle weights)
- Quadruped position (hands and knees): single-leg lift (progressed to simultaneous opposite arm and leg lift) attempting neutral spine; rising from quadruped into kneeling position
  - "Comparative" gait training:
    - Various devices are assessed for ability to control pain and optimize endurance while ambulating. Jose ambulates with his cane alone, with cane and lumbar support, and finally with only a walker.
    - Jose offers feedback on the level of pain control with various devices.
    - The therapist offers feedback on endurance capabilities with various devices.

Outcomes

"Comparative" gait training is necessary for the patient to experience dramatic improvements with endurance and pain reduction when using a walker. This approach helps pave the road to accepting the need for such a device and optimizing outcomes. Improvements as noted in this example are not unusual. After pain is managed with the walker, endurance limitations often result from deconditioning, which is easily remedied by walking more, or from arm fatigue in those with severe abdominal dystonia. Jose is motivated and has performed his exercises regularly. He has been hesitant to use a walker but understands the benefits. His walking endurance remains at 2 min with the cane because of pain at 8/10, but with the walker he is able to achieve his goal of walking 15 min with back pain at 3/10.

Drop-Head Posture

Drop-head posture is a downward-flexed posture of the head when the chin is almost resting on the chest (see figure 5.3, *a* and *b*). Drop-head posture affects swallowing capability and interferes with the ability to look up while walking, talking to someone, driving, or watching television.

Etiology

Dystonia in the anterior cervical musculature or myopathy of the cervical paravertebrals can result in drop-head posture. This condition tends to be more common in people with multiple systems atrophy (MSA) disorders, but it is also seen in people with PD (Askmark et al., 2001; Boesch et al., 2002; Rivest et al., 1990). People with PD can demonstrate a mix of dystonia of the anterior cervical musculature and weakness of the cervical extensors (Askmark et al., 2001; Fujimoto, 2006). No correlation seems to exist between disease severity and the severity of the drop-head posture (Yoshiyama et al., 1999). People with multiple systems atrophy who have this posture exhibit a greater propensity for having dystonia in the anterior musculature (Boesch et al., 2002; Fujimoto, 2006).

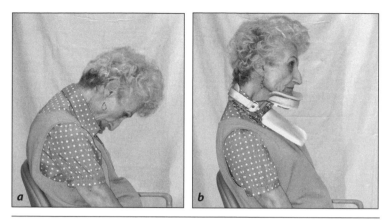

Figure 5.3 Drop-head posture *(a)* with no support and *(b)* with the support of an Oxford collar.

Management

Although medical management attempts to minimize the activity of dystonic muscles, the need to protect the spine and improve posture requires additional physical intervention.

Medical Management

Medications such as dopamine agonists tend to worsen this posture. Only some patients show improvement with L-dopa. Botox to the anterior neck musculature has limited results (Fujimoto, 2006). One of the side effects of Botox to the cervical musculature is dysphasia (swallowing problems), which is transient and lasts approximately 2 wk (Slawek et al., 2005).

Physical Management

As with camptocormic postures, strengthening interventions are marginally effective for drop-head postures to improve functionality, although the pathology is now the posterior cervical musculature instead of the lumbar region. Several interventions are included:

- Patient education
  - Patients sometimes voice expectations (or wishes) to correct their posture fully. They need to be advised to have realistic expectations from therapy interventions; they can expect to achieve only limited ability to lift the head, such as to hold it up long enough to perform brief functional activities.
  - Increase patients' awareness of the connection between poor posture and pain.
  - Inform patients of the importance of maintaining the flexibility and strength of the surrounding tissues for optimal bone and joint health and swallowing capability.
- Flexibility and strengthening exercises for the cervical, postural, and scapular musculature
  - Conditioning and shoulder ROM may need to be performed in supine to minimize dystonia or optimize comfort.
  - Focus should be on a home exercise program for long-term maintenance.

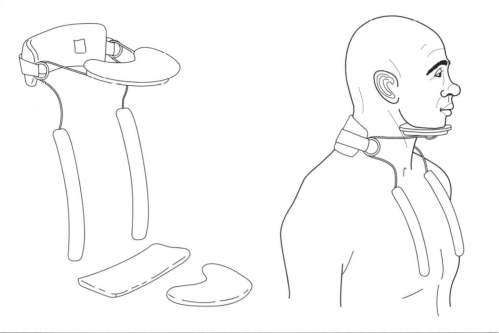

Figure 5.4   The Oxford collar improves cervical posture for those with drop-head posture.

- Orthotics
  - In my opinion soft cervical collars do not offer enough support to hold up the head. Patients report that these collars are often too warm when worn for extended periods. Over time, patients complain about the lack of effectiveness of soft collars.
  - Rigid collars may create greater pressure areas, especially for those with dystonia.
  - Depending on the severity of the dystonia, an effective orthotic for a drop-head posture is the Oxford collar (see figure 5.4). Made from foam and wire, this type of collar provides anterior support and allows cervical rotation. Improving cervical positioning reduces cervical strain and secondarily decreases pain experienced because of poor posturing. This collar is typically worn as needed for necessary activities or comfort.

Case Example: Drop-Head Posture

Barb has Parkinson's disease (Hoehn and Yahr stage 3). Drop-head posture developed approximately a year ago. X rays exhibit degenerative changes in the cervical spine. Barb exhibits a drop-head posture in the absence of dystonia.

Subjective Evaluation

Barb reports that she is able to lift her head for 10 s periods, typically in the morning and when not feeling fatigued. Later in the day, however, her chin rests on her chest

(continued)

and she needs to lift it passively. She uses a soft cervical collar or pillows to hold up her head when driving but states that this method is marginally effective. She complains of cervical achiness and pain at 7/10, which is alleviated to 2/10 by lying supine. She denies any pulling or tensing of her anterior musculature. Her goals are to continue to drive and be able to hold up her head to watch a movie. She states that she exercises regularly and does flexibility exercises for her neck. She is a community ambulator with a four-wheeled walker.

Objective Evaluation

Upon observation, Barb clearly has dropped head. The upper trapezius muscle is hypertrophied, particularly in the cervical region. Her passive cervical range of motion (ROM) is within normal limits. In sitting she is able to lift her head actively approximately 60% from a starting point on her chest. At end point, she lacks upper cervical extension (C1–C2), and her lower cervical spine is mildly kyphotic (C3–C7). Various muscle groups have been affected as follows:

Muscle strength:

- Suboccipitals: unable to fully lift head (no upper cervical extension) in prone or sitting. She is able to extend the upper cervical spine to 50% of full range when lying supine.
- Cervical paravertebrals: unable to establish a cervical lordosis unless supine.
- Scapular musculature is 3+/5 to 4–/5.

Muscle tightness is noted in

- scalenes,
- pectoral muscles, and
- latissimus dorsi.

Dystonia of anterior cervical musculature is absent. Barb is able to hold up her head for a maximum of 15 s while walking

Goals

The short-term goals established for Barb are to

- become independent with a home exercise program to address axial and shoulder girdle flexibility and strength to optimize posture and
- be able to hold her head up for 30 s, long enough to cross the street.

The long-term goals established for Barb are to

- reduce neck pain from 7/10 at worst to 3/10 at worst during sitting, standing, or walking and
- be able to keep her head up for driving and watching movies by using a cervical orthotic.

(continued)

Case Example   *(continued)*

Therapeutic Interventions

- Barb is instructed in an HEP to address the needs described earlier. Because Barb is unable to hold her head up for any substantial time, she needs to exercise in supported positions so that she can use proper form without adding undue strain. She is also educated about realistic expectations of her ability to lift her head and the relationship of poor posture and pain.

- To conform to the instructions, she will need to perform strengthening of the cervical paravertebrals, either supine or prone, with her head supported in the starting position or for the duration of the exercise (isometrics). As with campto-cormic postures, strengthening of the shoulder girdle can be performed supine with a Thera-band. Cervical ROM and stretching of the scalenes and latissimus dorsi can be performed supine, and stretching of the pectoral muscles can be performed side lying with the head comfortably supported. In addition, instead of taking medicine for her pain she may want to lie down or wear a supportive device to reduce neck strain and secondarily reduce pain. For functional activities, she should wear a cervical support for driving, watching television, or going to the movies.

Outcomes

Although gains in the strength of the cervical paravertebral musculature are typically marginal, maintaining flexibility of the cervical spine is necessary to preserve spinal integrity and maintain the ability to position the head for functional activities.

Ankle and Foot Dystonia in PD

Ankle and foot dystonia, which typically involves one foot but can affect both, pulls the foot into an equinovarus foot posture (inverted and plantarflexed), which is aggravated with walking and related to low dopamine levels (Melamed, 1992). Dystonia may be painful secondary to the sustained muscle contraction and joint stress. Considerable resistance is encountered when an attempt is made to return the ankle and foot passively to a neutral position. Patients may describe it as a charley horse.

Dystonia in the foot is more commonly seen in young onset PD (Tolosa & Compta, 2006). It typically improves with dopaminergic medications. In contrast, idiopathic PD can present with ankle and foot dystonia secondary to use of dopaminergic medications and occurs when dopamine levels are low or in "off" states. Early morning dystonia occurs in approximately 20% to 30% of the patients with PD from chronic use of L-dopa (Nutt, 1990; Steiger & Quinn, 1992), often before the first morning dose of L-dopa medication (Currie et al., 1998). After the first dose is taken the dystonia usually resolves. Some patients have repeated bouts of dystonia throughout the day, which are related to the wearing off of the medications. Other areas of dystonic postures are the toes—big toe extension or toe flexion of digits 2 through 5 (Uitti, 2000).

Medical and Surgical Management

Dystonia is initially addressed through medication adjustments to optimize the consistency of dopamine levels or other medications that can attenuate the severity of contraction.

Another medical approach involves botulinum toxin. When injected into a dystonic muscle, Botox reduces the muscle activity by locally blocking the release of acetylcholine (Abbruzzese & Berardelli, 2006).The effect of Botox is limited in duration. The greatest reduction in dystonia is usually experienced 2 to 6 wk following injection. Most benefits are lost approximately 3 mo postinjection. Repeated injections may be necessary every 3 to 6 mo (Huang et al., 2000; Wenzel, 2004). A study evaluated the effects of Botox for "off" state ankle and foot dystonia in 30 patients with PD. Although patients reported a reduction of dystonia, the greatest improvements were noted in pain reduction. The authors of the study thought that the underlying mechanism of dopamine levels should be addressed first before considering Botox (Pacchetti et al., 1995).

The efficacy of deep brain stimulation (DBS) surgery on dystonia depends on the nature of the dystonia. For example, if the dystonia worsens with lower dopamine levels and improves with dopaminergic medications DBS will likely improve "off" state dystonia. Bilateral DBS of the subthalamic nucleus (STN) can reduce dystonia related to L-dopa levels or "off" periods in people with severe diphasic and peak dose dyskinesias. In one study, "off" period dystonia was reduced by 90% and pain by 66% with bilateral STN (Krack et al., 1999).

Physical Management

Physical therapy cannot change the severity of dystonia. Altering the severity of dystonia is in the hands of the physician, who can use any of the medical interventions described earlier. Physical therapy for dystonia focuses primarily on maximizing joint ROM. Because standing or walking often triggers ankle dystonia, attempting to improve ankle dorsiflexion or eversion in the presence of dystonia during these activities will be counterproductive. If the ankle and foot dystonia improves with L-dopa medication, the patient should exercise the joint when the dystonia is minimal or absent. Focus should be on flexibility to avoid deformities.

On rare occasions, severe and unrelenting ankle dystonia can result in inability to ambulate. In such cases the ankle can become fixed in the plantarflexed and inverted position. The patient will be unable to place the foot flat on the floor for functional gait or standing transfers.

For maximum effectiveness with foot and ankle dystonia, the patient should follow these guidelines:

1. Focus on flexibility to avoid contractures.
2. Do not attempt to stretch in the standing position if dystonia is triggered.
3. If dopaminergic medications reduce ankle dystonia, stretching should be performed when the effects of medications are optimal.

Summary

1. Parkinsonian postures are not always stereotypical.
2. Camptocormic and drop-head postures result from myopathic changes in the paravertebral muscles or dystonia of the anterior musculature and tend to be resistant to medical treatment, surgical intervention, and physical management.

3. Physical management should focus on minimizing secondary musculoskeletal impairments.

4. Postural improvement is typically achieved with supportive devices to reduce disabilities.

   • Walkers should be used for people with camptocormic postures for functional ambulation and minimization of back strain or pain.

   • Cervical orthotics can reduce neck strain or pain in drop-head postures.

5. A home exercise program is needed for long-term maintenance of impairments and mobility.

6. Foot and ankle dystonia can be position sensitive or dependent on dopamine levels.

7. Physical therapy for foot and ankle dystonia should focus primarily on maximizing joint ROM.

6

Tremors

Tremor is a "rhythmical, involuntary oscillatory movement of a body part" (Deuschl et al., 1998). It is the most common movement disorder (Habib ur, 2000). Approximately 5 to 10 million people are affected by tremor in the United States alone (Pahwa & Lyons, 2003). The prevalence of essential tremor is reportedly 5 to 10 times higher than the prevalence of Parkinson's disease (PD) ("Essential tremor," 2004). Thus, people with PD can also exhibit an essential tremor (Giladi et al., 2001). However, some people with PD may never develop any tremor. The severity of disability from a tremor is relative to the amplitude of movement. All tremors can be aggravated with emotional or physical stress and disappear when sleeping. Alcoholic consumption can help buffer essential tremors temporarily, and people with essential tremor are at no greater risk to drink excessively or become alcoholics than the general population (Hubble, 2000). Tremors can be associated with various pathological conditions, but the most common tremors are essential and resting tremors (see figure 6.1), which are the focus of this chapter.

Essential and Resting Tremors

Essential tremors can be described by when the tremor occurs. Kinetic tremor occurs with voluntary muscle contraction as when actively moving a body part. Postural tremor occurs during active muscle contraction to maintain a body part in a postural position that is not fully supported against gravity. For example, when sitting or standing, the head may exhibit what is called a yes-yes tremor or a no-no tremor. Katherine Hepburn presented with such a tremor. Holding the arm at shoulder level and maintaining that position may exhibit a postural hand and forearm tremor. Most people with postural tremors also have kinetic tremors (Matsumoto, 2000). People with Parkinson's disease may exhibit essential tremor and resting tremor.

• **Essential tremor**. Essential tremor can present with a varied combination of both kinetic and postural tremors (Pahwa & Lyons, 2003). The inclusion criterion for essential tremor is the bilateral presence of postural or kinetic tremor of the hands and forearms, or isolated head tremor without evidence of dystonia. The exclusion criterion for essential tremor is the presence of other neurological signs (Deuschl et al., 1998). Essential tremor typically occurs in the upper extremities but can also occur in the head, face, voice, trunk, and lower extremities (Pahwa & Lyons, 2003). Because essential tremor occurs with motion or while attempting to maintain a position in which a body part is not fully supported

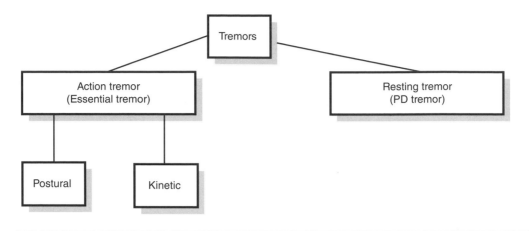

Figure 6.1 Categorization of tremors.

against gravity, it can significantly affect functional activities such as eating, drinking, fine motor coordination, dressing, handwriting, typing, or using a computer mouse. The presence of essential tremors can affect legibility of handwriting in those with PD. But the progressively smaller handwriting strokes are due more to bradykinesia and the difficulty of performing sequential movements than to tremors. The small handwriting seen in PD is called micrographia.

• **Resting tremor**. Resting tremor is associated with PD and occurs at rest even when the body part is fully supported. It can be more noticeable after an activity. Tremor amplitude abates with active movement and therefore does not interfere with ADLs. Pure resting tremor alone is uncommon, and signs of kinetic or postural tremors may also be seen (Deuschl et al., 1998). People with PD who exhibit resting tremor will initially present with unilateral symptoms, whereas essential tremor has a bilateral presentation.

Medical treatment for essential and resting tremors is not curative. The two main drugs for essential tremor are propranolol (Inderal) and primidone (Mysoline) (Whitney, 2006). Medications such as gabapentin (Neurontin), toparimate (Topamax), and benzodiazepines are also used (Raethjen & Deuschl, 2007). Approximately 50% of patients show improvement of their tremor with medications (Lyons et al., 2003). Deep brain stimulation (DBS) is an effective option for tremor control and has been shown to help 90% of the patients with essential tremor (Lyons et al., 2003). The thalamus is targeted for tremor control on the contralateral side. To be considered for DBS surgery for tremor control, a person needs to have a tremor of sufficient magnitude to be functionally disabling. Because this site does not improve other PD symptoms, it is most commonly used for people with essential tremors only (Alesch et al., 1995). Although DBS can be an effective option, it has risks. Dopaminergic medications may improve resting tremor, but responses are inconsistent (Deuschl et al., 2007).

Physical Management of Tremors

Therapy is based on compensatory strategies and the use of adaptive devices to improve ADL abilities. The following suggestions may help patients cope with tremors.

Case Example: Tremors

Marie is 80 yr old and has Parkinson's disease (Hoehn and Yahr stage 1.5). She has both resting and essential tremors.

Subjective Evaluation

Marie complains of worsening of her tremor, especially when she is trying to write and eat. When drinking she reports that she spills some of her drink. Her eating utensils have extremely thin handles. She states that her doctor is going to adjust her medications to help reduce tremor.

Objective Evaluation

Marie demonstrates a mild resting tremor. Essential tremor dominates, and she requires assistance to fill out her history form.

Goals

The goals for Marie are to

- be able to drink without spilling,
- report reduced difficulty with using eating utensils, and
- demonstrate increased awareness of various adaptive devices to assist in self-management.

Therapeutic Interventions

- Because physical management has no direct effect on tremors, adaptive equipment is recommended.
- Patient education on available equipment is the focus of therapy. Marie is advised to use a cup with a lid that has an opening for drinking and to increase the thickness of her pen grip and the handles of her eating utensils.

Outcomes

The effectiveness of adaptive equipment depends on the severity of her tremor and the ability to manage her tremor medically.

- Computer devices can be helpful for patients with PD.
  - An assistive mouse adaptor (figure 6.2) filters out tremor oscillations when the person with PD manipulates the mouse. The movement of the curser on the monitor is smoother and controlled. The filter can be adjusted to the amplitude of the tremor. Adjustments can also be made to filter out unintended clicks of the mouse. No additional software is needed, the adaptor can be connected with a standard USB port, and it can be turned on or off for different computer users. The adaptor, invented by IBM researchers, is available from the British electronics company Montrose Secam. For more information see www.montrosesecam.com.
  - A computer voice activation program eliminates the need for typing.

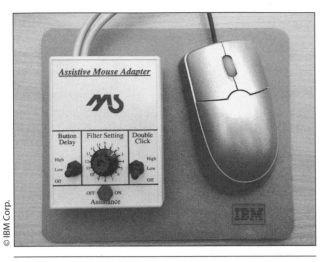

© IBM Corp.

Figure 6.2 Assistive mouse adaptor to filter out tremor oscillations when using a computer mouse.

- Adaptations for eating can involve both devices and physical strategies.
  - Use cups with lids.
  - Large-handle utensils can reduce strain with gripping.
  - Try wrist weights to buffer the tremor.
  - Weighted plates or bowls may reduce shifting.
  - Place a rubbery material between the plate and the table to reduce shifting.
  - Stabilize the arm by pressing the elbow into the waist while attempting to use the hand.
  - Attempt to use the nontremor hand or the hand with less tremor.

Summary

1. Essential tremors are more prevalent than resting tremors.
2. Essential tremors are more disabling than resting tremors.
3. All tremors are aggravated with emotional stress or physical stress and disappear when sleeping.
4. Therapy interventions focus on educating patients in the use of adaptive equipment.

BALANCE

The hallmark of PD Hoehn and Yahr stage 3 is the impairment of postural reflexes. The etiologic contributors to the impairments of postural reflexes are discussed in chapter 7, "Postural Instability," which also includes evaluative procedures and treatment interventions specific to postural instability. Chapter 8, "Balance Evaluation," addresses balance deficits in a broader sense by looking more at the interrelationship of balance and function. The effects of L-dopa and fall risk factors that contribute to imbalance are reviewed. A variety of balance tests are discussed to help the clinician choose the most appropriate tests for her or his patients. Appendix B contains balance tests and procedures; appendix C contains sample subjective and objective evaluation forms and sample goals. Appendix D includes the section "Problem-Oriented Treatment Interventions" pertaining to balance for quick referencing and implementation.

Postural Instability

Postural instability is a characteristic of Parkinson's disease (PD) that occurs later in disease progression. Postural instability is typically in the backward direction. Standing postural stability is described by the ability to control the relative motion between the body's center of mass (COM) and its base of support (BOS). A loss of balance occurs when the instantaneous position and velocity of the COM exceed the stability limits of the BOS and a new BOS is necessary to reestablish balance (Pai, 2003). People with PD who demonstrate a loss of trunk flexibility and trunk-righting capability can have difficulty maintaining the position of the COM over the base of support. Secondarily, greater reliance on stepping strategies will be necessary to establish a new base of support.

The velocity of the COM can also affect stability, which can be demonstrated by comparing recovery capabilities at various gait speeds. The forward momentum of the body with slow walking is minimal, and any destabilizing forces should take little effort to correct when attempting to stop. On the other hand the forward momentum of the body when running can be destabilizing during a sudden stop. A quicker and larger stepping response will be necessary to maintain stability. This chapter discusses adult postural responses compared with the responses seen in people with PD and the evaluation and treatment of deficient areas for fall prevention.

Definitions

The following terms are important for understanding issues of postural instability in Parkinson's disease:

• **Base of support (BOS)**—the area of the object that is in contact with the support surface (Shumway-Cook & Woollacott, 2001). A person's base of support is the feet. The position of the feet can either increase or decrease stability. Assistive devices can improve the base of support. A narrow base of support, which is more common in later stages of PD, is destabilizing, especially laterally (Dimitrova et al., 2004).

• **Center of mass (COM)**—the point located in the center of the total body mass, established by finding the weighted average of each body segment. The center of mass in the adult is at the L5–S1 level (Shumway-Cook & Woollacott, 2001).

• **Center of gravity (COG)**—the vertical projection of the COM. For example, with static standing the center of gravity falls between the feet.

- **Limits of stability**—the relative outermost point on the base of support where the forces of the COM can go before a stepping strategy is necessary. If perturbations are of a higher velocity, stepping strategies are initiated sooner, with less COM displacement. High-velocity perturbations will result in stepping strategies that can occur before the COM exceeds the BOS, but they are velocity dependent (Pai, 2003; Rogers et al., 2003). The limits of stability are not fixed, and they are influenced by many variables such as ROM or strength impairments, velocity, the type of activity, and environmental factors.

- **Loss of balance**—occurs when a change in the BOS is required to regain stability and prevent a fall. Changing the BOS could mean either taking a protective step or grabbing an object to regain stability. When I ask patients whether they lose their balance, they often think that I am asking them whether they fall. To avoid miscommunication or misrepresentation of balance deficits, the best approach is to describe to patients what a loss of balance is. Note, however, that an intentional stepping response may occur without a loss of balance in people who have a fear of falling (Pai, 2003). These people have an altered perception of danger concerning their balance ability.

- **Fall**—a sudden unintended change in position (displacement) that causes a person to land inadvertently at a lower level on an object, floor, or ground (Pai, 2003). You may observe a person with PD falling back into a chair. Do you consider this action a fall? Technically, the answer would be yes. For therapeutic interventions, falling back into a chair and falling onto the floor should be documented and addressed as two separate issues. For example, Mary has fallen three times in 6 mo because of rushing and tripping, but she tends to fall back into her chair approximately 15 times a day. So would you say that Mary falls 15 times a day? If you did, then it would sound as if Mary has a serious balance problem. You could paint a more accurate picture by stating, "Mary has fallen three times in 6 mo and has difficulty controlling descent with chair transfers." Therapeutic interventions for the two types of falls are different. Consideration should be given to defining a fall relative to clinical implications.

Postural Control Strategies

Healthy people use various postural control strategies to maintain balance while standing, depending on the destabilizing forces and environmental factors. To counter progressively higher disturbances, people use ankle strategies, then hip strategies, and finally stepping strategies. People with PD have greater difficulty implementing effective postural control strategies.

Healthy Adult Strategies for Postural Control

Each strategy uses a particular muscular activation and movement pattern to optimize balance in various conditions. The ultimate goal of the central nervous system (CNS) is to maintain balance by controlling the COM in relation to the BOS. The following is a hierarchy of balance strategies that normal healthy adults use to maintain balance:

- **Ankle strategy.** This strategy is used with quiet standing to control anterior and posterior body sway so that the body remains within the limits of the base of support; no change in BOS is necessary (feet-in-place strategy). The axis of motion occurs at the ankles. Synergistic muscle activation patterns occur to maintain balance depending on the direction of required stabilization. Muscle activation is from distal to proximal. To control a backward sway (to prevent loss of balance backward), the muscles attempt to pull the body forward. The muscle activation pattern is anterior tibialis first, quadriceps second, and abdominal muscles third. To control an anterior sway (to prevent loss of balance forward), the muscles attempt to pull the body backward. The muscle activation pattern is gastrocnemius first, hamstrings second, and paravertebral muscles third (Horak & Nashner, 1986).

• **Hip strategy.** This reaction occurs with a greater destabilizing force or when the BOS is limited, as when standing on a support surface smaller than the feet; no change in BOS is necessary (feet-in-place strategy). The axis of motion is at the hips. Muscle activation to control a backward sway (to pull the body forward to prevent loss of balance backward) begins proximally with the abdominal muscles and then uses the quadriceps. To control a forward sway, the paravertebral muscles and then the hamstrings are activated (Horak & Nashner, 1986).

• **Protective stepping strategies.** These maneuvers occur when balance can no longer be maintained unless a new base of support is established. Stepping strategies can be either anterior–posterior or lateral. Among older people, the stepping strategy is the most commonly used strategy to maintain balance (Mille et al., 2003). Older people demonstrate a delay in lateral weight shift to free up the stepping leg as well as a delay in the stepping response itself. Step initiation times and execution times are greater than those of younger adults (Mille et al., 2003; Rogers et al., 2003). Clinically, protective stepping strategies are the focus when evaluating and treating postural balance responses.

- **Anterior–posterior stepping strategy.** When older adults are subjected to destabilizing forces of similar magnitudes, stepping strategies are more commonly initiated as the balance strategy in the backward direction than in the forward direction. The increased incidence of posterior stepping may be due to the perceived risk of injury with backward falls (Pai et al., 2000). This stepping pattern has also been noted in young healthy adults (Rogers et al., 1996). The increased inclination of healthy young and older adults to step posteriorly to protect against a fall only further accentuates the posterior stepping deficits observed in people with PD, which can be delayed or absent.

- **Lateral stepping strategy.** This strategy relies heavily on trunk ROM and trunk-righting capabilities and the power strength of the hip abductor and adductor muscles to be effective (Mille et al., 2003). The most efficient strategy is trunk rotation and lateral trunk bending away from the direction of the perturbation and a sidestep in the direction of the perturbation. For example, if someone pulls you to the right, ideally your trunk should side-bend left to unload your right foot to take a step (figure 7.1, *a–c*). Typically, younger adults use this type of stepping strategy.

- The crossover step is a modified type of lateral stepping strategy that occurs because of limited trunk reactions. Limited trunk reaction interferes with the ability to unload the intended stepping foot. This stepping strategy is less effective in balance recovery, resulting in a greater probability of falls (Mille et al., 2003). This step is more commonly seen in older adults (figure 7.2, *a–c*).

Clinically, protective stepping strategies should be the focus when evaluating and treating postural balance responses.

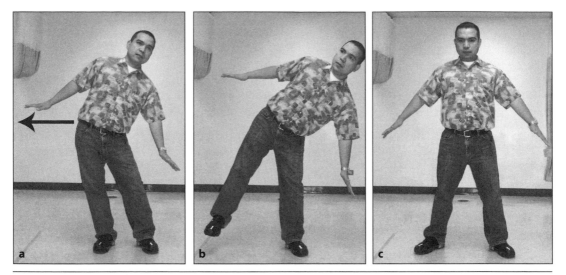

Figure 7.1 *(a)* Trunk sidebending to the left to counteract destabilizing forces to the right; *(b)* trunk response resulting in unloading the right foot for a single sidestepping strategy; *(c)* ending in a stable stance position.

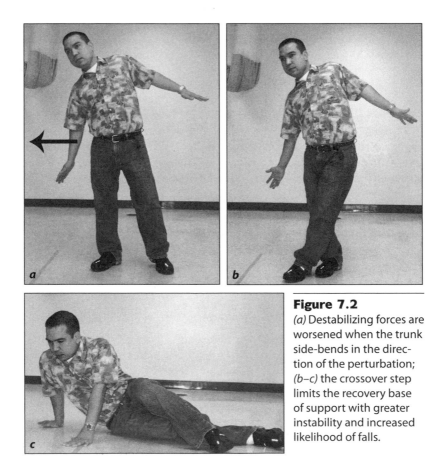

Figure 7.2

(a) Destabilizing forces are worsened when the trunk side-bends in the direction of the perturbation; *(b–c)* the crossover step limits the recovery base of support with greater instability and increased likelihood of falls.

Factors Influencing Postural Responses in PD

In those with PD, muscle activation patterns appear to be intact, but impairments are noted in the timing and magnitude of contraction of agonist and antagonist muscle groups.

"On" Versus "Off" States

Postural responses differ depending on the effects of L-dopa medication alone or in combination with other anti-Parkinson's medications. An "on" state refers to a period when dopamine levels are optimal, PD symptoms decrease, and mobility improves. An "off" state occurs when dopamine levels are less than optimal, increased PD symptoms are apparent, and mobility may be more difficult. See chapter 2, "Medical and Surgical Interventions," page 16.

Muscle activation while "off"

Dimitrova and colleagues (2004) compared the postural responses of people with PD in their "off" mode with healthy age-matched controls in response to low-amplitude multidirectional surface translations in two stance positions—narrow-based stance and wide-based stance. The researchers found the muscle activation synergies to be similar between the subjects with PD and controls, but the magnitude of muscle activation of the agonist muscles in those with PD was below those of the controls except for the trunk musculature, which exhibited higher than normal muscle activation. For example, to control backward sway (to prevent a loss of balance backward, the muscles attempt to pull the body forward), the group with PD activated the anterior tibialis first, the quadriceps second, and the abdominal muscles third, as would be expected in norms, but the magnitude of activation varied in comparison with controls. In addition, the muscle activation of the antagonist muscle groups was of a larger magnitude and with earlier onset when compared with controls. Therefore, during a backward sway, the antagonists (the gastrocnemius, hamstrings, and especially the erector spinae) were activated sooner and with relatively larger magnitudes, resulting in cocontraction.

Although evidence is limited, is it possible that the increased activation of the erector spinae can contribute to the propensity of backward postural instability in people with PD? When changing from a wide base of support to a narrow base, both groups exhibited increased magnitude of muscle activation, but the group with PD remained below normal levels. Ultimately, the relative activation imbalance of the agonistic muscles and the antagonist muscles results in cocontraction and reduced adaptability to postural changes.

Muscle activation while "on"

Another study evaluated postural responses in people with PD and compared the differences in postural responses in the "on" state versus the "off" state. Subjects were asked to rise on their toes while postural responses were measured. The results showed that L-dopa can improve the magnitude and relative timing of postural muscles, although not to the level of normal values (Frank et al., 2000).

Impairment of Postural Reflexes

Postural reflex impairments are resistant to dopamine replacement medications (Bloem, 1992). Difficulties begin with the inability of the postural muscles to respond rapidly and with enough magnitude to destabilizing forces. In fact, L-dopa has been shown to worsen postural responses by decreasing tone. Tone would otherwise act passively to reduce the amount of sway (Horak et al., 1996).

Depending on disease progression, various synergistic stepping strategies (or lack thereof) in response to perturbations can be observed. These responses can range from taking a few steps with the ability to self-correct to having no response when the person starts falling like a tree and needs to be caught. In addition, stepping strategies tend to be delayed and underscaled (Beckley et al., 1993). L-dopa medication improves step length and accuracy in people with moderate and severe PD, but these improvements are not consistent (Jacobs & Horak, 2006). A person with PD may be categorized in different Hoehn and Yahr stages depending on improvements in stepping from L-dopa. A person may be in Hoehn and Yahr stage 3 during an "off" state and in Hoehn and Yahr stage 2 during an "on" state.

Proprioception and Anticipatory Postural Adjustments

People with PD tend to lack accurately scaled movements because of inability to integrate proprioceptive inputs centrally. Therefore, they must rely more heavily on visual input to optimize movements. This reliance increases with disease severity (Keijsers et al., 2005). The underscaled movements found in stepping strategies are caused partly by impairments of central proprioceptive integration (Jacobs & Horak, 2006).

When performing volitional activities, people with PD demonstrate impairment in the preparatory postural set preceding an activity (Bazalgette et al., 1987; Frank et al., 2000; Kaneoke et al., 1989; Rogers et al., 1987). A study on lateral stepping strategies found that people with PD did not activate anticipatory postural adjustments (APAs) 56% of the time before stepping. The lack of APAs or trunk-righting ability contributes to reduced ability in balance recovery (King & Horak, 2008).

In summary, postural instability in people who have PD is multifactorial and is related to disease severity. Several neurological impairments influence postural responses:

- Lower-extremity cocontractions cause reduced adaptability to postural changes.
- Reduced magnitude of agonistic muscle activation patterns in the lower extremities produces an underscaled stepping strategy.
- Postural reflex impairments result in a delayed stepping strategy or no stepping strategy.
- Proprioception integration impairments centrally can result in underscaled or inaccurate stepping strategies.
- Impairments in anticipatory postural adjustments result in reduced trunk-righting ability and lower extremity responses, causing greater difficulty in maintaining the COM over the base of support for balance.

Evaluation of Postural Stability

To permit evaluation of postural stability, the balance challenge must be of sufficient magnitude to cause instability, thereby forcing the person to react in some way to regain balance. Because the reactions of destabilizing forces are unpredictable, the use of a gait belt is recommended during the evaluation and interventions. The ability to maintain postural stability is important for fall prevention regardless of direction, but the emphasis here is on posterior stability and lateral stability. Anterior stability can be evaluated with the functional reach test or with various components of the Berg balance test. See chapter 8, "Balance Evaluation," pages 105–106.

Posterior Stability

Evaluating postural stability in people with PD requires creating a loss of balance in the posterior direction and observing recovery capability. Three tests can be used to evaluate posterior stability. The expected retropulsive test and the Nutt unexpected retropulsive test are both referred to as the pull test. The difference between the two pull tests is that in one of them the patient is forewarned and is expecting to be pulled off balance and in the other one there is no forewarning. The third test is the push and release test. These tests are designed to determine whether the person with PD is at Hoehn and Yahr stage 2 (bilateral disease, balance intact) or stage 3 (mild to moderate bilateral disease, some postural instability, physically independent). The execution of these tests and the position of the patient and therapist are important to obtaining accurate results.

Expected Retropulsive Test

This test procedure is required in the Unified Parkinson's Disease Rating Scale (UPDRS) and is typically performed by a neurologist. Because patients are aware that they are going to be pulled backward during the test, they can prepare their postural set or alter their base of support so that they can pass the test. Inaccurate results can occur because in a home environment people are usually not warned in advance when they are going to lose their balance. The unexpected nature of falls is what makes them dangerous. Thus, I do not recommend using the expected retropulsive test.

Nutt Unexpected Retropulsive Test

When executed once, this test has a higher overall predictive accuracy when compared with the expected test (Visser et al., 2003), and it yields the most accurate results for appropriate therapeutic intervention. If executed more than once, the element of surprise (or unexpectedness) is gone and the results will be less definitive (Visser et al., 2003). Technically, the protocols for retropulsive tests are performed by pulling backward on the shoulders (see figure 7.3, *a* and *b*). Because of the wide variety of recovery abilities and for safety concerns, using a gait belt and pulling backward on the gait belt using the following method is recommended:

Technique

1. The therapist stands behind the patient.
2. The patient's feet are positioned comfortably apart and parallel (not one ahead of the other).
3. Without warning, the therapist pulls the patient briskly backward using sufficient force to create a loss of balance that requires a stepping response.

Common errors in the patient's position are

- bracing forward or
- standing with an increased base of support.

Common errors in the therapist's position or execution are

- pulling continuously and steadily (which does not create the element of surprise needed or the velocity that would facilitate a stepping strategy sooner),
- not pulling with sufficient force to elicit a stepping strategy, or
- standing too close to the patient, limiting the patient's space and ability to react (Munhoz et al., 2004).

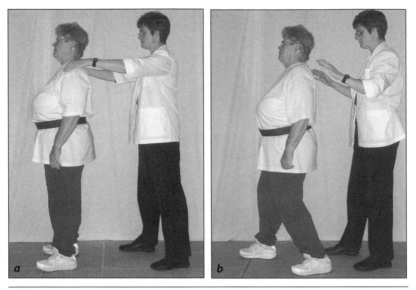

Figure 7.3 The *(a)* starting and *(b)* end positions of the pull test. The clinician allows enough space behind the patient to allow responses without interference.

Rating Scale

0 = Normal; may take two steps to recover

1 = Takes three or more steps and recovers unaided

2 = Would fall if not caught

3 = Spontaneous tendency to fall or unable to stand unaided (test not executable)

This scale indicates the patient's response to regain an unexpected loss of balance. Normally, a person is expected to take a sufficiently sized step or two to regain balance. Any response outside the norm is cause for therapeutic interventions.

Push and Release Test

The push and release test was found to be a more sensitive instrument than the expected pull test in detecting postural instability in people who felt less confident in their balance determined by the Activities-Specific Confidence (ABC) Scale (Jacobs et al., 2006). But it was determined to be less specific in determining postural instability in those who had high balance confidence (Jacobs et al., 2006). In other words, the push and release test may be negative in people with high balance confidence when impairment exists. The administration of the push and release test was also found to be more consistent regarding perturbation forces (see figure 7.4, *a* and *b*).

Technique

1. The therapist stands behind the patient.

2. The patient is instructed to do whatever is necessary, including taking a step, to regain balance.

3. The therapist places the palms of his or her hands against the patient's scapulae.

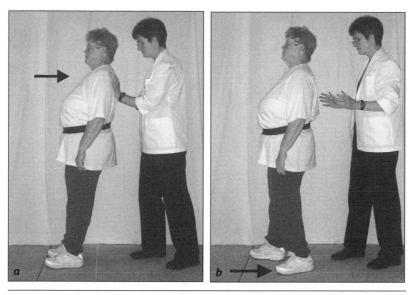

Figure 7.4 *(a)* In the push and release test, the patient actively pushes back while the clinician allows enough trunk movement to create an unstable stance position; *(b)* the removal of the counterpressure by the clinician requires the patient to take a step to regain balance.

4. The patient is instructed to push backward against the palms of the therapist's hands.

5. The therapist flexes his or her elbows just enough to allow slight backward movement of the patient's trunk while supporting the patient's weight in the hands.

6. The therapist monitors the force and positioning as the patient pushes back The patient should not push so hard that the heels rise off the ground. The patient is not allowed to lean back passively into the therapist's hands.

7. When the patient's shoulders and hips have moved to an unstable position just behind the heels, the therapist suddenly removes the hands, requiring the patient to take a step to regain balance.

Rating Scale for Push and Release Test

0 = Recovers independently with one step of normal length and width

1 = Takes two or three small steps backward but recovers independently

2 = Takes four or more steps backward but recovers independently

3 = Steps backward but needs assistance to prevent a fall

4 = Falls without attempting a step or unable to stand without assistance

This scale describes possible patient responses to an unexpected loss of balance. Therapeutic interventions are indicated for ratings 1 through 4.

Lateral Stability

Lateral stability can be problematic for people with PD because of the progressive narrowing of their base of support with disease progression in combination with reduced ability to right the trunk and maintain the COM over the BOS. A typical stepping strategy in older people is a crossover step (Mille et al., 2003). King and Horak (2008) compared lateral balance responses in healthy older people with the responses of people with PD in their "off" and "on" states. Subjects stood on a movable platform and wore a harness without tension. Perturbations were performed with lateral platform translations. Each subject underwent seven trials. Both controls and PD subjects commonly used the lateral sidestepping strategy. The incidence of falls was higher in the people with PD who used the crossover stepping strategy. The highest incidence of falls was in those with PD who lacked any stepping strategy. PD subjects in their "off" state demonstrated greater delay in initiating stepping. Step size was smaller, and steps were slower. This study also demonstrated improved step size in the PD subjects in their "on" state after repeated trials, which indicates possibilities for therapeutic intervention. People with PD who varied their stepping strategy also had a higher fall rate than those who did not. This finding was attributed to the inability to elicit a consistent response, which resulted in delayed step initiation.

A Caveat

My experience suggests that lateral waist pulls can impede trunk righting and may even facilitate a crossover stepping response, but the ability to self-recover remains the main objective. Tandem standing can offer greater insights into trunk-righting ability, lateral stability, and stepping strategies (see chapter 8, "Balance Evaluation," page 105). The procedures for the lateral waist pull are of greatest benefit when addressing interventions for lateral stability.

Lateral Waist Pull Test

The lateral waist pull can be a means of evaluating lateral stability.

Technique

Here are the steps the therapist follows for the lateral waist pull test:

1. The therapist stands to the side of the perturbation direction.
2. The patient's feet are positioned comfortably apart and parallel (not one ahead of the other).
3. Without warning, the therapist pulls the patient briskly toward the side using sufficient force to create a loss of balance that requires a stepping response.

Possible responses

Observed responses to lateral perturbations may include but are not limited to the following:

- Normal; recovers unaided
- Lack of trunk righting
- Crossover stepping
- Delay in step initiation
- Underscaled stepping
- No steps; must be caught

The patient may exhibit more than one of the responses. No rating scale has been established for lateral waist pulls, but the observed responses can guide physical interventions.

Interventions for Postural Instability

The first line of defense in fall prevention is to make the standing base of support more stable. The goal is to avoid loss of balance in the first place. This section discusses the effect of foot placement during standing on stability and intervention guidelines.

Altering the Base of Support

If stability is established during static standing, reliance on a protective stepping strategy should be reduced. But simply increasing the width of the base of support does not protect a person from anterior–posterior instability. Likewise, standing with one foot ahead in a narrowly based stance does not protect against lateral instability. To illustrate this, think about how people orient their feet when they are standing on a moving bus or train that is alternately stopping and starting. The people facing the front of the vehicle will have one foot ahead of the other for greater anterior–posterior stability. The people facing the side of the vehicle will have a wider base of support to improve their lateral stability when the vehicle stops (figure 7.5, a and b).

Kirby et al. (1987) looked at the influence of foot position on standing balance. They found that a narrow base of support created increased medial–lateral instability. Widening the stance improved lateral stability, but not anterior–posterior stability. But when one foot was placed ahead of the other, both anterior–posterior and medial–lateral stability improved. The interventions that follow are based on this finding.

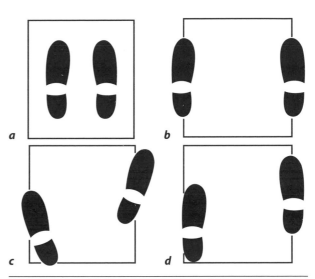

Figure 7.5 *(a)* Normal stance width; *(b)* wide-based stance; *(c)* staggered stance for optimal anterior stability; *(d)* staggered stance for optimal posterior stability.

Intervention to Enhance Patient Stability

It is not unusual to note posterior postural instability with static standing and not with ambulation, probably because the forward momentum of walking counteracts posterior instability. A person with such symptoms would be at greater risk of falling with static standing activities than with ambulation. Most patients with balance issues gain more understanding of how foot position affects standing stability if you enable them to experience the following activity:

- Review with the patient the principles of altering the base of support to improve stability and fall prevention.

Walking on Ramps

Walking on ramps can be extremely destabilizing. Patients commonly exhibit a step-to gait when walking on ramps, especially when fearful of falling. The step-to gait can further compound their instability. A step-through gait, in which one foot always passes the other, offers greater stability (as in the staggered-stance position) (Kirby et al., 1987).

- Have the patient experience feelings of anterior–posterior instability by standing with a wider base but with feet even (toes of both feet touching a line on the floor). Gently move the patient anteriorly and posteriorly with sufficient force to allow visible ankle strategies or feelings of instability.

- Ask the patient to use the same stance width but to slide the right foot back so that the toes of that foot are about even with the arch of the other foot (left foot). Repeat the gentle anterior and posterior perturbations and assess for increased feelings of stability. Increase the magnitude of the anterior and posterior waist pulls to confirm feet-in-place standing stability.

- Have the patient repeat the procedure with the left foot more posterior than the right foot. Repeat the gentle anterior and posterior perturbations and assess for increased feelings of stability. Increase the magnitude of the anterior and posterior waist pulls to confirm feet-in-place standing stability.

- Some people are more stable with the left foot ahead; others are more stable with the right foot ahead.

- Fine-tuning of foot placement may be necessary to maximize feelings of steadiness. The stance position should feel natural.

- Staggered standing with the feet pointed out offers greater anterior stability (wider anterior base of support).

- Staggered standing with the feet pointed forward can offer improved posterior stability.

- Advise patients to use their most stable stance position with all standing activities.

- If appropriate, review lifting body mechanics with staggered standing.

- Issue a patient education handout on staggered stance positions (see "Staggered Standing," appendix D).

- During follow-up visits observe whether the patient uses the new staggered-stance position. The person will typically need reminders. Ask informed family members to remind the patient.

Stepping Strategy

Older adults exhibit longer delays in step initiation and need more time to complete a step when compared with young adults (Rogers et al., 2003). These delays are accentuated in people with PD. As mentioned earlier, it is possible to elicit an earlier stepping response with higher velocities of the COM in relation to the BOS. (The faster the

COM moves in relation to the BOS, the sooner the step response occurs.) When treating patients, a perturbation of higher velocity can facilitate an earlier step response for fall prevention.

We also know that the predominant balance strategy for older adults is the stepping strategy. Fine-tuning and capitalizing on this strategy can yield effective results. People with PD tend to underscale their postural response, which is especially apparent when they take ineffective small steps as their COM quickly moves beyond their BOS. Educating the patient and practicing modifications of step size and location and trunk positioning can improve stability. If the inability to step quickly is caused by muscle weakness, this is an area that we can truly rehabilitate. When working with people who have PD, attention strategies (see "Voluntary Stepping," appendix D) can facilitate and improve stepping responses (Behrman et al., 1998; Farley & Koshland, 2005).

Studies have been performed on the effects of step training to improve protective stepping responses. One study demonstrated that training improved the time required to initiate a step and the time required to complete a step in both young and older healthy adults. Two types of training were performed. One group underwent induced stepping training (destabilizing large waist pulls), and the other group performed voluntary stepping to a small waist pull. Training sessions were two times a week for 3 wk. Both groups improved significantly in their step initiation times. The induced step training, however, yielded greater improvements (Rogers et al., 2003).

Another study focused on step training with subjects who have PD. Training was performed for 10 d, twice a day for 20 min. Training consisted of repetitive pulls backward and pulls and pushes sideways to the left and right of sufficient magnitude to induce stepping. Verbal feedback that emphasized taking larger steps was given as needed. Initial training was performed in a predictable direction. Later, the directions of perturbations were random. Results demonstrated improved step initiation and improved step length. Subjects maintained these improvements for 2 mo following training (Jobges et al., 2004).

Clinically, I too have found the combination of voluntary compensatory stepping and induced step training to improve the effectiveness of stepping in those with PD. In my opinion, however, the ability to learn and apply stepping strategies depends on the cognitive integrity of the patient and the severity of PD. Voluntary stepping is reviewed and practiced in the clinic initially, but ultimately it becomes part of a home exercise program. Induced stepping with greater destabilizing forces is performed in the clinic.

Intervention Guidelines for Compensatory Stepping

These guidelines are supported by the previously mentioned studies and my clinical observations. The goal is to make step training understandable, optimally effective, and meaningful to the patient.

Preliminary Matters

Two preliminary issues that you should consider for every patient are patient education and the amount of upper-extremity support. Every person with PD should have a basic understanding of postural and other reflexes. Upper-extremity support may or may not be required.

• **Patient education.** Patients seem to benefit from an explanation of what postural reflexes are and how they protect the body. Helpful examples include the reflexes that respond to touching a hot stove or stepping on a sharp object. Patients need to learn that taking a step to protect their balance no longer occurs automatically. They now need to think about taking a step for it to happen. Patients must also understand that short steps are usually ineffective in fall prevention.

• **Upper-extremity support.** Patients have different levels of confidence when they practice quicker and larger steps. Initial practice may therefore require bilateral upper-extremity support so that patients can focus on their feet without fear of falling. Typically, support by one hand is sufficient. Patients should use hand support only for balance, not to control the momentum of stepping.

Strategies for Improving Dysfunctional Stepping

Many subcomponents of stepping strategies must be addressed to improve balance recovery. These include step location, weight shifting, speed of the step, and trunk control. Each component builds on the next to improve ability.

Step location

Step length and foot positioning of the stepping foot is the initial focus. Foot placement can be critical in fall prevention. An overlarge step can be further destabilizing or take too much time to complete. If the step is too narrow, which is often the case, additional lateral instability results. Another common problem is that patients step backward without shifting their weight to the back leg. Stepping errors may be due to centrally impaired proprioceptive integration, but stepping can improve with practice. At times visual targets can initially guide people to appropriate step size and location (figure 7.6, *a* and *b*). These targets are positioned to allow a natural and effective step position.

Weight shift

When practicing stepping strategies, having patients shift their weight in the direction of the "loss of balance," or in the direction of the stepping foot, more closely simulates a real loss of balance. As shown in figure 7.6*b*, body weight should be transferred to the back leg and not remain on the front leg. Encourage patients to shift their weight every time they take a step. During this phase of training, speed is not an issue. Patients can practice in one direction (backward) with one foot until they demonstrate understanding of foot placement and proper weight shifting. Then they move to the next foot, same direction. The focus should be in the direction of greatest instability.

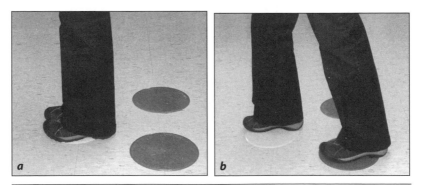

Figure 7.6 Use of visual targets to improve step size and location in voluntary stepping interventions: *(a)* starting position; *(b)* ending position to stabilize a backward loss of balance.

Speed

Use attention strategies to focus on speed. To facilitate the urgency or speed of the step-ping response, ask patients to think of a word or action that will cue them to step quickly. They continue to practice their stepping and use attention strategies to facilitate the speed of the step. Some words that patients have chosen are "Charge" (as in charging to battle), "Step," and "Quick." An example of an action that they can visualize would be squishing a bug, which can also facilitate weight shifting. When working on speed, verbal cuing may be needed initially to create the urgency of the step. Continue to reinforce proper step size and weight shifting as needed during this phase of training.

Trunk control

Some patients may need to incorporate trunk strategies to improve trunk control. For example, many patients tend to lead with their shoulders in the retropulsion test so that the trunk is hyperextended beyond their base of support, a position that is extremely desta-bilizing. Patients are usually unaware that this motion affects their balance. Attempting to maintain some degree of forward leaning with posterior perturbations can make a significant difference in balance recovery. Abdominal strengthening exercises may be necessary. Advise the patient to contract the abdominal muscles when experiencing posterior destabilizing forces to improve balance control.

Voluntary and induced stepping

Voluntary stepping is performed when the patient volitionally steps in the absence of any threat to stability. Any destabilizing forces are low in magnitude. This type of stepping is performed as a home exercise program (see "Voluntary Stepping," appendix D) to maintain both the optimal stepping strategy and the readiness to take a protective step.

Induced stepping occurs when a destabilizing force of sufficient magnitude creates a loss of balance that requires a step to prevent a fall. Induced stepping forces the patient to react, revealing true response deficits that can then be fine-tuned to increase effectiveness. Induced stepping should be performed in an open area because patients tend to grab for stability instead of stepping. Grabbing is not a bad thing if it prevents a fall, but the emphasis here is to encourage lower-extremity responses. In real life there will not always be something to grab. Two approaches can be used for induced step training:

- **Magnitude and direction of perturbations.** This approach initially involves adjusting the magnitude of waist pulls so that the patient needs to take a step but can successfully regain balance without assistance. This activity can build confidence and morale. As the patient improves, larger amplitude waist pulls can be implemented. As in the study of induced stepping, starting with unidirectional waist pulls and later implementing random directional waist pulls is a good progression. Unidirectional perturbations are performed until consistent and effective responses are established. Perturbations in unpredictable directions, although expected, place greater demands on postural adjustments to improve responsiveness in stepping strategies. Predictable adaptability (learning phase) to unpre-dictable adaptability (real life applications) is a logical progression.

- **Reduction in base of support to facilitate stepping.** In this approach, the practitioner alters the support surface or base of support to create sufficient instability to require a step. Often, when working on balance training, the emphasis is on maintaining balance without taking a step, such as with ankle or hip strategies. When doing balance training to facilitate stepping strategies, however, balance equipment with compliant or smaller surface areas can be used. For example, to facilitate lateral stepping, the patient can stand on a half foam

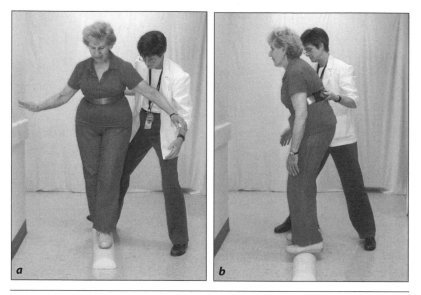

Figure 7.7 *(a)* Altering the support surface to facilitate lateral stepping strategies and *(b)* anterior–posterior stepping strategies.

roll in tandem (figure 7.7*a*). To facilitate anterior and posterior stepping, the patient can stand perpendicularly on the half foam roll (figure 7.7*b*).

When the emphasis of balance training is to facilitate a stepping strategy, the definition of a successful recovery is different than it is for a hip or ankle strategy. When doing balance stepping training, patients need to be informed of the rules of balance training, which emphasize stepping strategies, and the responses that are considered successful, as follows:

- It is OK to lose balance (this is not a bad thing).
- When losing balance, patients need to take a step and catch themselves (this is a good thing, which is encouraged).
- The more often that patients are able to catch themselves and the less often that the therapist needs to assist, the better their scores are.

If the rules are not explained, patients may feel that every time they lose their balance they have done poorly, even if they were able to catch themselves. As with all step training in this population, teaching attention strategies to maximize the location and speed of stepping is encouraged (see "Voluntary Stepping," appendix D). As balance with a smaller base of support improves, mild perturbations in these stance positions can be added.

Figures 7.8 and 7.9 provide a summary of general treatment intervention guidelines based on the direction of instability.

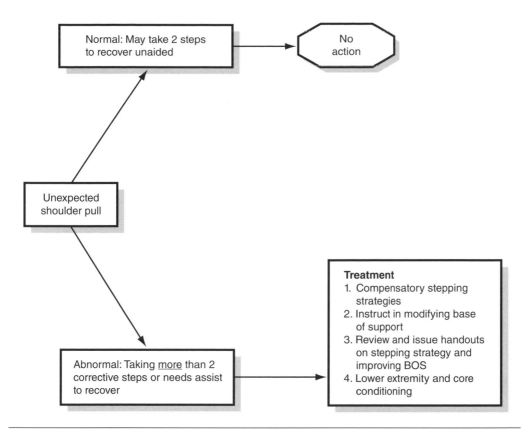

Figure 7.8 Posterior instability.

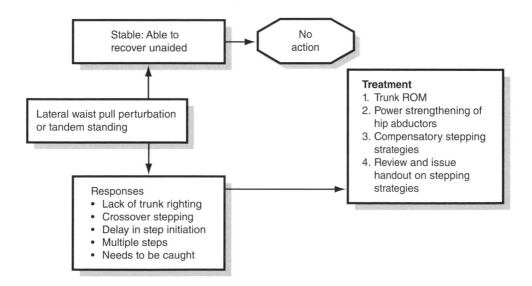

Figure 7.9 Lateral instability.

Jack has PD (Hoehn and Yahr stage 3). He has no history of orthostatic hypotension and is generally healthy.

Subjective Evaluation

The patient reports that he feels unsteady with static standing. When reaching over-head or backing up out of his closet, he states that his feet start moving fast and he falls backward. Jack admits to falling two times a week because of losing his balance while standing. He denies any unsteadiness with walking.

Objective Evaluation

The patient presents with overall good flexibility and strength except for weakness in the abdominal muscles. The Berg balance score of 53/56 demonstrates good balance, but the Nutt unexpected retropulsive test is positive; he needs to be caught to prevent a fall. Tandem standing exhibits good lateral stability. Jack's proprioceptive awareness of when he feels that he is losing his balance is intact.

Goals

The goals for Jack are to

- reduce incidence of falls to once a month,
- improve stability with static standing with a modified base of support to reduce the risk of falls,
- demonstrate understanding of effective stepping strategies to prevent back-ward falls, and
- become independent in an HEP to improve abdominal strength for balance recovery and to prevent deconditioning or loss of flexibility.

Therapeutic Interventions

Postural instability is primarily addressed with compensatory strategies. Conditioning and flexibility exercises focus on rehabilitation and prevention to optimize balance.

• Jack is taught that postural reflexes are intended to protect him from falls and that his postural reflexes are no longer automatic. He is taught that he can use compensatory strategies such as altering the base of support and consciously taking a large step backward to regain balance.

• Staggered standing for optimal stability is assessed. Jack's most stable standing position is with his right foot more forward than his left, and he is advised to capital-ize on this position for stability and to perform reaching and standing activities in a staggered-standing position to reinforce and confirm stability.

• Voluntary stepping in combination with attempting to lean forward with his trunk is reviewed and practiced. Handouts regarding modified base of support and stepping strategies are issued (see appendix D for reproducible handouts).

(continued)

Case Example   *(continued)*

• Jack is instructed in an HEP for general conditioning and flexibility exercises. Abdominal strengthening is targeted because this activity may help with balance recovery. In addition, making a conscious effort to avoid leaning back with his trunk is reemphasized. He is advised to practice voluntary stepping at home and to observe foot positioning for stability with standing activities.

• In therapy he is put through a rigorous program of induced stepping using waist pulls and balance equipment to facilitate stepping strategies. Retrowalking with emphasis on taking large steps and maintaining balance is practiced to minimize retropulsion. He is advised to stop during this activity or attempt to lean forward to counterbalance to establish better control in the backward direction in the presence of feelings of backward instability.

Outcomes

Jack should fall less often if he continues to recognize that he must consciously modify his stepping strategies and habitually stands with the appropriate staggered-feet position. His HEP program is targeted for general conditioning and flexibility. It should help him preserve his ability to maintain balance, which would otherwise be affected by deconditioning. If Jack were to lack the proprioceptive sensation of when he is losing his balance, he would require an assist device for fall prevention and possibly closer supervision when performing standing activities.

Summary

1. In the later stages of PD, posterior postural instability is common.

2. Lateral instability is common in those with Parkinson's disease. Factors that influence lateral stability are limited trunk flexibility and anticipatory postural adjustments, narrow base of support, and deconditioning of hip abductors.

3. Compensatory strategies such as modifying the BOS with standing or using attention strategies with protective stepping can help in fall prevention.

4. Interventions that focus on effective stepping strategies are effective in people with PD.

5. Rehabilitation of stepping strategies should initially be direction specific and then be progressed to random directions for adaptability.

6. Patients may need to modify trunk movements with stepping to improve effectiveness further.

Balance Evaluation

Appropriate therapeutic intervention for fall prevention can be implemented after balance deficits are determined. The evaluation of balance in the older population can be a complex issue. When adding a diagnosis of PD to this age group, more investigation is often necessary to establish needs. Many balance tests and questionnaires have been developed to assess fall risk. Typically, a combination of tests is necessary for balance assessment because no balance test, given in isolation, can cover fall risk comprehensively, particularly in the PD population in the presence of motor fluctuations.

The basis of evaluating balance is twofold:

• First, specific areas of imbalance need to be determined so that interventions can target deficits. To identify impairments and dysfunctions, the patient is asked about occurrences and causes of instability. One study demonstrated that repeated fallers often have etiological patterns that cause their falls (Rudzinska, 2007). The determination of etiological patterns can refine interventions. In other words, establishing a common precipitating factor in falls can help target therapy or other rehab strategies. Patients are not always aware of patterns, but detailed questioning can often expose them.

• Second, a baseline of balance abilities needs to be established to evaluate the effectiveness of interventions.

The goal is to reduce the risk of falls and, in some severe cases, to reduce the frequency of falls. Evaluating postural reflexes (chapter 7) should be an integral part of determining balance deficits in all patients with PD. Balance tests can indicate whether a person is at risk of falls but may not establish why they are at risk. We must also consider multifactorial issues such as impairments in vision, proprioception, neuropathies, vestibular deficits, muscle weakness, limited flexibility, cognition, other medical problems, and the effects of medications. This chapter discusses how L-dopa can affect balance ability in the PD population. Fall risk factors are reviewed. Some of these factors occur in the general older population, and some are more specific to people with PD. Both the clinician and the patient should be aware of modifiable and nonmodifiable fall risk factors to maximize therapy interventions and maintain realistic expectations.

Parkinson's Disease Fall Risk Factors

People with PD can be at risk of falling for many reasons. Some may be at greater risk of falls depending on where they are in their anti-Parkinson's medication cycle. Gait disturbances, impaired cognition, medications for other medical conditions, and inactivity can affect the risk of falls. Some factors are treatable through physical interventions, whereas other areas are more resistant.

Effects of L-Dopa on Balance and Performance

Balance in people with PD can vary dramatically depending on where they are in the medication cycle. People with PD can exhibit improved balance when medications are working optimally ("on" state). Worsening of balance can be seen during the "off" state. A study of 23 people with PD in Hoehn and Yahr stage 3 and motor fluctuations were evaluated regarding the effects of L-dopa on balance. The mean Berg balance test score was 42.7 during the "on" state and 31.7 during the "off" state (Nova et al., 2004). The higher score demonstrates improved balance during the "on" state.

Another study addressed the repeatability of gait parameters during "on" and "off" states. When tested during their "on" state, participants demonstrated good repeatability of gait parameters, even from one day to the next. But low correlations of repeatability were found when comparing gait parameters during the "on" and "off" states. Participants demonstrated increased gait variability during "off" states (Morris et al., 1996). Repeatability of measures is important to making accurate assessments of therapeutic interventions. Typically, outpatients are seen during their "on" states, but if fluctuations are erratic, periods of "off" states may be observed. Balance issues occurring during both "off" and "on" states need to be evaluated and addressed separately.

A person at low risk of falling during the "on" state may not be at low risk during the "off" state. The evaluation of "off" states in an outpatient clinic tends to come more from subjective patient reports than from clinical observations. Home health professionals, however, may have the advantage of seeing patients during their "off" state.

Debate has occurred about whether people with PD exhibit improved postural stability when "on" versus "off." On the one hand,

- L-dopa tends to increase postural sway without improving postural reflexes, which can result in greater instability;
- people with PD tend to be more active during their "on" state because moving is less difficult; and
- people with postural instability can be at higher risk of falls when they become more active.

On the other hand,

- L-dopa can improve the ability to respond to destabilizing forces by reducing bradykinesia and rigidity (Nova et al., 2004); and
- L-dopa can improve the relative timing and the magnitude of postural responses (Frank et al., 2000).

People with PD may exhibit increased sway during their "on" state, requiring small adjustments to regain balance, but they will demonstrate improved stepping strategies in response to induced stepping interventions. During "off" states, reduced sway often occurs in static standing, but stepping strategies exhibit greater impairments, such as greater delay in step initiation, smaller scaled steps, and greater variability in stepping responses. Postural instability tends to be more apparent with standing activities than with gait. Impairment of postural stability in the backward direction is the hallmark of Hoehn and Yahr stage 3. During static standing or overhead reaching activities, instability can be observed. When ambulating, the forward momentum of the body appears to counteract posterior forces. This circumstance can be observed when applying posterior perturbations to a walking patient. No instability will be observed, but this same person will exhibit impairments during the retropulsive test.

Common Fall Risk Factors

People with PD share fall risk factors with the older adult population but have additional unique risk factors. Studies on the prediction of falls have varying results. (Part of this variance may be due in part to differences in the focus of each study.) Several conclusions, however, can be drawn.

The areas of greatest consensus in the prediction of falls are a history of repeated falls, disease severity of PD, dementia, and use of benzodiazepines. Many of the additional fall risk factors mentioned here tend to be interdependent with other risk factors. For example, urinary incontinence is likely associated with rushing to get to the bathroom. Rushing or making abrupt movements is considered a risk factor that becomes more evident in the presence of postural instability and difficulty with making appropriate postural adjustments to stabilize before moving. Many falls in PD have been noted to occur when turning, standing up, or bending or are the result of stumbling because of reduced ground clearance or shuffling gait (Willemsen et al., 2000).

The percentage of people with PD who fall ranges between 38% and 68% (Balash et al., 2005). The greatest number of falls seems to occur in people with moderate disease. This phenomenon has been attributed to their continued mobility in the presence of reduced stability. People with more severe PD who have reduced their activities in part because of their fear of falling have a lower incidence of falls (Bloem et al., 2001b). The number of falls, therefore, should be associated not only with the level of instability but also with the level of activity. Here is a summary of common fall risk factors in people with PD:

- **History of recurrent falls.** Recurrent falls are defined as having two or more falls in a 12 mo period, which places the patient at a higher risk of future falls (Ashburn, 2001).

- **Disease severity.** Disease severity is a contributing factor to increased fall risk but is not considered an independent fall risk (Ashburn et al., 2001; Bloem et al., 2001a). As noted previously, greater disease severity results in reduced activity level and a lower incidence of falls.

- **Dementia.** Not all people with PD have dementia. A systematic review has demonstrated that 24% to 31% of people with PD have dementia, but PD is not necessarily the cause. Of people with PD who have dementia, only 3% to 4% have dementia because of PD (Aarsland et al., 2005). The severity of dementia can be as varied as other symptoms of PD. Regardless of the cause, dementia is considered a fall risk factor. When communicating with a person with PD, bradyphrenia (slowness of thought) should not be confused with dementia. A person with bradyphrenia may take longer to respond, but the responses will be appropriate and accurate.

- **Use of benzodiazepines.** Benzodiazepines are a class of drugs that may be administered for anxiety, seizures, insomnia, restless leg syndrome, and panic disorders. Benzodiazepines also have muscle relaxant properties. These drugs increase the risk of falls regardless of whether a person has PD (Bloem et al., 2001a; Sgadari et al., 2000).

- **Motor fluctuations.** Dyskinesias and unpredictable "on-off" episodes are considered a fall risk factor (Ashburn et al., 2001). Unpredictable "on-off" episodes result in abrupt changes in mobility. Minimizing motor fluctuations requires medical management through medication adjustments or deep brain stimulation. The therapist should be aware of such fluctuations so that mobility and balance issues specific to both the "on" state and the "off" state can be addressed.

- **Freezing.** This experience can be destabilizing, especially when coupled with postural instability. The unpredictability of known freezing triggers such as start hesitation, turning, and narrow spaces only adds to the difficulty of maintaining balance. Freezing has been associated with disease progression and urinary incontinence (Giladi et al., 1997). Stride variability has been associated with freezing and festinating gait (speeding up of gait) (Hausdorff et al., 2003b).

- **Difficulty turning.** Patient reports of difficulty with turns while ambulating are often associated with freezing and falls (Stack et al., 2006).

- **Stride time variability.** When ambulating, a person's stride length or stride time can vary from one step to the next, resulting in an arrhythmical gait. This variability leads to increased fall risk (Schaafsma et al., 2003). Gait variability has also been correlated with disease duration and severity and cognitive changes (Hausdorff et al., 2003a). As noted earlier, stride variability is also associated with freezing.

- **Urinary incontinence.** In a study of 230 nondemented people with PD, urinary incontinence was cited as a strong risk factor associated with falls (Balash et al., 2005). My observations suggest that falls likely result from the combination of freezing and rushing, which can easily derail a patient's stability.

- **Gait deviations.** Reduced ground clearance is a significant hazard for tripping or can simply result in the foot sticking to the floor with secondary forward loss of balance (Bloem et al., 2001b). Because of the increased reliance on vision resulting from abnormal central processing of proprioceptive input (Jacobs & Horak, 2006), the risk of tripping increases in poorly lit areas.

- **Deconditioned state.** Increased feelings of unsteadiness lead to a fear of falling and a reduction in daily activities (Bloem et al., 2001a). Inactivity leads to secondary loss of strength and flexibility. Loss of lower-extremity strength adversely affects balance, gait, and mobility (Scandalis et al., 2001; Seynnes et al., 2004). Thus, the ability to recover from a loss of balance declines when a person is deconditioned.

- **Abrupt movements.** Performing abrupt movements in the presence of postural instability and underscaled or delayed postural responses can easily result in a loss of balance or falls (Bloem et al., 2004; Willemsen et al., 2000). My experience is that abrupt movements such as rushing or quickly changing direction when ambulating are difficult to treat because there seems to be at least in part a personality trait or a lack of safety awareness. Some people, however, can modify their behavior to some degree and reduce their fall risk. Interventions in this area are primarily patient education.

An extreme example that comes to mind is a female patient with PD who was falling at least 10 times a day primarily because she was always rushing and somewhat impulsive. She did not use a walker for balance in her home, although its use was highly recommended. Repeated counseling helped her make the connection between her behavior and the incidence of falls, and she was able to reduce her falls to an average of twice a day.

A male patient with PD who was ambulatory with a rolling walker had a similar history of falls caused by rushing. When he rushed, however, he froze and was not able to stop the walker. In addition, his turns with the walker were abrupt. The walker turn far exceeded his capability to turn his feet and keep up with the walker. This person had never seen a physical therapist for his PD and bought a walker on his own without any gait training. He reduced his falls to three times daily with therapy intervention. Although the goal is to avoid any falls, these people are now at relative lower risk of becoming injured.

• **Dual tasking.** Trying to do two things at once—for example, walking and attempting to count money in a wallet or look for something in a purse—contributes to greater gait variability (Hausdorff et al., 2003a) and secondarily increases the risk of falls (figure 8.1). Dual tasking (motor or cognitive tasks) can decrease postural control during quiet standing in people with PD and is more destabilizing in people who already have a history of falls (Marchese et al., 2003).

Interventions for Fall Risk Factors

The balance evaluation process requires the identification of intrinsic fall risk factors (factors related to the patient) that are treatable and those that are resistant to change. The patient should be educated on the risk factors that are difficult to treat and be advised on compensatory options to maximize safety (which may include modification of environment-related extrinsic factors). Generally, people with PD have more intrinsic fall risk factors than those without the condition (Bloem et al., 2004; Willemsen et al., 2000). Therapeutic interventions should address both intrinsic and extrinsic factors to reduce the risk of falls.

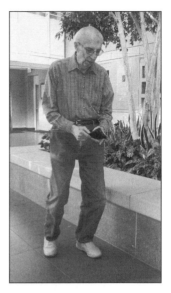

Figure 8.1 Tasks that are second nature to a person without PD can contribute to the risk of falls for the person with PD who has difficulties with dual tasking.

Environmental changes to deal with difficult-to-treat risk factors may include altering the home environment, changing shoe wear, or adding an ambulatory assist device. Treatable factors, such as deconditioning or stride length, require the patient's full cooperation for the best results.

Treatable Risk Factors

Physical intervention can improve strength and stride length. People who are deconditioned lose some of their ability to maintain or prevent a loss of balance. Reduced stride length can limit gait velocity, which can affect functional ambulation. If a person is at greater risk of falls because of inability to change intrinsic risk factors, changes in the home environment can be recommended.

• **Deconditioned state.** Many people with PD have become deconditioned from being sedentary. The effects of deconditioning can be reversed with conditioning exercises. For long-term maintenance, a home exercise program should be emphasized. Review chapter 3 for details about how to construct a home exercise program and how to enhance adherence.

• **Stride length.** Improving stride length with rhythmic auditory stimulation (RAS) can be an effective modality. But in the presence of lateral instability because of a narrowly based gait, improving stride length can be difficult and unsafe. Lateral stability may improve with conditioning exercises but the use of an ambulatory assist device to widen the base of support may still be needed. After lateral stability is established (pages 83–84), the patient can safely start on a walking program with RAS (see chapter 13, "Compensatory Strategies for Gait Interventions").

Difficult-to-Treat Risk Factors

Some gait characteristics tend to be more resistant to improvements from physical interventions. In my experience, the narrow-based gait is most resistant. Depending on the person's motivation and the severity of the condition, ground clearance and freezing can be improved.

- **Narrow-based gait.** A narrow-based gait contributes to lateral instability. The use of a walker offers improved lateral support and stability.

- **Ground clearance.** Ground clearance can improve with improved stride length and is enhanced with either attention strategies or rhythmical auditory stimulation. But this response is highly variable, depending on the patient's presentation or disease severity. If this factor is nonmodifiable, the patient should be advised about appropriate footwear. Shoes with low-friction soles help reduce the friction between the sole and the ground surface. This modification often reduces the frequency and severity of the feet sticking to the floor (see chapter 16, "Walkers, Canes, and Footwear").

- **Freezing.** Freezing is considered a fall risk and needs to be addressed by reviewing relevant compensatory strategies (see chapter 14, "Freezing"; "Problem-Oriented Treatment Interventions" in appendix D; and a reproducible patient handout on freezing in appendix D). One of the ways to reduce freezing is to accentuate lateral weight shift to unload the stepping foot. A person's base of support can be so narrow that any increase in amplitude of lateral weight shift is destabilizing. Using a walker allows an increase in lateral weight shift and secondarily helps with freezing. Patients should be aware that although freezing will continue to occur, its frequency and duration are modifiable (see "Freezing of Gait Questionnaire," appendix A).

- **Environmental measures.** Home modifications may be necessary to reduce the risk of falls. Ideally, an occupational therapist would go to the patient's home and offer comprehensive recommendations to reduce the risk of falls.

Case Example: Interventions for Fall Risk Factors

Josh has PD Hoehn and Yahr stage 3.

Subjective Evaluation

Josh has reportedly become sedentary secondary to fear of falling. He states that he currently ambulates without an assist device but has had recurrent falls because of freezing, turning while ambulating, and catching his feet. Falls are typically forward but also occur sideways.

Objective Evaluation

Josh comes into therapy with a significantly narrow-based gait. His gait also exhibits reduced ground clearance, short shuffling steps (reduced stride length), and intermittent

(continued)

freezing. His foot intermittently becomes stuck on the ground. He marginally recovers his balance after a stumble. Mild rigidity is noted in both lower extremities. Josh has become deconditioned and is exhibiting ROM limitations in the lower extremities. Gait velocity is significantly slower than his age-matched norms (see chapter 12, "Gait Deviations and Instability," pages 147–148).

Goals

The goals for Josh are to

- become independent in an HEP to improve strength and flexibility,
- understand how wearing shoes with low-friction soles can reduce the likelihood of catching his feet and lower the risk of losing balance,
- achieve steady ambulation with a walker and demonstrate proper use,
- understand antifreezing compensatory strategies to minimize frequency and duration of freezing episodes, and
- improve gait velocity by 10% from baseline.

Therapeutic Interventions

Comprehensively, interventions are intended to enable Josh to ambulate safely and more functionally. Conditioning should be an integral part to restore strength and prevent deconditioning.

- Josh is advised about the adverse effects of deconditioning and the need for proper footwear for fall prevention. He is informed that therapy is not effective in improving the width of his base of support and that he will need additional support (walker) for steady ambulation. He should know that compensatory strategies (RAS and weight shifting) and the use of a walker and proper shoes can improve freezing episodes but not eliminate them.

- Therapeutically, narrowness of gait in a person with PD is highly resistant to physical interventions. Therefore, the focus is on increasing Josh's base of support with safe use of a walker. Antifreezing strategies are reviewed and practiced (see "Freezing" in appendix D). Josh is instructed in a comprehensive HEP for conditioning and flexibility. Gait training with RAS is initiated after Josh demonstrates proper use of a walker (see chapter 13, "Compensatory Strategies for Gait Interventions").

Outcomes

By changing footwear and using a walker, Josh is able to improve gait stability and lateral weight shift. Secondarily, he is able to reduce freezing and improve walking endurance. Improved stride length and, secondarily, improved gait velocity can be expected with use of RAS, and his HEP can improve strength and flexibility.

Balance Evaluation and Treatment

The more we learn from a patient regarding the causative nature of falls or feelings of instability and the more objective data we collect from balance testing, the better we can serve the person by targeting those issues with appropriate interventions. The sample subjective and objective evaluation forms in appendix C provide questions that target the PD population. This section discusses unique considerations regarding the subjective evaluation and various balance tests and suggestions for interventions.

Subjective Evaluation

Patients usually perform better during balance testing in the clinic than they do in real situations because they are giving full attention to their effort, their medications are likely to be working properly, environmental conditions tend to be optimal, and they are not multitasking. Therefore, obtaining a thorough history focused on balance and mobility is paramount.

Besides obtaining standard subjective information about items such as barriers in the home, current physical abilities, use of an ambulatory assist device, social or family support, pain, other medical issues, and medications, several questions may be unique to this population regarding balance:

- If a person is taking L-dopa, questions should be asked about potential motor fluctuations.
- The nature and cause of falls should be established to guide therapeutic intervention.
- Questions relative to balance should address
  - feelings of instability,
  - frequency and direction of loss of balance or falls,
  - ability to get up from the floor,
  - difficulties with turning and freezing, and
  - whether the patient participates in a regular exercise regime for prevention and maintenance.

As mentioned previously, a history of falls is an indication of future falls. Note, however, that a lack of fall history does not indicate that the person is not at risk of future falls. A meta-analysis demonstrated a 3 mo follow-up fall rate of 21% among people with PD without a previous history of falls (Pickering et al., 2007).

Obtaining accurate, comprehensive information from the patient can be challenging. Intentionally or unintentionally, the patient may omit information, minimize symptoms, or answer questions vaguely in an attempt to hide deficits. For example, Lina reports that she is ambulatory without an assist device and admits to owning a rolling walker. She may have acquired the walker after having a total joint replacement that required its temporary use. The other possibility, which may be revealed only by more prodding, is that the doctor or a previous therapist recommended a walker for stability and Lina was noncompliant in its use. Having the patient's spouse or family member present during the subjective evaluation can help obtain information that is more comprehensive. Sometimes the spouse or other family member may observe problems that are not apparent to the patient. This additional information can be helpful for therapy interventions.

The patient's report of stability may be inconsistent with the objective exam. For example, you may ask a patient whether she or he feels unsteady when walking. The patient denies any feelings of unsteadiness, but you observe this person reaching for walls to maintain balance while walking. Although inconsistencies can be expected because of variations in mobility in response to anti-Parkinson's medications, patients may underreport falls or feelings of instability for various reasons:

- Cognitive impairments may interfere with the recollection of falls or feelings of unsteadiness.
- The patient may lack safety awareness and not regard feelings or occurrences of instability as an issue.
- The patient may be concerned that the therapist may recommend an assistive device.

Many patients voice the concern of "going downhill" when the need for using an assist device is discussed. From the patient's perspective, the onset of unsteadiness is not sudden, but its potential progressive nature can create concern. Over time the patient has already made adaptations in response to unsteadiness, such as limiting activities or relying on furniture for additional balance support. The therapist should clear up the misconception of "going downhill" when a patient voices concerns about using an assist device. Becoming deconditioned by limiting activities will only accelerate impairments, resulting in greater disability. If a patient is able to become more active—safely—the likelihood of becoming deconditioned can be reduced. Thus, using the assistive device can prevent and reverse the downhill trend. This point should be made clear.

On the other hand, the patient may not be psychologically ready to hear about the possible need for an assist device. In such cases, the discussion may need to wait, but it should not be forgotten. Establishing rapport with the patient and working on other fall prevention issues before addressing the possible need for an assistive device can pave the way for acceptance and compliance.

Objective Evaluation and Treatment

As mentioned previously, no single test can determine a person's risk of falls. Selection of the most appropriate balance tests can be facilitated by observing the patient's mobility when entering the clinic and by obtaining a thorough subjective evaluation. To ensure appropriateness and save time, selectiveness is necessary when choosing balance tests. For example, Josie, who is unable to remain in a standing position without holding on to her walker, does not require a pull test to establish postural instability, and she does not qualify for the Berg balance test because it requires the patient to be ambulatory without a device or at least be able to perform the test without an ambulatory device. She would, however, be appropriate for the timed up and go (see appendix B). In addition, performing perturbations during ambulation and while standing with her walker will establish whether she is safe and steady with her current ambulatory device. Reassessment of balance will indicate the effectiveness of interventions and offer guidance for future needs.

Various tests for assessing the risk of falls are discussed in the following sections. The most common tests used are the Berg balance test, timed up and go (TUG), functional reach, and tandem standing. Other tests such as the Tinneti performance-oriented mobility assessment (POMA) and the stop walking while talking test are discussed but not recommended because they are not appropriate for this population. The recommended tests are followed by suggestions for interventions. "Statistical Terms" will aid in understanding the appropriateness of the various tests.

Berg Balance Test

The Berg balance test has shown strong correlations with valid and reliable PD scales such as the Unified Parkinson's Disease Rating Scale (UPDRS), Hoehn and Yahr, and the Modified Schwab and England Activities of Daily Living Scale (S&E ADL Scale) (Qutubuddin et al., 2005). A study of people with PD Hoehn and Yahr stage 2 (bilateral involvement and intact postural reflexes) has demonstrated good correlations of the Berg balance test with the UPDRS, timed up and go (TUG), functional reach, and gait speed. The researchers concluded that the Berg balance test is a good measure of functional performance in people with PD in Hoehn and Yahr stage 2 (Brusse et al., 2005). The Berg balance test (see appendix B) can bring out specific deficits to target in therapy.

Suggested interventions: Therapeutic interventions that address or mimic activities found deficient in the Berg balance test can improve balance. For example, a person who has difficulty with alternate stepping on a stool can perform this activity as an exercise using progressively less upper-extremity support, depending on safety. Balance exercises that can be performed safely should be performed as a home exercise program. Balance activities that require assistance should be done in the clinic with the therapist until the patient can safely perform them at home. Long-term maintenance is ultimately the patient's responsibility.

Timed Up and Go

The timed up and go (TUG) is a highly reliable test for people with PD. The test can detect changes in performance between "on" and "off" states with L-dopa use, and it can detect differences between people with PD and age-matched controls (Morris et al., 2001). Increased fall risk in people with PD was associated with increased times of TUG (Balash et al., 2005). The TUG can detect performance improvement following therapy. The greatest area of difficulty in test performance for people with PD is getting out of the chair and turning (see appendix B for the procedure).

Suggested interventions: Therapeutic interventions should focus on turning strategies and body mechanics involved in sitting down and standing up (see chapter 9, "Chair Transfers"). Both activities may need to be broken down and repeatedly rehearsed with cuing.

Statistical Terms

These terms will help with the understanding and appropriateness of various tests discussed in this section.

specificity—a measure of the validity of a test based on the probability that a person not at risk of falls will test negative

sensitivity—a measure of the validity of a test based on the probability that a person with a risk of falls will test positive

validity—the degree to which a test measures what it is intended to measure

reliability—the degree of consistency or reproducibility of a test or rater in measuring a variable

> ### What Does Functional Reach Measure?
>
> Functional reach measures anterior stability, or the ability of a person to reach beyond her or his base of support. It should not be used alone to predict the risk of falls. For example:
>
> - Specificity: 92%. These results demonstrate with 92% accuracy that if a person with PD is able to reach 10 in. (25 cm) or more, he or she has no history of falls.
> - Sensitivity: 30%. These results show that even though the person with PD can reach 10 in. (25 cm) or more, which is a negative result, he or she still has a high likelihood of having a history of falls.

Turning technique may improve with rhythmical auditory stimulation (RAS) by reducing stepping variability (Willems et al., 2007) (see chapter 13, pages 151–160). By addressing foot advancement during turns, a reduction in freezing and improvements in turning abilities can be appreciated (see chapter 15, "Turning While Ambulating," pages 179–181).

Functional Reach

Functional reach is "the maximum distance one can reach forward beyond arm's length while maintaining a fixed base of support in the standing position" (Duncan et al., 1990). But as shown in "What Does Functional Reach Measure?" this test is not a sensitive instrument for predicting fall risk in PD (Behrman et al., 2002).

Functional reach may not be a sensitive instrument to predict falls in PD, but it does exhibit a measure for anterior stability or perhaps a confidence level with reaching. Improved strength and flexibility or confidence can allow greater reaching capability. The functional reach test can detect improvements in balance from rehabilitation in other populations (Weiner et al., 1993) (see appendix B for the procedure).

If functional reach is less than 10 in. (25 cm), conditioning and range of motion exercises of the lower extremities, shoulders, and trunk may be needed depending on areas of impairment (see chapter 3). People with PD tend to lack hip balance strategies when performing the functional reach test (figure 8.2, *a* and *b*). Without the counterbalance from the hips, loss of balance occurs sooner. Exercises that target reaching in combination with counterbalancing of the hips are recommended (figure 8.3). Functional activities that require forward reaching and a counterbalancing hip strategy will improve awareness of how to self-monitor balance. Foot position may need to be adjusted to improve the base of support for stability (Kirby et al., 1987) (see chapter 7, "Postural Instability," page 85).

Tandem Standing

Tandem standing should not be performed as the sole balance test, but it can offer insight to lateral trunk-righting capabilities and the ability to self-recover in the event of a loss of balance. Timing the tandem stance and noting balance responses can offer objective data for goal setting. For example, Karen was able to tandem stand for 10 s with close supervision but then needed to be caught because trunk-righting capability and stepping strategy were absent.

Suggested interventions: The treatment goal is to improve lateral balance and reduce fall risk, demonstrated by the ability to tandem stand for 15 s and self-recover with an effective stepping strategy. The primary focus is on power strengthening of the hip abductor muscles,

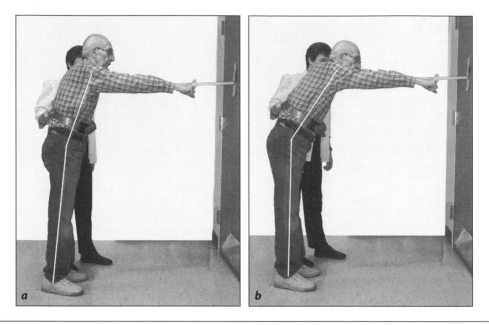

Figure 8.2 *(a)* Functional reach without hip strategy, resulting in limited reach and reduced stability; *(b)* functional reach with hip strategy, resulting in a greater reach and improved stability.

increasing trunk flexibility, and facilitating lateral stepping strategies (see chapter 7, "Postural Instability," pages 87–90).

Clinical Test Combinations

Smithson et al. (1998) studied 10 fallers with PD, 10 people with PD but no history of falls, and 10 controls. The ability of various tests to predict fall risk was evaluated. The following tests, in combination, were found to be sensitive in discriminating between people with PD who fell and people with PD who had no history of falls: tandem stance, single-limb stance, functional reach test, and pull test (see chapter 7, "Postural Instability," for details on the pull test, also known as the retropulsive test). Tests were performed in the peak dose L-dopa cycle ("on" state). Clinically, this combination of tests is both practical and efficient when time is limited. It addresses areas of potential instability anteriorly, posteriorly, and laterally.

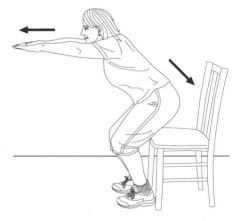

Figure 8.3 This exercise can be used to improve body mechanics while reaching (facilitation of hip strategy), strengthen the leg and postural musculature, and build confidence in reaching. The person squats while reaching. The chair is used for a safety backup.

    Suggested interventions: Refer to separate sections in this chapter on tandem standing and functional reach for interventions. See chapter 7, "Postural Instability," for interventions regarding a positive pull test. Although improvements in single-leg stance tend to be limited, it has been my experience that any improvement is more the result from lower-extremity conditioning and power strengthening than from balance training (see chapter 3, "Exercise and Rehabilitation Considerations," pages 35–38).

Tinneti Performance-Oriented Mobility Assessment

This test was developed to screen for balance and mobility deficits in the older population and to determine the probability of falls. There are two testing sections. The first section, called balance tests, consists of nine test items. Four of these items address performance related to standing up and sitting down. These items are helpful in qualifying this activity and could be incorporated into the mobility part of an evaluation (see "Objective Evaluation" in appendix C). The second section, called gait tests, evaluates seven components of gait. This section is not sensitive to change in people with PD who are moderately affected and therefore is not recommended as an evaluation tool for this population (Behrman et al., 2002).

Stop Walking While Talking

"Stop walking while talking" is considered a good predictor of falls in frail institutionalized older people who have depression or cognitive impairment (Lundin-Olsson et al., 1997) but is a poor predictor of falls in those with PD whose cognition is intact and who are not depressed. Results of a study of 38 people with PD and 35 controls without PD, with no cognitive impairments or depression in either group, yielded a sensitivity of 14.3% and a specificity of 91.7% in discriminating between PD fallers and PD nonfallers (Bloem et al., 2000). This test seems to be a better indicator of fall risk in those who are cognitively impaired than in those who are not.

Balance Assessment During Gait

Because of the potential effects of Parkinsonian gait deviations on balance, an additional balance examination is necessary for walking. The effects of dual tasking on gait and balance should also be examined. Dual tasking can exacerbate deviations and place the patient at greater risk of falls. Chapter 12 discusses the examination of and interventions for gait instability.

Summary

1. People with moderate PD who remain active in the presence of reduced stability have the greatest risk of falls.

2. Subjective and objective balance evaluations are equally important when establishing fall risk factors and appropriate treatment interventions.

3. Balance tests should be patient specific:
   - Berg balance test: higher-level patients, performed without assist device
   - TUG: patients with assist device
   - Combination: tandem stance, single-limb stance, functional reach, and pull test—efficient and sensitive in predicting PD fallers and PD nonfallers

4. Evaluation of postural reflexes should be an integral part of balance evaluation in the movement disorder population (see chapter 7, "Postural Instability").

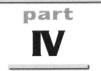

part

IV

TRANSFERS

Difficulties in chair transfers, bed mobility, and floor transfers are often multifactorial. Disease severity can make sequential movements difficult. This part of the book addresses both the neurologic and secondary musculoskeletal impairments that contribute to transfer difficulties. Chapters are organized by problem area. Theory as well as evaluative and treatment procedures are discussed.

Chair Transfers

Chair transfers can be inherently difficult for the Parkinson's disease (PD) population. The ability to get in and out of a chair can be further reduced by muscle weakness resulting from deconditioning or limited flexibility or arthritis in the lower extremities. Psychological factors, such as the fear of falling when getting out of a chair, can prevent a person from leaning sufficiently forward with the trunk when attempting to get up.

Activity Analysis

Chair transfers can be categorized as two separate activities: standing up from a seated position and sitting back down. Excluding factors related to the type of chair, both activities rely heavily on body positioning as well as strength and coordination.

- Sit to stand begins with scooting to the edge of the chair to allow proper foot placement. The feet need to be positioned under the knees and apart to stabilize and ease the transition from one base of support (the seat) to the final base of support (the feet). Sufficient hip flexion is needed to bring the trunk forward over the feet before liftoff, which is necessary for stability in the transition. During initial standing, the feet function as the stabilizing base. If the feet are positioned too close together before standing, stability with initial standing will be compromised. Postural responses and a person's strength should work as the stabilizing guide wires for initial standing. Instability can result from the inability of the body to keep the center of mass (COM) over the base of support (BOS), which may occur when postural reflexes or strength is impaired. Orthostatic hypotension can also cause instability with initial standing, but that topic will not be addressed in this chapter (see chapter 2, "Medical and Surgical Interventions," pages 19–20).

- Stand to sit involves approaching the chair and sitting down. Simply approaching a chair can be problematic for people who freeze (feet stick to the floor). Freezing that occurs when approaching objects is called destination hesitation. After the chair has been approached, the turning arc can range from 90° to 180° depending on the approach angle. People with PD do not turn as far as controls do (Huxham et al., 2008), which may explain why this population can be observed to side-sit on a chair. Turning can precipitate freezing or become destabilizing because of difficulty with coordinating foot placement. If the person has turned prematurely, backing up to the chair is necessary. For some this is not an issue, but for those who experience retropulsion (an involuntary backward stepping with progressively smaller steps and increasing momentum), this movement can create a high risk of falling. Finally, how does the person sit down? Is it a controlled descent? Does the person fall back into the chair or use the hands on the armrests to control descent? If the person has a walker, does she or he let go of the walker to reach for the chair? Cognitive safety issues may also arise. Does the person attempt to sit before fully backing up to the chair? Does the person attempt to line up with the chair before sitting (to the left or right)? Any combination of these suboptimal movements can make chair transfers more difficult or potentially unsafe.

Chair Transfer Kinematic Patterns

A great deal of research has addressed kinematic patterns going from a sitting position to a standing position. This emphasis is appropriate because if a person cannot get out of a chair, disability implications are much greater. To stand up from a chair, a person needs to have enough strength to raise the body against gravity. When sitting down, gravity works to the person's advantage. Falling into a chair still allows a person to sit down, although this technique is not recommended or safe. This section compares the kinematic patterns of chair transfers of healthy adults to the patterns of people with PD and relates these patterns to difficulties encountered. A better understanding of the kinematics can offer insights to interventions for a more individualized approach.

In Healthy Adults

Going from a seated position to a standing position initially requires horizontal forces of the trunk followed by vertical forces. In other words, the trunk leans forward with sufficient magnitude of force before vertical forces begin to lift the buttocks from the chair (liftoff). A study compared the maximum horizontal velocity of the trunk in healthy young adults with the same in healthy older adults. The maximum horizontal velocity was less in the older people, resulting in a posterior shift of the COM when the buttocks lifted up from the seat. This discrepancy was further accentuated when vision was impaired (Mourey et al., 2000). The posterior shift of the COM could account for some of the falling back into the chair, which is seen at times in older people when they attempt to stand up. When compared with younger adults, older adults demonstrate reduced hip flexor torque and less horizontal momentum but increased ankle dorsiflexion torque during liftoff, which has been postulated to be a strategy to maximize postural stability and prevent loss of balance (Mak et al., 2003).

In a study of more than 600 healthy older people, Lord et al. (2002) looked at various physical and psychological factors that contribute to the vertical forces of sit to stand. Although many factors play a part, the greatest contributor is the strength of the quadriceps muscle. Muscular forces have been noted to increase in magnitude, and the vertical forces occur sooner with increased speed. Horizontal forces, however, do not increase proportionately to vertical forces with increased speed (Pai & Rogers, 1991). In other words, as someone attempts to stand up more quickly, the momentum of the leg muscles increases significantly, yet the horizontal momentum of the trunk does not show this relative change. This may be the body's attempt to keep the COM—the trunk—over the BOS with increased velocities to prevent forward loss of balance.

A study by Pai & Lee (1994) supported the hypothesis that the inherent postural control mechanisms were more tightly restrained with increased velocities to guard against a loss of balance. The researchers had healthy adult subjects perform sit to stand under three conditions: sit to stand at normal speed, sit to stand as quickly as possible without the availability of a supportive bar to grab in the event of a loss of balance, and sit to stand as quickly as possible with a bar available to assist in recovery from a loss of balance. The horizontal forward movement of the trunk was much less in the group without a support bar.

Finally, a review of 39 sit-to-stand studies found three mechanical factors that have a strong influence on the ability to stand up from a seated position (Janssen et al., 2002):

- **Seat height**. A higher seat height can reduce the forces needed by approximately 60% at the knee and up to 50% at the hip. When sitting in lower chairs, people may rely more on momentum to stand up.
- **Foot position**. Positioning of the feet more posteriorly can reduce the forces needed at the hip.
- **Armrests**. A person can push up on armrests while attempting to stand. This technique distributes the stress across more muscles and joints, reducing the required lower-extremity forces.

These mechanical factors can be individually adjusted when considering therapeutic interventions. Depending on individual needs, positioning can be optimized to reduce difficulty or altered to encourage strength gains. For example, someone who has bilateral knee arthritis may need to rely on a higher seat and be encouraged to use armrests to minimize knee irritation and preserve the knee joints. On the other hand, someone who is deconditioned can use a lower chair without armrests to force the legs to work harder.

In People With PD

The kinematic patterns seen in norms and in people with PD are similar during sit to stand and start with hip flexion to bring the trunk forward, followed by hip extension, knee extension, and ankle dorsiflexion. Upon initial standing, ankle plantarflexion torque helps to control the forward momentum of the body. Although the sequential kinematics may be similar, the timing of these movements may be altered. The joint angle displacements or force productions can also vary from norms. Difficulties with going from sit to stand depend on the severity of PD and the effectiveness of the Parkinson's medications.

For example, a person with PD Hoehn and Yahr stage 2 (bilateral involvement, balance intact) who is in an "on" state can stand up from a chair much like someone without PD. A person with PD Hoehn and Yahr stage 2 who is in an "off" state can exhibit lower peak knee extensor torque and require more time to stand up. People with mild PD regardless of "on" or "off" state exhibit greater anterior COM displacement before liftoff from a chair. During liftoff, however, there tends to be a reversal of the anterior displacement when compared with norms. When this reversal occurs in combination with a peak knee extension torque just before liftoff, the ease of getting up can be hampered (Inkster & Eng, 2004). Normally, the peak knee extension torque occurs just after liftoff when the COM is well over the base of support. Exaggerating and maintaining a forward-leaning trunk during liftoff can help reduce these difficulties.

Someone with PD Hoehn and Yahr stage 3 (mild to moderate bilateral disease, some postural instability) will have greater problems when attempting to stand up. People with moderate PD have increased difficulties with motor unit recruitment. They need additional time to develop peak muscle forces. In addition, peak muscle forces are significantly lower than norms. Increased cocontraction of antagonists further impedes abilities. These factors contribute to reduced horizontal and vertical forces when standing up. Peak hip extensor torque occurs just before liftoff, and knee extension occurs just after liftoff but sooner than norms (Inkster & Eng, 2004; Mak et al., 2003). Clinically, what is frequently observed is insufficient forward leaning of the trunk and a disproportionate amount of hip extension during liftoff. As with mild PD, greater hip flexion to bring the trunk forward will not only help maintain the COM over the BOS but also discourage premature hip extension, which can contribute to backward loss of balance.

In people with PD, the speed of standing up from a chair can significantly affect the ability to stand up. When performing sit to stand at a natural speed, people with PD have impaired ability to switch from horizontal to vertical forces (Mak & Hui-Chan, 2002; Mak et al., 2003). A study compared the ability of people with PD to stand up from a chair at normal and fast speeds with the same ability in healthy age- and sex-matched controls. When the speed of sit to stand was increased, the subjects with PD were able to increase force production and their rate of force production was similar to what the controls could accomplish (Mak & Hui-Chan, 2005). This study helps explain why a person with PD may have difficulty standing up, perhaps requiring more than one attempt even when using the hands, and only moments later can perform the chair stand test and quickly stand up and sit down without upper-extremity support 10 times in 30 s without flaw. Adjusting sit-to-stand speeds may be an additional consideration in therapeutic interventions to minimize difficulties. Both safety and function should be assessed when advising a patient to stand up quickly as a functional solution.

Fear of falling can limit forward excursion of the trunk when attempting to stand up. Objects located in front of the person may help or impede sit to stand. For example, if a patient has a walker in front of him or her, standing up may be easier. Knowing that support is available if needed may increase the forward leaning of the trunk. On the other hand, a patient may report increased difficulty standing up from a couch when facing a coffee table but have no difficulty when the coffee table is removed. The person may view the table as an obstacle for injury, or the table may be a visual trigger that impedes movement.

Controlling velocity when sitting down becomes difficult with a more posteriorly positioned COM in combination with impaired postural reflexes. Greater hip flexion to position the trunk more over the base of support will improve controlled descent. Impaired cognition can accentuate difficulties and reduce safety awareness. Repetition of activities in the clinic followed by repeated practice at home can facilitate proper technique.

Evaluation of Chair Transfers

The subjective evaluation helps uncover difficulties with chair transfers that occur at home but are not observed in the clinic. This evaluation will be especially important if the patient experiences motor fluctuations because of dopaminergic medications. The focus is to find out whether chair transfers are easy or difficult. The patient is asked whether he or she is having difficulties getting in or out of a chair. If yes, is it sometimes or all the time? Does the person need assistance with chair transfers? If yes, is assistance needed sometimes or all the time?

Objective evaluation is primarily through observation. As mentioned earlier, the strength of the quadriceps muscle is a key contributor to the ability to stand up. Lower-extremity power strength and endurance can be evaluated with the chair stand test. The test is valid in predicting age-related declines and differentiating between sedentary and active independent older adults. Norms for this test were established from a sample of over 7,000 independently living older adults (Rickli & Jones, 2001). Chair stand norms can be used for goal setting. This test can be highly motivational. Patients can see how they measure up against age- and sex-matched norms. Patients seem to understand the practicality of the movement as a test and as a home exercise program. As a home exercise program, repeatedly standing up and sitting down can be modified for maximal benefits and safety (see appendix B for chair stand test procedure and norms).

Therapeutic Interventions

Improvements with sit-to-stand or stand-to-sit capabilities often require the synergistic effects of optimal body mechanics and greater strength in the leg muscles. Interventions will target both areas.

Interventions to Improve Sit to Stand

Educating the patient or caregiver in proper body mechanics to reduce the degree of difficulty with sit to stand is an initial consideration. Although strength training will greatly enhance ability, some people must rely solely on body mechanics because of comorbidities such as bilateral knee arthritis.

Body Mechanics Instruction

Standing up from a seated position can be broken down from one sequential movement into a series of simple movements (Kamsma et al., 1995) (see the patient handout "Standing Up From a Chair" in appendix D.) The ordering of body mechanics is as follows:

1. Scoot to the edge of the chair.
2. Slide the feet back so that the toes are under the knees.
3. Lean forward with the trunk while standing up.

If necessary, the caregiver can be instructed how to assist a patient with sit to stand. Sometimes, all that is needed is downward pressure on the upper back to maintain a forward-leaning position. The caregiver places one hand between the patient's shoulder blades. After the patient leans forward in the attempt to stand up, the caregiver applies enough pressure to maintain this forward-leaning position while the patient stands up. Caregivers are often reluctant and skeptical, but with practice they begin to appreciate the benefits. Caregivers should be advised not to stand in front of the patient and pull the person up by the hands. This technique creates greater stress on both, develops bad habits, and hampers learning of the proper technique. An alternative is to use a gait belt and have the patient use armrests and maintain some forward flexion while standing up. The patient and the caregiver should repeatedly practice body mechanics in the clinic until they understand the technique.

Strength Training

Separate from the instruction of body mechanics is the implementation of an exercise program that targets strength enhancement. The primary exercise to improve sit to stand requires repeatedly standing up and sitting down. The standing-up portion should be performed quickly to facilitate concentric power of the quadriceps. Sitting down should be performed slowly to develop eccentric strength and control. Regardless of the level of progression, standing up quickly and sitting down slowly will produce the greatest gains. As mentioned earlier, people with PD were able to increase force production and rate of force production similar to what controls accomplished when the speed of sit to stand was increased. Like any exercise, this exercise should be modified or discontinued if performing it is painful.

Seat height, foot positioning, and arm position can be adjusted to control the difficulty of the exercise (Janssen et al., 2002). The intensity of the exercise should be adjusted so that the rate of perceived exertion (RPE) is "somewhat hard" or "moderate." Ten repetitions are sufficient for strength gains (see chapter 3 for strengthening guidelines). If the patient cannot demonstrate proper form throughout the exercise, difficulty should be reduced by adjusting seat height or arm position. Initially, the exercise should be easy enough so that the patient can perform it successfully but difficult enough to facilitate gains in strength and function. The therapist helps determine the optimal therapeutic positions and initiates progression when appropriate, but the patient is responsible for working on this at home. Guidelines for adjusting the variables in the exercise follow.

Seat height

As mentioned earlier, a higher seat reduces the effort needed at the knee by approximately 60% and at the hip by up to 50%. Seat height can be critical in a successful chair transfer for those who are significantly deconditioned or have arthritic problems. Increasing the seat height may be needed initially.

Foot positioning

This factor is not as simple to adjust as seat height is. Keep these factors in mind as you instruct your patient on foot positioning:

- Weakness in the hip extensors from disuse is not uncommon. As mentioned earlier, positioning the feet more posteriorly can significantly reduce the effort required of the hip extensors when standing up.
- Before the feet can be placed more posteriorly, room must be available for them to be placed back. The type of chair (open or closed at the base) determines how much the patient needs to scoot to the edge for proper foot positioning.
- Training the patient to scoot habitually to the front half of the chair before standing, regardless of the type of chair, will facilitate greater consistency for carryover and adaptability.
- Foot positioning is also important in stability with initial standing. Positioning the feet approximately shoulder-width apart offers improved lateral stability. Having one foot farther back can improve anterior and posterior stability (Kirby et al., 1987).
- To assume the staggered-foot positioning, patients often slide one foot forward instead of sliding one foot back. The forward foot is then at a mechanical disadvantage, which can make standing up more difficult. Patients can achieve optimal foot placement by choosing a reference foot. If a plumb line were dropped from the knee, the toes of the reference foot would be just behind the plumb line. The other foot should be placed farther back from the reference foot. To demonstrate this to the patient, use a cane or pole as the plumb line (figure 9.1).

Arm positioning

Hand and arm position can be used as a progression with a home exercise program (figure 9.2, *a* and *b*). The patient should be successful yet challenged. Three positions can be used:

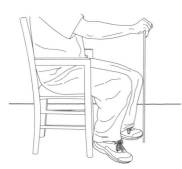

Figure 9.1 To improve a staggered-foot position for stability with initial standing, a cane or stick can be used to guide the patient in placing the reference foot when getting into position to stand up. The other foot is placed posterior to the reference foot.

- Hands on armrests
- Arms reaching forward
- Arms crossed against chest as in the chair stand test

Here are suggestions to progress the difficulty of the sit-to-stand exercise:

- high seat and hands on armrests to normal-height seat and hands on armrests, to
- high seat with arms reaching to normal-height seat with arms reaching, to
- high seat with arms crossed against chest to normal-height seat with arms crossed.

As patients become stronger they can try to get in and out of chairs at home that are lower, softer, and more difficult to use, usually the ones that they have been avoiding in the past. Arm position can be modified so that the difficulty level remains at a RPE of "somewhat hard" or "moderate," but balance and safety are always the first priority.

Interventions to Improve Stand to Sit

The focus of going from standing to sitting is on controlling the descending motion and avoiding a fall into the chair.

Body Mechanics Instruction

Studies have focused primarily on going from a sitting position to a standing position, but the body mechanics of going from a standing position to a sitting position are similar in some ways. Less forward leaning of the trunk and reduced hip and knee flexion tend to

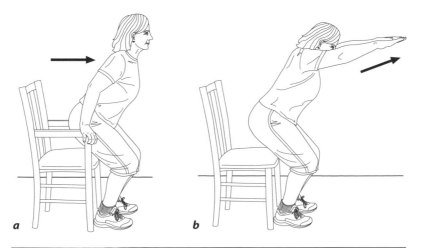

Figure 9.2 The progression of difficulty going from (a) sit to (b) stand by modifying hand positions.

occur, which can contribute to backward loss of balance. Some patients also have difficulty flexing their knees, which makes lowering more difficult and unstable.

People with PD who have this problem typically are not aware that their knees are not flexing sufficiently. To improve stability, therapy interventions should target normalization of kinematics. The first step is to increase the patient's awareness that her or his knee flexion is insufficient and that this condition affects stability. Some patients respond to cueing such as "Let your knees relax" or "Let your knees bend as you sit down." Other patients respond better to the indirect approach. For example, advising the patient to attempt to sit in the back of the chair when sitting down offers a visualization that promotes greater hip flexion and forward trunk leaning, which can indirectly promote knee flexion. Repeated practice is necessary, and it needs to be reinforced with daily activities as well as with the sit-to-stand exercise.

Chair Approach

People with PD who report difficulty with turns frequently experience freezing or falls (Stack et al., 2006). Greater turning angles tend to be more destabilizing. One study demonstrated greater freezing with 360° turns than with 180° turns (Schaafsma et al., 2003). Another study demonstrated greater turning impairments with 120° turns compared with 60° turns (Huxham et al., 2008). With this in mind, adjusting the angle at which a chair is approached is of clinical significance for those who have difficulty turning. Normally, a person approaches a chair directly and must make a 180° turn to sit down. By approaching the chair from the side, however, the person needs to make only a 90° turn, thereby reducing the turning angle by 50%.

A significant reduction in freezing or difficulty with turning can be achieved by using a side approach. People who become unstable when backing up to a chair because of retropulsion also benefit from approaching a chair from the side. (Retropulsion is an involuntary backward stepping with progressively smaller steps and increasing momentum and instability.) Any backward stepping before sitting should be minimized. Approaching the chair from the side can accomplish this goal. With one leg against the chair and one hand on the armrest, the patient can steadily step back with the opposite foot and pivot safely into the chair (figure 9.3, a–d).

Case Example: Sit to Stand

Sue is 80 yr old and sedentary. She has PD Hoehn and Yahr stage 2 and is mildly affected by PD.

Subjective Evaluation

The patient reports that she is having difficulty getting out of chairs and is relying heavily on her hands to get up. She avoids low chairs.

Objective Evaluation

Sue is unable to perform any repetitions based on the standard chair stand test criteria. The seat height is adjusted to 20 in (50 cm). Following the same testing position and procedures, she is able to perform five repetitions in 30 s when the seat height is 20 in (50 cm).

(continued)

Goals

Sue has one short-term goal and two long-term goals.

- The short-term goal for Sue is to demonstrate improved lower-extremity strength by being able to stand up and sit down without upper-extremity support 10 times in 30 s with seat height at 20 in. (50 cm).
- The long-term goals for Sue are to verbalize improved ability with getting up from a chair and to perform 9 reps in the chair stand test (her age- and sex-matched norm is 9 to 14 reps).

Therapeutic Interventions

Body mechanics are monitored and muscles are progressively challenged.

- Instruct in repeated sit to stand.
- Progress difficulty of repeated sit to stand.

Outcomes

Sue was having difficulties because she was deconditioned. She had no other comorbidities, so we can expect significant strength improvement and secondarily less difficulty getting out of chairs.

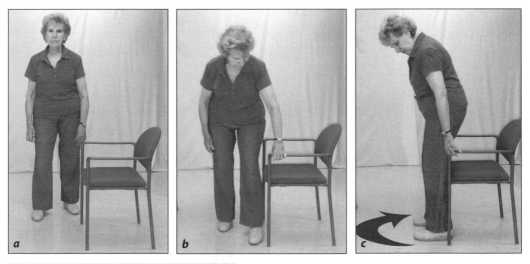

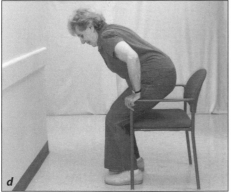

Figure 9.3   *(a)* Approaching the chair from the side reduces turning needs; *(b)* placing one leg against the chair and one hand on the armrest promotes stability; *(c)* pivoting without needing to step back can prevent instability; *(d)* optimal body mechanics prevents backward loss of balance or missing the chair.

Summary

1. Difficulty with sit to stand is multifactorial, but quadriceps strength plays a significant role, particularly if a person is deconditioned.

2. People with moderate PD have difficulty with force production and transitional movements with sit to stand.

3. Difficulty with sit to stand can be modified by seat height, foot position, and hand and arm position.

4. Breaking down sit to stand into the following three simple sequential movements can improve performance:
   - First, scoot;
   - second, slide feet back; and
   - third, lean forward while standing up.

5. Difficulties with standing up or sitting down can be caused by suboptimal kinematics.

6. Chair stand test norms can be used for goal setting.

7. People who have problems with turning or who exhibit instability because of retropulsion can improve their stand-to-sit ability by modifying their chair approach angle.

10

Bed Mobility

Difficulties with bed mobility have been correlated to low dopamine levels, disease duration, and disease severity. This conclusion was demonstrated in a study that evaluated the effects of L-dopa in subjects with PD ranging from Hoehn and Yahr stage 1 through stage 5 and their ability to turn in bed. After dopamine withdrawal, increased axial rigidity and extremity bradykinesia were noted in all stages, but the condition was most pronounced among those in the advanced stages. During their "off" state, some patients were unable to turn. Others changed their strategy, such as by sitting up, to enable them to lie on the side. When dopamine was reinstituted, the ability to turn in bed returned to close to normal. The difficulty noted with turning in bed was also attributed to lack of ability to perform sequential movements (Steiger et al., 1996). The basal ganglia are responsible for the automaticity of learned movements (Seitz & Roland, 1992), and the supplementary motor cortex is responsible for sequential movements of multiple muscles at multiple joints (Morecraft & Hoesen, 1996). Underactivation of the supplementary motor cortex has been noted in people with PD during movements (Turner et al., 2003). When dopamine levels are deficient, both the automaticity of movement and the ability to perform sequential movements are impaired.

People with mild PD may have little or no difficulty with bed mobility. People with moderate PD, however, experience a nocturnal "off" state (Rye & Bliwise, 2004). Controlled-release L-dopa taken later in the evening can relieve nighttime akinesia in advanced PD (Jansen & Meerwaldt, 1988). Managing nighttime PD symptoms, however, can be delicate because high doses of L-dopa can cause difficulty with falling asleep and result in disrupted sleep for the first half of the night (Bergonzi et al., 1974; Bergonzi et al., 1975).

Bed mobility requires a multitude of sequential movements. Reviewing sequential movements early on with people who have mild PD can be beneficial. When patients are moderately to severely impaired, however, focusing on compensatory strategies such as using a bed transfer rail is a better utilization of resources. When patients are seen in the clinic, dopamine levels are higher than they are at night. If a patient is unable to perform effective sequential movements when dopamine levels are optimal, we cannot expect improved performance at night. The effectiveness of therapeutic interventions depends on the patient's or caregiver's feedback concerning their successes or failures. Recommendations can be modified based on reported continued difficulties.

Bed Mobility Assessment

Assessment of bed mobility is accomplished partly by the patient's or caregiver's history and partly by observation. Patients typically report that they have better bed mobility during therapy than they do at night, most likely because of the effects of medications, not having to contend with blankets and sheets, and the firm surface of a mat table when compared with a softer bed mattress. The most effective and efficient way to assess bed mobility is to have the patient explain any areas of difficulty and demonstrate how he or she gets into and out of bed at home. I have observed patients entering their beds on hands and knees. This technique may be a compensatory method to minimize sequential movements or an attempt to reduce difficulties when the bed is too high. Some people show a significant difference in ability when getting into bed on one side versus the other. In such a case, the patient may benefit from sleeping on the other side of the bed. Patients (and significant others) can be resistant to giving up their side of the bed, but this change may be negotiable if it means extra sleep for the significant other and greater independence for the patient.

Therapeutic Interventions

Physical interventions to improve bed mobility are needed because of the limitations of medical management. The patient or the caregiver often recognizes improvements in bed mobility, although the changes are not necessarily observed in the clinic. The following sections offer recommendations about equipment and bed height and compare interventions for mild PD versus moderate and severe PD.

Environmental Changes

The physical management to improve bed mobility in the moderately to severely impaired patient with PD focuses on environmental changes. Making changes earlier rather than later can help establish less difficult movement patterns and improve safety.

Bed Assist Rail

To improve rolling capability, visual input can be added to enhance hypokinetic arm-reaching movements. If a patient looks at her or his hand when reaching toward a visual target, movement errors when reaching are reduced (Adamovich et al., 2001). Visual cues also improve the initiation of movement (Praamstra et al., 1998). I have found that the bed assist rail improves the initiation and magnitude of reaching ability in people with moderate PD, possibly because of the addition of this visual feedback.

Unfortunately, the term *bed assist rail* is not universal, although it may be the most frequently used. Other terms are *bed cane, transfer handles, freedom grip,* and *bedside valet assist* (see figure 10.1). The bed assist rail is a device mounted to the side of the bed (just below the pillow) and is approximately 12 in. (30 cm) wide. It enables people to swing in and out of bed on their own when they previously needed assistance, and it can reduce the amount of help required from the caregiver. Bed assist rails should be stationary and safely secured to the bed in a manner appropriate to the patient's size and weight. Bed assist rails that swivel should be avoided because of safety implications.

As with any device that aids mobility, a patient can view the bed assist rail as a sign of "going downhill" or deem it aesthetically unpleasing. The level of acceptance is usually directly related to the level of difficulty that the patient is having with bed mobility. The following information may be useful in persuading patients to use the bedrail when they are initially resistant to the idea:

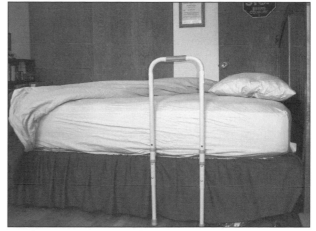

Figure 10.1 Bed assist rail.

The bed assist rail offers the following benefits when going from supine to sitting:

- provides greater visual input, allowing for improved reaching capability;
- allows easier rolling by having a rail to pull on;
- reduces sequential movements by offering the ability to pivot from a lying position to a sitting position; and
- offers additional support to
  - prevent falling back into the bed when initially sitting,
  - facilitate going from a seated position to a standing position, and
  - achieve balance during initial standing.

The bed assist rail offers the following benefits when going from sitting to supine:

- reduces sequential movements by offering the ability to pivot from a sitting position to a lying position and
- reduces lying down on a diagonal in the bed, which can be difficult for the patient or caregiver to correct.

Practicing bed mobility in the clinic with and without such a rail can offer insight into its value and help with acceptance. Because outpatient clinics typically do not have beds with bed assist rails, training can be performed by placing a pickup walker next to a mat table, which is anchored by the therapist while the patient uses it as if it were a bed assist rail (see figure 10.2, *a–c*).

People with greater disease severity may need assistance to reach the bed assist rail. This inability is multifactorial but may be aggravated by visual integration deficits associated with increased disease severity (Keijsers et al., 2005).

Bed Height

The height of the bed may need to be adjusted to reduce difficulty and improve safety. Beds tend to be too high, which makes getting into bed more difficult. At the other extreme, a bed that is too low increases the effort required to make the transition from sitting to standing. Neither case is optimal because of the potential risk of falls, especially in the presence of orthostatic hypotension when morning blood pressure drops can be worse when initially getting out of bed (Mathias & Kimber, 1998). Some patients accommodate to a high bed by adding a stepstool, which only adds to the risk of falls. The optimal bed height is at knee level or slightly higher so that when the patient is sitting on it, the feet are flat on the floor and the knees are at a 90° (or slightly greater) angle.

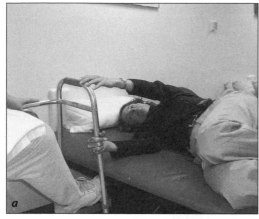

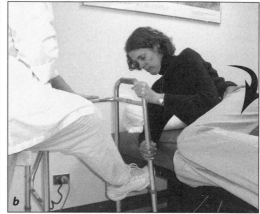

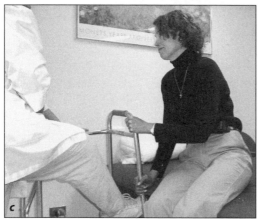

Figure 10.2 *(a)* Visually guided reaching to facilitate rolling before sitting up; *(b)* use of rail to pivot into sitting and minimize sequential movements; *(c)* hand position on rail when going from sitting to lying.

Several methods can be used to lower a bed to a more suitable height:

- Remove the bed frame.
- Replace the box springs with a piece of plywood and place the mattress on the plywood.
- Replace standard box springs with low-profile box springs.

Blanket Support

Some patients may complain of increased difficulty moving in bed because their legs become tangled in the sheets. The sheets may also interfere with getting in or out of bed. Others may report that the weight of their blankets creates problems with moving. A blanket support is a frame that is anchored at the foot end of the bed. The sheets and blankets are draped over this frame to allow greater freedom of movement for the legs. Blanket supports vary in size. Some are adjustable, and others are not. An adjustable frame allows greater customization (see figure 10.3).

Overhead Trapeze Bar

The therapist should know which items not to recommend. An overhead trapeze bar is fine for scooting laterally and up and down in bed, but I do not believe that it offers the best assistance in going from a lying position to sitting position or from a sitting position to lying position, because the movement creates suboptimal body mechanics for both the patient and the caregiver. I have found that people who initially use a trapeze bar to assist in sitting up and lying down but are later unable to use it because of increased difficulties have greater problems learning new and more effective strategies.

Draw Sheet

For those with severe disability who are unable to assist, a draw sheet can reduce caregiver strain. The draw sheet can be used by a single caregiver to roll a person on to his or her side to aid in transfers or repositioning. It can also be used to assist in scooting up in bed, although this task will require the assistance of two people.

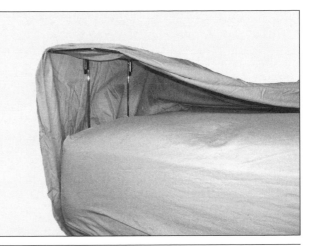

Figure 10.3 Blanket support.

Bed Mobility Interventions

Because people at different stages of Hoehn and Yahr do not have the same difficulty with bed mobility, interventions focus on several aspects of bed mobility. Interventions for people with mild PD are not as comprehensive as those for people with moderate or severe PD.

Mild PD

Sequential movements are usually not problematic in patients with mild PD. This group may report increased difficulty with bed mobility but not to the point where it would interfere with their independence. Recommendations on improving body mechanics can be made based on observations. Typically, instructing a patient to reach while log rolling onto one side and swinging the legs off the bed while pushing with the upper extremities into a seated position is sufficient.

Moderate and Severe PD

The difficulty of sequential movements is compounded by rigidity and bradykinesia. Assistance may be necessary with any aspect of bed mobility. Great difficulties are reported in repositioning in bed to get comfortable. When getting into bed, patients typically lie diagonally in relation to the bed, a position that usually requires cumbersome or impossible readjustment. Thus, therapists must instruct people with PD and their caregivers how to avoid getting into this position. The best solution is to use the bed assist rail.

In my experience, patients who are having this level of difficulty are looking for advice to improve their ability or level of independence. Caregivers have voiced their appreciation for any information that will make their caregiving less demanding. Although advice is welcomed, the thought of using a bed assist rail can be psychologically difficult for some. An alternative is to place a chair with open armrests next to the bed so that the person can pull on the armrest while swinging the legs off the bed. If this technique is successful

Case Example: Bed Mobility

Jerry has PD Hoehn and Yahr stage 3.

Subjective Evaluation

Jerry reports having increased difficulty with bed mobility. Jerry's wife reports that she helps him into bed every night: "I help him with his legs." She also states that she has to get up at night to help him sit up in bed.

Objective Evaluation

Jerry and his wife are asked to demonstrate how they maneuver at night when getting in and out of bed. When Jerry is lying down, his wife demonstrates good body mechanics when assisting with his legs. Both admit that Jerry always ends up lying diagonally. When Jerry is getting out of bed, his wife starts to pull him up by his hands but has to let him back down so that she can move his feet. She then goes back to pulling him up by grabbing his hands.

Goals

Jerry and his wife are each given a goal:

- Jerry will demonstrate understanding of proper body mechanics with bed mobility by using the bed assist rail and receiving no assistance from his wife.
- Jerry's wife will use proper body mechanics in assisting Jerry should he need it.

Therapeutic Interventions

To facilitate carryover from therapeutic interventions, Jerry needs to have a bed assist rail in place or a chair with arms. Any residual problems can then be discussed and modified.

- Jerry and his wife are educated about the need for a bed assist rail. They are told that their current method of working together to get out of bed is inefficient and places undue strain on the wife. They are given information on the bed assist rail so that they understand what to buy.
- Jerry is taught how to use the bed rail properly so that he can more easily pivot in and out of bed and reduce his tendency to lie on a diagonal. His wife is present during this training so that she can reinforce the information if needed. After Jerry demonstrates good understanding, his wife is trained in how to guide and assist him.

Outcomes

Outcomes depend on a person's cognitive status, disease severity, and adherence to recommendations. Jerry bought a bed assist rail and has been using it every time that he gets in and out of bed. He proudly reports that he can now get in and out of bed on his own. His wife states that she is now getting a good night's sleep.

at home the patient will not have to buy a bed assist rail. Some patients are more open to this method because they find it humiliating or discouraging to have a bed assist rail attached to their bed.

For someone who needs assistance with all aspects of bed mobility, the focus of therapy should be on educating the caregiver. Reviewing log rolling and practicing the use of the bed assist rail with the caregiver can result in improved ability. The following are recommended areas to review or advise as appropriate:

- Assisted log rolling
- Use of the bed assist rail supplemented by the assistance of the caregiver to help pivot the patient into or out of bed
- Use of a draw sheet
- Reducing friction between bedding and the patient, perhaps by using satin sheets or pajamas

Summary

1. Nighttime bed mobility can be difficult because of lower dopamine levels.
2. Bradykinesia, rigidity, and reduced ability with sequential movements negatively affect bed mobility.
3. A bed assist rail helps with bed mobility and reduces strain on the patient and caregiver.
4. Proper bed height can reduce the difficulty of getting in and out of bed.
5. A bed that is too high can be a safety concern.

Floor Transfers

PD is associated with increased risk of falls and injury. People with PD may not experience increased fall risk until later in disease progression, at Hoehn and Yahr stage 3, indicating bilateral involvement with some postural instability. Early postural instability is an indication of a movement disorder other than PD (Sethi, 2003). People with PD exhibit a higher rate of hip fractures compared with wrist or forearm fractures (Williams et al., 2006). Hip fractures in people with PD may result from limited trunk adaptations and reduced upper-extremity response during a loss of balance (Grimbergen et al., 2004).

A common concern for patients and their caregivers is the patient's ability to get up from the floor after a fall (Davey et al., 2004). Some patients do not have a history of falls but when asked whether they have trouble getting up from the floor may reply, "I don't know because it's been so long since I've been on the floor." Floor transfers (referring to the ability to get up from the floor) should be reviewed with anyone who is at risk for falling or looks at the floor as an alien domain. Practicing getting up and down from the floor in therapy may need to wait until the patient becomes more conditioned and flexible. But floor transfers may be an immediate priority for the patient or caregiver, in which case it should be addressed sooner rather than later. A gait belt should be used when reviewing floor transfers.

Successful Floor Transfers

The ultimate goal is fall prevention, but anyone at risk of falls should know how to get up from the floor. Various methods of performing floor transfers may need to be considered, depending on upper-extremity strength, arthritis, back problems, or other comorbidities. Active people may need to know how to get up without external support. Some people may need to use furniture (or their walker if it is stable enough) for support to get up. Others will need the support of furniture and the assistance of another person, in which case both the caregiver and the patient should be trained in floor transfers.

Consideration should be given to the easiest and most comfortable method of getting up from the floor, which may include the assistance of another person. Assessing the patient's capability to perform floor transfers or the caregiver's ability to assist can help determine whether a medical alert system is needed (see chapter 4, "Equipping Caregivers"). The patient who knows how to get up from the floor or has a medical alert system can avoid the devastating and humiliating experience of lying on the floor for hours (or days) if alone. A medical alert system provides the patient a greater sense of independence and gives comfort to both the patient and his or her family.

Patients who exhibit difficulty with mobility and their caregivers are generally appreciative of learning what to do. On occasion, after reviewing floor transfers in therapy, the patient proudly reports at the next therapy visit of being able to get up from the floor after a fall. Of course, further questioning is needed about the circumstances of the fall to prevent another from occurring. Limited knee flexion or quadriceps tightness can interfere with the ability to get up from the floor. These impairments should be addressed to optimize abilities (see ROM exercises for lower extremities in chapter 3, "Exercise and Rehabilitation Considerations," pages 32–34). The following sections demonstrate the various components of floor transfers. They are not all inclusive, but they incorporate the most common methods that I have encountered from years of practicing these procedures.

The following equipment is needed to practice floor transfers:

- Cushioned floor mat
- Chair
- Gait belt

Unassisted Floor Transfer Techniques

The ability to get up from the floor without the help of another person allows greater independence. People with PD who exercise to optimize their strength and flexibility and have mild or moderate PD can typically manage without assistance. Exceptions are those with comorbidities unrelated to PD, which may hamper mobility. This section reviews methods of getting up from the floor without the assistance of another person. Floor transfers from the all-fours position is discussed with and without the use of furniture.

- **Side lying to hands-and-knees position.** Going from side lying to the hands-and-knees position is the most common method of initiating floor transfers. People who are mildly affected by PD often demonstrate equal ability from the left and right side when going from side lying to an all-fours position. Others, who may have significant scoliosis or unilateral musculoskeletal impairments, may have greater ability to get up from one side or the other. When patients practice going from side lying to the all-fours position, they should try getting up from both sides so that they can identify the easier method. The hips and knees should remain flexed before rolling onto all fours to avoid rolling into a prone position (figure 11.1, *a* and *b*). Some patients may be fearful of getting down on the floor. Going from side lying to the all-fours position can be reviewed initially on a mat table for those who are fearful or debilitated.

- **Prone to hands and knees.** This alternative for going from side lying to the hands-and-knees position needs to be evaluated on an individual basis. This infrequently used method is the best choice for some people. Good arm strength is needed because the method mimics a modified pushup. This method may cause back irritation depending on comorbidities. In such cases alternative methods of getting up are recommended (figure 11.2, *a* and *b*).

- **Half kneeling to standing.** The patient's stronger side and least painful method can be established by practicing standing up twice from half kneeling. On one attempt, the right foot should be placed flat on the floor before standing up. The patient then tries again starting with the left foot flat on the floor (figure 11.3, *a* and *b*). This method may

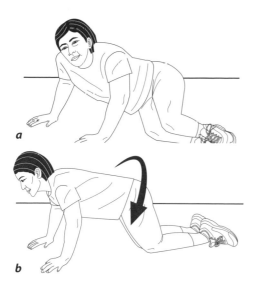

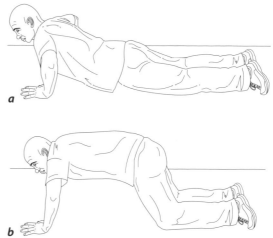

Figure 11.1 *(a)* Maintaining hip and knee flexion to *(b)* facilitate rolling into the all-fours position.

Figure 11.2 *(a)* Prone to *(b)* all fours requires good arm strength.

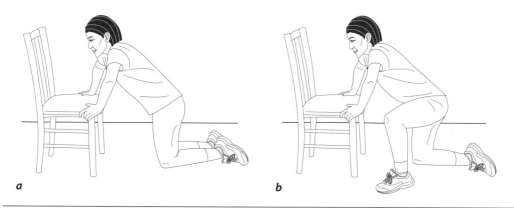

Figure 11.3 *(a)* When using furniture for support the support surface should be approximately waist high or a bit lower for better leverage; *(b)* placing the foot flat on the floor offers greater stability.

be too difficult for patients who have bilateral knee problems. When using an armchair to get up, patients often place their hands on the armrests instead of the seat of the chair. If the hands are on the armrests, the arm is in a poor mechanical position that will deter the person from getting up. Placing the foot flat on the floor rather than on the toes offers greater stability when standing up.

• **Kneeling position to standing.** This method tends to be more comfortable for people with bilateral knee problems, although limited ankle dorsiflexion and toe extension may make this difficult. The method should be assessed on an individual basis (figure 11.4, *a* and *b*).

• **Standing up without external support.** This method can be considered for people who are ambulatory without an assist device and may have an occasional mild loss of balance (figure 11.5, *a–c*).

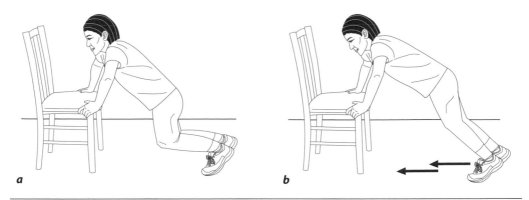

Figure 11.4 *(a)* From a kneeling position both knees are raised simultaneously to avoid placing too much pressure on one knee. Weight bearing is through the hands and toes; *(b)* after the knees are raised, the feet are walked toward the chair.

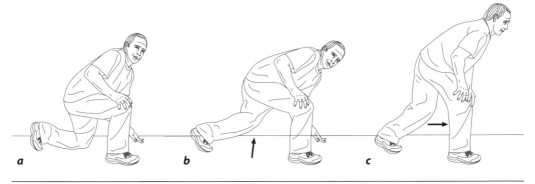

Figure 11.5 *(a)* One hand is placed on the knee for added support, and the other hand is placed on the floor for stability; (b) the back knee is raised while the person maintains upper-extremity support; (c) both hands are placed on one knee while the person brings the leg forward into a standing position.

Assisted Floor Transfer Techniques

When the caregiver helps the patient up from the floor, both must be kept safe. If this is not possible, additional help such as a medical alert system may be needed. If possible, the gait belt should be snug for better leverage. Transfers should be coordinated between the patient and caregiver to ensure simultaneous maximal effort and to minimize strain on both. The caregiver can accomplish this by giving instructions such as "On the count of three try rolling onto your hands and knees" or "On the count of three try to stand up." Because of Parkinsonian symptoms, the patient may not initiate movement at the count of three. The caregiver should be advised of this possibility so that she or he can delay giving assistance until the patient starts. Coordination of effort will avoid placing excessive strain on the caregiver. Caregivers should be encouraged to use optimal lifting body mechanics. I have found the following methods to be effective ways of getting up from the floor. Some patients may have unique restrictions that do not allow them to be supported in these areas. In such cases modifications of hand placement or gait belt placement will be necessary.

• **Assisted side lying to hands-and-knees position.** The optimal hand placement of the caregiver is to position one hand under the bottom hip and the other hand under the gait belt. The caregiver pulls up on the patient's hips as if turning a big wheel (figure 11.6, *a* and *b*). The caregiver should flex the knees to facilitate lifting with the legs rather than the back.

• **Assisted prone to hands and knees.** If the patient has strong arms, the caregiver (with proper body mechanics) can straddle the patient, grab the gait belt, and lean back while pulling up on the belt. At the same time the patient pushes with the arms (figure 11.7). As the patient walks her or his hands backward, the caregiver walks backward and guides the hips into the all-fours position.

• **Assisted half kneeling to standing.** The caregiver stands on the side of the patient that requires greater support. This positioning allows the patient to assist with his or her strongest side, which reduces difficulties in general. The caregiver places one hand on the gait belt and the other arm under the patient's axilla (figure 11.8).

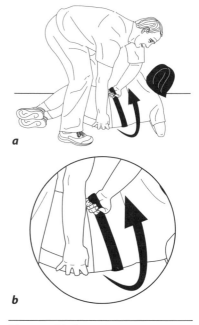

a

b

Figure 11.6 Assisted *(a)* positioning; *(b)* position of caregiver's hands.

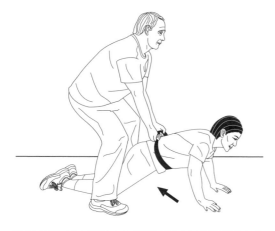

Figure 11.7 Alternative method to obtain an all-fours position.

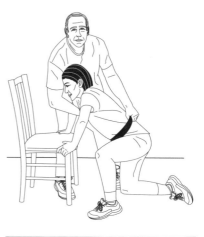

Figure 11.8 Assisted half kneeling to standing.

What to Do After a Fall

Patients often want to get up from the floor immediately after a fall. This desire may be due to the embarrassment of falling or their concern about their ability to get up. Sometimes patients do not think about the fact that after they have fallen, they cannot fall any farther

Joe has moderate PD, Hoehn and Yahr stage 3. He has a history of spinal stenosis and arthritis in the lumbar spine.

Subjective Evaluation

Joe walks with a walker but when he forgets to use it, he loses his balance and falls. He falls approximately twice a month. Joe's wife, Sue, states that she needs to help him up from the floor. She reports that doing this is difficult because of the amount of assistance that he requires. Sue works part-time, leaving Joe alone in the home 3 d a week for 4 h. Sue worries that her husband will fall when she is at work. She is the sole caregiver, and her children live too far away to help. Sue and Joe have tried using a cell phone in case of an emergency, but half the time he forgets to carry it with him. During the evaluation Joe denies having any pain. He admits to being sedentary and does not exercise. Ambulation is primarily in the home.

Objective Evaluation

Joe is generally deconditioned. Reduced flexibility is noted primarily in the lower extremities and trunk. Poor balance requires him to use the walker full time. His gait with the walker is steady. Assessment of floor transfers is deferred during the evaluation because of time constraints and Joe's deconditioned state.

Goals

The goals for Joe are the following:

- He and his caregiver will obtain a medical alert system.
- Joe will demonstrate (with or without the assistance of the caregiver) understanding of a conditioning and flexibility program to improve transfers.
- He will to be able to get up from the floor with minimal assistance.
- Joe's wife will be able to assist him using proper body mechanics to minimize strain.

Therapeutic Interventions

Joe is reluctant to lie down on the floor. The first component of the floor transfer is therefore practiced on a mat table (lying on his side and rolling onto his hands and knees). The second component (kneeling to standing) is performed on the padded floor. On the day of the evaluation Joe and Sue are educated about the benefits and logistics of medical alert systems (see chapter 4, "Equipping Caregivers," and appendix D for a patient handout about medical alert systems). They are advised about the importance of exercise and walking more to improve mobility. They are educated about using a gait belt during floor transfers and are advised to buy one.

Follow-up visits include instruction in an HEP for general strengthening and flexibility. When deemed appropriate (depending on the urgency of the patient or caregiver and conditioning) floor transfer training is initiated. First, various methods of getting up from the floor are tried. Through trial and error it is determined that Joe can get

(continued)

Case Example   *(continued)*

up with the least difficulty from his right side-lying position to all fours and is able to stand up from kneeling to full standing by bringing up his right foot. Using these optimal positions, Sue is instructed how to assist Joe in getting up from the floor. They are given patient handouts that demonstrate the optimal positions for them. They are not required to practice floor transfers but are advised to study the informational handouts. However, practicing floor transfers in therapy or at home can be used as a means of conditioning if no provocation of back symptoms occurs.

Outcomes

Joe now wears a medical alert wristband. Sue states that she is less anxious about going to work now that they have the medical alert system. With conditioning and flexibility exercises, Joe demonstrates significant improvement in his ability to get up from the floor. He now needs only minimal assistance with getting up, which Sue reports is manageable.

and should be in no hurry to get up. Bystanders occasionally offer a helping hand, but their help may cause greater destabilization or irritate an already arthritic joint. Educating the patient about how to guide bystanders will help minimize these problems. Here are some general guidelines about what to tell your patient:

1. Do not try to get up right away.
2. Before attempting to get up, mentally note whether any areas feel injured. If you suspect injury, seek medical attention.
3. Attempt to relax for a moment before getting up.
4. If you are in your "off" medication state and are not very mobile, wait until medications are working before getting up. If you are not alone, someone can make you comfortable in the meantime with a pillow or other soft item.
5. Before attempting to get up, someone should bring a chair close to you if needed so that you can use it for support to get up.
6. An additional chair could be placed behind you if you have difficulty turning. After you are standing, you can sit on the chair without having to turn.

Appendix D contains the handout "What to Do After a Fall" that you may photocopy for your patients. Items 1, 2, and 3 are applicable to all patients. Items 4, 5, and 6 are for patients with individual needs or greater mobility problems. When you give the list to a patient, cross out any items do not apply to that person.

Summary

1. Patients should be instructed in floor transfers (getting up from the floor) if they
   a. have a history of falls,
   b. are at risk of falls, or

    c. have not been on the floor in such a long time that they do not know whether they are capable of getting up.

2. Limited knee flexion or quadriceps tightness may interfere with floor transfers.

3. Caregivers should be an integral component of transfer training when appropriate.

4. Patients should understand how to instruct untrained persons to help them up if that is the only option available.

GAIT

This part of the book is dedicated exclusively to gait. The ability to walk contributes significantly to quality of life and is a critical component of cardiopulmonary, bone, musculoskeletal, and psychosocial health. The qualitative and quantitative assessment of gait is addressed. Theory, benefits, and procedural guidelines for physical interventions regarding compensatory strategies are reviewed with emphasis on improving stride length and ultimately walking endurance. Freezing of gait, when present, can be disruptive and destabilizing. Unique treatment interventions to reduce its severity and frequency as well as theories on the potential causes of freezing are reviewed. Alterations in turning ability while walking have been noted even early on in patients with PD. Turns have been cited as destabilizing and as a cause of falls, especially in people who exhibit freezing. To help the clinician improve patients' stability when turning, the dynamics of turning and ways of altering these dynamics are discussed. An ambulatory assist device or alterations of footwear may be necessary when patients' intrinsic abilities prevent them from walking safely or limit their endurance. Guidelines and considerations for various devices are reviewed. Sample documentation can be found in appendix C. For a quick overview of intervention recommendations regarding gait, see appendix D, which houses "Problem-Oriented Treatment Interventions."

12

Gait Deviations and Instability

Gait deviations in people with PD may seem similar, but on close examination you will see many variations of this stereotypical gait. Some people exhibit mild shuffling. Others present with severe freezing of gait. Forward-flexed postures can interfere with balance and result in involuntary speeding up of gait. Some people have choreatic-type movements, and others exhibit a relatively normal gait pattern. Deviations resulting from basal ganglia dysfunction can be further compounded by general deconditioning or unrelated comorbidities such as neuropathies, arthritis, or other musculoskeletal impairments.

Evaluation of gait is primarily through observation. People with PD can have many deviations; the key is to focus on deviations that present as potential fall risk hazards. In addition, dual tasking while ambulating is inherently more difficult in this population because of the increased attentional demand required during ambulation. Secondarily, dual tasking can lead to falls. Gait velocity should be assessed when attempting to optimize functional ambulation. People with PD tend to have slower gait velocities than their age-matched norms because of reduced stride length and decreased amplitude of movement (Morris et al., 1996; Sofuwa et al., 2005). Cadence tends to be preserved and does not need to be assessed unless rhythmic auditory stimulation is being considered as a treatment intervention (see chapter 13, "Compensatory Strategies for Gait Interventions").

Gait deviations that can cause instability or falls are not always observed in the clinic. People with PD may have motor fluctuations from L-dopa therapy and present with a relatively stable gait when being evaluated. A thorough subjective evaluation can help bring out gait issues that are not evident in the clinic (see "Subjective Evaluation," appendix C.)

L-dopa improves stride length, increases gait velocity, and reduces the percentage of the gait cycle in double-limb support. L-dopa does not, however, improve timing of stepping related to the arrhythmicity of gait (Blin et al., 1991). Arrhythmicity of gait can contribute to gait deviations such as freezing and festination of gait, which can lead to falls (Kemoun & Defebvre, 2001; Nieuwboer et al., 2001). After long-term use of L-dopa and worsening of disease severity, the benefits of L-dopa diminish, and dyskinesias (primarily choreatic-type movements but also dystonic movements) become more apparent, which may or may not be destabilizing or disabling. Disease progression is highly variable from one person to the next. People can have PD for 20 or 30 yr and continue to function independently.

Interventions for Gait Deviations

There is no standard Parkinsonian gait. Each patient presents a combination of common deviations. Some patients display most of these deviations, whereas others display only a few. This section describes Parkinsonian gait deviations, their clinical relevance, and suggestions for treatment interventions. One of the gait deviations, freezing, is not covered here but is discussed in detail in chapter 14. Although gait deviations or balance impairments may necessitate use of a walker, using it properly requires additional training (see appendix D, table D.3, Gait Training Strategies When Using a Walker, page 263).

Reduced Ground Clearance

Reduced ground clearance of the foot during the swing phase also involves increased forefoot loading in stance phases (Kimmeskamp & Hennig, 2001).

• **Clinical relevance.** Reduced ground clearance with increased forefoot loading in the stance phase increases the likelihood that the forefoot will catch on the walking surface. People with this gait deviation tend to trip on uneven surfaces or catch their feet on compliant surfaces such as thick carpeting. Tripping typically results in a forward loss of balance or a fall because of the forward momentum of the center of mass (COM) during ambulation.

• **Treatment.** Modifying footwear to reduce friction between the sole of the shoe and the ground can help stabilize gait to some degree by reducing the frequency or severity of catching the foot (Warshaw, 1999) (see chapter 16, "Walkers, Canes, and Footwear," page 201).

Reduced Stride Length

Reduced stride length is the most common deviation and the most treatable from a physical management standpoint.

• **Clinical relevance.** This deviation has a direct effect on gait velocity and can cause greater anterior instability.

• **Treatment.** Rhythmic auditory stimulation (RAS) is the most effective therapeutic intervention when attempting to improve gait velocity by increasing stride length (Lim et al., 2005). Attentional strategies can also be helpful with improving stride length, but they are most effective in people who are mildly affected by PD. Both RAS and attention strategies are discussed in chapter 13, "Compensatory Strategies for Gait Interventions."

Gait Variability

Gait variability is a measure of inconsistency and arrhythmicity of stepping and arm movement. The arrhythmicity of stepping can be manifested as inconsistent step length, which can be observed unilaterally or bilaterally.

• **Clinical relevance.** Gait variability is associated with freezing and increased fall risk (Hausdorff et al., 2003b). It can be related to impaired cognitive function, disease severity, or disease duration (Hausdorff et al., 2003a).

• **Treatment.** RAS has been shown to improve rhythmicity of gait.

Festination

Festination is a shuffling gait combined with involuntary speeding up of gait in a forward direction and progressive shortening of stride length.

- **Clinical relevance.** Festination is associated with imbalance and falls and is caused in part by an increased forward-flexed posture while the person is attempting to catch up with his or her center of gravity, resulting in a propulsive gait (Dewey, 2000). More severe cases are unable to stop without falling.

- **Treatment.** Treatment for this gait deviation is challenging.

  - When evaluating walkers, the ability to control the speed of the walker itself can be a balance issue. Walker recommendations depend on the person's ability to control the speed of the walker. A pickup walker may occasionally be needed for severe cases. A two-wheeled walker or a four-wheeled walker with slowdown brakes will usually be appropriate for moderate problems. See chapter 16, "Walkers, Canes, and Footwear," for detailed information about walkers.

  - A patient can often sense the initial onset of festination before it has escalated to the point of being unstable. To improve control of festination, patients should stop as often as necessary when they first perceive that they are speeding up. Some people may need to do this frequently, which can be frustrating, but stopping will help them keep this momentous instability in control.

  - Gait training with rhythmical auditory stimulation to facilitate improved stride length and rhythmicity of gait has offered improvement in gait festination for those who are mildly impaired. Some difficulties with festination control can be caused by deconditioning. Treatment interventions may include the following:

    1. In stop-and-go drills, the patient walks at her or his natural speed and then must make a sudden stop when cued. Foot position at the time of the stop is important for stability. If the feet are even and parallel at the time of stopping, the smaller anterior–posterior base of support will create greater instability. A more stable base of support results from stopping with the feet in staggered positioned, with one foot positioned ahead of the other. During stop-and-go drills, gait velocity can be increased as the patient progresses. This activity also conditions the hip extensors and paravertebral muscles to control the forward momentum of the trunk.

    2. Performing a repeated sit-to-stand exercise can further develop eccentric strength of the quadriceps when the focus is to sit down slowly. The patient stands up quickly from the chair and sits down slowly (see chapter 9, "Chair Transfers," pages 115–117).

    3. Strengthening of the calf muscles can help improve festination control (see chapter 3, "Exercise and Rehabilitation Considerations").

Narrow-Based Gait

Varying degrees of severity of this deviation can be observed. Although uncommon, severe cases demonstrate scuffing along the medial aspects of the shoes.

- **Clinical relevance.** A narrowed-based gait (figure 12.1a) causes lateral instability and interferes with effective lateral weight shift. This condition is resistant to both medical and physical interventions.

- **Treatment.** Because of the narrowness of the base of support, an assistive device is typically required to improve lateral stability and weight shift for ambulation. Some people do well with a cane. On the other hand, a cane can interfere with ambulation because using it requires dual tasking. Ultimately, a walker may be necessary for fall prevention.

Reduced Arm Swing and Trunk Rotation

Reduced arm swing (figure 12.1b) may be observed unilaterally (Hoehn and Yahr stage 1) or bilaterally (Hoehn and Yahr stage 2 or greater). Reduced trunk rotation may be observed in Hoehn and Yahr 1.5 or greater.

- **Clinical relevance.** Because dual tasking can be difficult for people who have PD, attempting to improve arm swing or trunk rotation may be difficult for a patient who needs to focus on improving ground clearance to minimize the potential for tripping. Walking requires increased conscious effort. Focusing on the less essential parts of gait will distract from the more critical components. Focusing on arm swing has been shown to improve stride length 18%, but focusing on the legs has been shown to improve stride length 38% to 47% (Behrman et al., 1998). This finding reinforces the need to prioritize attention strategies to the lower extremities.

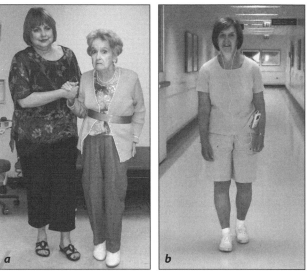

Figure 12.1 (a) Narrow-based gait requiring additional lateral support; (b) reduced bilateral arm swing. Rhythmic auditory stimulation with music focuses on lower-extremity parameters.

- **Treatment.** The only gait deviation for some patients may be reduced arm swing. They can be advised to focus on arm swing provided they are able to maintain a normal lower-extremity gait pattern. Arm swing spontaneously improves in some patients in response to rhythmic auditory stimulation without sacrificing lower-extremity movements. As with arm swing, trunk rotation should not be addressed if it interferes with lower-extremity movements.

Forward-Flexed Trunk

Flexing the trunk forward during gait may result in a forward imbalance that causes the patient to walk more on the forefoot. This posture often occurs at the hips. Less often, the forward-leaning posture occurs from the ankles (similar to a leaning tree).

- **Clinical relevance.** A forward-leaning posture that occurs from the ankles tends to be more disabling. Unfortunately, the forward-flexed posture in general tends to be resistant to physical, medicinal, or surgical interventions.

• **Treatment.** Therapy needs to address existing or potential orthopedic impairments (preventing loss of flexibility and maximizing strength of the postural muscles) and compensatory strategies (the need for an ambulatory assist device for fall prevention if needed). Patients should not be given false hopes of correcting this posture, but they should be educated about the importance of exercising to optimize spinal and hip flexibility and strength for spinal health and comfort, balance, respiratory capacity, and sleeping postures. Both the family and patient should be advised about the difficulty of treating this problem. I have observed that when patients and families focus on this problem, frustration can occur for everyone involved.

Shuffling Gait

Shuffling gait is seen after PD has progressed to bilateral involvement (Hoehn and Yahr stage 2). This kind of gait shows bilateral deviations of reduced stride length, reduced ground clearance, and diminished or no heel strike.

• **Clinical relevance.** Shuffling gait is different from festinating gait, and the terms should not be used interchangeably. Festination of gait exhibits involuntary speeding up (propulsion) of gait, which is not a characteristic of shuffling gait.

• **Treatment.** People who are mildly affected by PD may need only to resort to attention strategies to improve stride length and ground clearance. Rhythmic auditory stimulation has been shown to improve these types of deviations for Hoehn and Yahr stages 1 through 4 (Nieuwboer et al., 2007).

Examination of and Interventions for Gait Instability

Although the gait deviations mentioned in the preceding section can be a cause of imbalance, further assessment of gait stability is necessary. The person's ability to recover or maintain balance in response to additional imposed mental and physical demands is the focus of this section. Although imbalance caused by turning while ambulating is an aspect of gait instability that needs to be addressed, it will be reviewed in chapter 15, not here.

Dual Tasking

People with basal ganglia dysfunction require greater concentrated effort to perform automatic movements such as walking. Their concentration can be at a level similar to that required when learning how to perform a new task such as tying a shoe or typing. Every submovement demands greater concentration. Performing two activities effectively at the same time (dual tasking) becomes more difficult when the activities are demanding. The amount of concentration required for walking varies, but this is an area of concern because the potential changes in gait can cause imbalance.

The ability to dual task can be further hampered by impaired cognition, depression, and instability (Rochester et al., 2004). When dual tasking, people with PD place lower priority on gait stability compared with healthy age-matched controls (Bloem et al., 2006). Lower priority given to balance can lead to loss of balance or falls.

How much is the patient concentrating on gait outside the clinic? During evaluation of a person's gait, a family member often remarks, "He never walks that well at home." Typically, patients concentrate more on gait when they know that they are being evaluated. An easy way to expose gait deviations is to ask the patient to count backward (aloud) from 50 by 3s while he or she is walking. Many patients show only subtle changes in their gait pattern, whereas others demonstrate significant deterioration. With other methods of assessing the effects of dual tasking, the level of deterioration may depend on the complexity of the motor task or the presence of cognitive impairment (Yogev et al., 2005). Common gait deviations during dual tasking are reduced stride length, increased asymmetry, and reduced gait speed (Bond & Morris, 2000; O'Shea et al., 2002).

Patients who show changes in gait should be educated about how dual-tasking activities can change the way that they walk and affect their steadiness. The greater the deterioration that occurs with dual tasking, the greater the emphasis should be on paying attention to walking and avoiding abrupt movements (rushing) because both are related to increased fall risk (Willemsen et al., 2000). Rushing does not allow a person time to focus on movements.

In one study, researchers compared the effects of dual tasking on gait in people with mild to moderate PD. The aim of the study was to establish how various attention strategies during dual-tasking conditions would affect gait. Without receiving specific instructions, the subjects initially walked hands free and then while carrying a tray with glasses. They were later asked to walk with the tray and glasses under two attention conditions. During one of the walking conditions the attention focus was on the tray with glasses. In the second condition the focus of attention was directed to the walking, not the tray. The results showed that gait deteriorated more when the focus was on the tray with glasses. When subjects focused on their feet while carrying the tray with glasses, their gait was similar to the gait that they used when walking hands free and their ability to carry the tray was not compromised (Canning, 2005).

Interventions similar to the one used in this study can improve the patient's awareness and further determine whether she or he can focus on the feet when carrying something. The patient who cannot focus on the feet and becomes unsteady when carrying items should be advised to use a walker with a basket or tray. Shoulder bags can also help keep the hands free.

In another study, researchers looked at the effectiveness of rhythmic auditory stimulation (RAS) on gait during dual tasking. Dual-tasking activities were performed with and without rhythmical cues in subjects with PD. Under dual-tasking conditions, stride length with RAS improved by 19% when compared with ambulating without RAS (Rochester et al., 2005). My observation is that patients tend to be more talkative when listening to a musical tape (RAS) and to exhibit less deterioration of gait. This type of treatment has the potential of reducing fall risk during dual tasking, but further research is needed.

A person who is unable to dual task or becomes unsteady because of cognitive impairments may require a walker for fall prevention. On the other hand, prioritizing the feet while walking when dual tasking may be all that is needed to maintain stability for the cognitively intact. Either case should be evaluated on an individual basis.

Note: When challenging the ability of a person to recover from a loss of balance, a gait belt should be used for safety.

Lateral Stability

Perturbations caused while the patient ambulates can provide information about the patient's recovery capabilities. To test lateral stability, perturbations should be performed while the patient is walking. Lateral perturbations can be performed even if a patient is using an ambulatory assist device. The effectiveness of the ambulatory assist device (typically a cane) can then be established. The therapist should use sufficient force to interfere with the patient's usual gait pattern and cause him or her to react to prevent loss of balance. Perturbations are performed to the left and right while the patient is walking with the usual ambulatory assist device, if any.

If the patient does not consistently use an ambulatory assist device, causing a perturbation when the patient is both with and without the device may offer additional information about stability that can be useful for patient education and recommendations.

For example, Joe has PD, takes L-dopa medication, and has motor fluctuations and a narrow-based gait. He uses a cane intermittently for stability. He has told his therapist, "I don't like using this cane because it makes me look old." Objectively, Joe is "on" during the exam (his mobility and dopamine levels are optimal).

Performing lateral perturbations both with and without his cane allows both Joe and the therapist to see whether he can reasonably stop using this assistive device. Without his cane and without perturbations, Joe tends to veer to the left and right. Lateral perturbations cause a loss of balance that requires assistance to prevent a fall. When using a cane, however, Joe is stable during lateral perturbations and veering is minimal. These objective findings provide a strong basis for Joe's education.

Joe needs to be educated about the need to use his cane regularly for fall prevention. Causes of lateral instability are typically multifactorial. Contributing factors should be reviewed with Joe to help him understand and self-manage problems. Common causes of lateral instability are hip abductor weakness, lack of trunk-righting ability, narrow-based gait, axial musculoskeletal impairments, and impaired postural reflexes. These potential contributors should be evaluated, and impairments should be addressed.

Anterior Stability

People who freeze, have a festinating gait, or are deconditioned tend to have greater difficulty with anterior stability. The patient is asked to walk at normal walking speed, as fast as she or he can (safely), and then is asked to walk slowly. Observe for adaptability and variations of gait patterns. Although some people have a slower gait because of basal ganglia dysfunction, others walk slowly because they had an experience of losing balance from walking briskly. A person may have caught a foot on something, resulting in inability to recover from a forward loss of balance. The patient should also be asked to walk briskly and then stop suddenly on command. Observe for anterior instability and foot positioning.

Patients often perform sudden stops with feet even and parallel, causing greater anterior instability. If the person alters foot position during a sudden stop so that one foot is ahead of the other, stability against forward momentum improves significantly. The width of the stance position may also need to be addressed because a narrow base can create additional lateral instability. Lower-extremity conditioning and stop-and-go drills can further improve stability with sudden stops.

Posterior Stability

Evaluation of posterior stability during gait activities requires the patient to walk backward. Although you may wonder who walks backward, many people do, even if only for short distances such as to back away from the refrigerator before closing the door, open any door that needs to be pulled open, back up to a chair, or back out of a closet. Any of these circumstances can present a serious fall risk for a person who exhibits retropulsion when backing up. Retropulsion is an involuntary speeding up in the backward direction, which can lead to momentous falls. Detection of retropulsion is important for fall prevention and therapeutic interventions

A perturbation in the backward direction while the patient walks forward is typically not performed to assess backward stability, because ambulation creates forward momentum. Backward stability relative to gait activities is more effectively evaluated during backward walking. While the patient walks backward, observe balance, speed control, and guardedness; note stride length and compensatory forward leaning to maintain balance.

In severe cases, the best treatment is to avoid backing up altogether. In those rare cases in which backing up cannot be avoided, the person must have the assistance of another person to keep balance in check. Approaching a chair from the side instead of backing up to it is one strategy to avoid imbalance (see chapter 9, "Chair Transfers," page 119).

The U-Step walker offers greater posterior support than other walkers and can prevent or reduce the likelihood of backward falls. Some patients may exhibit a compensatory forward-flexed posture to counteract posterior instability. Both the patient and family may need to be educated that this posture should not be discouraged because it serves to preserve balance.

People with milder deficits can benefit from backward walking drills that they repeat until they exhibit improved mechanics and balance control. From a practical standpoint, you can guide the patient how to back out of a closet and how to step back when opening a door and cue them regarding step size, leaning forward, and using additional upper-extremity support as needed. The following activities can teach patients how to keep their balance in better control:

- Retro walking while altering posture as necessary (leaning forward) to provide counterbalance and to stop themselves when they detect an imbalance.
- Retro walking stop-and-go drills with emphasis on foot position. Feet should be staggered, one behind the other, for improved base of support.
- Exaggerating stride length while walking backward.
- Increasing the base of support for static standing activities to help reduce susceptibility to a backward loss of balance (see chapter 7, "Postural Instability").

Gait Velocity

Gait velocity is a measure of gait speed, which is a function of distance covered per unit of time. Commonly used measures are meters per second or meters per minute. The ultimate goal of therapy is to ensure that the person's gait velocity is optimal in comparison with age-matched velocities for functional gait. A gait velocity above 0.8 m/s, equivalent to 1.8 mph, allows a person to walk more functionally in the community (Perry et al., 1995).

Gait Parameters Affecting Velocity

The primary gait parameters that influence functional gait speed are stride length and cadence. Gait velocity is the product of these parameters. Stride length is not a necessary measure for therapeutic interventions and is not needed to calculate improvements in gait velocity. Although improvement in gait velocity typically results from increased stride length, the critical measure for establishing functional ambulation is gait velocity. Stride length in people with PD tends to be on average just above two-thirds of age-matched norms (Morris et al., 2001). Average stride length norms are 1.46 m in men and 1.28 m in women (Perry, 1992). Because the calculation of cadence is necessary only when implementing RAS, it is discussed not here but in chapter 13, "Compensatory Strategies for Gait Interventions," page 156.

Norms

Norms have been developed for age-specific walking velocities (Bohannon, 1997; Oberg et al., 1993; Steffen et al., 2002). These studies were compared with a larger national study whose purpose was to establish normative fitness values for older people and ultimately to establish a valid and reliable senior fitness test. One of the measures evaluated was the distance walked in 6 min. This study involved over 7,000 independent-living older adults ranging in ages from 60 to 94 (Rikli & Jones, 2001). The senior fitness test study included norms for walking speed at 5 yr intervals. The other studies showed average norms by the decade (every 10 yr instead of every 5). When the 5 yr incremental values were averaged to the decade norms in the Steffen study, the results were almost identical for women's comfortable walking speed. The men's norms, however, were somewhat faster in the senior fitness test study.

The values of the 6 min walk in the senior fitness test study have been converted to velocities in meters per second, meters per minute, miles per hour, and kilometers per hour. These values can be used as a reference for goal setting (see appendix B for walking velocity norms for males and females). The Bohannon and Oberg studies included walking velocity norms of younger populations, which may be a beneficial reference if treating a younger patient.

Calculating Gait Velocity

To determine gait velocity, the patient must walk a specified distance. The interval required to do this is timed. Procedures for the 10 m walk test are reviewed, and sample calculations to help with goal setting are provided.

When measuring velocity make sure that you are measuring constant velocity. To do this, have the patient start walking and continue to walk beyond the distance timed. If you know the number of meters that your patient walks and divide by the number of seconds walked, you can refer to the chart with velocity norms to see where your patient rates in comparison (see tables B.2 and B.3 in appendix B).

Procedures for the 10 m walk test to establish gait velocity (figure 12.2) are as follows. To calculate gait velocity,

1. Mark off a 10 m (32.8 ft) distance

2. The patient should start walking 0.6 m (2 ft) or more before the marker to allow for acceleration.

3. The patient needs to continue to walk 0.6 m (2 ft) or more beyond the 10 m (32.8 ft) point to allow for deceleration.

4. Only the distance covered from one marker to the next is timed (see figure 12.2).

5. The patient's gait velocity is 10 m (32.8 ft) divided by the number of seconds needed to complete the distance.

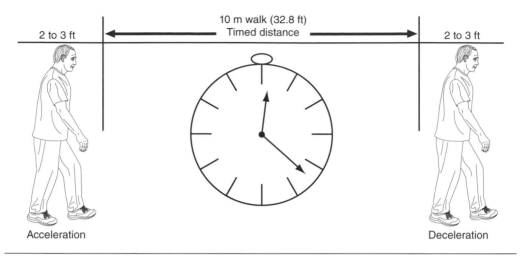

Figure 12.2 A 10 m (32.8 ft) walk to establish gait velocity. To ensure a measure of constant velocity, allowance for acceleration and deceleration is needed.

Because the standard is measured in meters per second, if you have your patient walk a distance measured in feet rather than meters, you will need to convert that distance into meters. To do so, you need to know that

$$1 \text{ ft} = 0.3048 \text{ m}$$

Thus, you simply multiply the number of feet by 0.3048 to convert to the number of meters. For example, suppose that you had your patient walk 50 ft and she did so in 20 s. Now you want to know how fast she walked in meters per second. You multiply the number of feet (50) by the fraction of a meter (0.3048) that is in each foot:

$$50 \times 0.3048 = 15.24$$

Then you divide 15.24 (the number of meters that your patient walked) by 20 (the number of seconds in which she walked those meters). The result is her gait velocity in meters per second:

$$15.24 \div 20 = 0.76 \text{ m/s}$$

Here are other metric-to-English equivalents that may be useful in similar conversion operations, depending on the units in which you prefer to work:

- 1 m = 39.37 in.
- 1 m = 3.2808 ft

Sample Gait Velocity Goals

Goals are targeted to optimize gait velocity for functional ambulation as well as prevention of falls.

- Increase gait velocity from 0.90 m/s to 1.08 m/s (norm for the patient's age and sex is 1.17 m/s).

Sample Problems: Determining Gait Velocity

Use the preceding information to solve the following sample problems.

Case Example: Gait Velocity #1

Lori is 68 yr old with a shuffling gait. She walked 10 m in 11 s.

1. 10 m divided by 11 s = 0.91 m/s.
2. Lori's gait velocity is 0.91 m/s.
3. The norm gait velocity for Lori's age- and sex-matched control is 1.43 m/s.
4. (0.91 m/s ÷ 1.43 m/s) × 100 = 64%
5. Lori's gait velocity is 64% of her age- and sex-matched norms.

Lori will benefit from gait training with RAS (rhythmic auditory stimulation) to help her gait deviations and gait velocity. RAS is discussed in detail in chapter 13, "Compensatory Strategies for Gait Interventions."

Case Example: Gait Velocity #2

Dan is 80 yr old. He walked 50 ft. in 20 s (acceleration and deceleration factors have been taken into consideration.) To determine gait velocity, feet per second was converted to meters per second.

- The gait velocity for Dan's age- and sex-matched norm is 1.32 m/s.
- Dan's gait velocity is 58% of his age- and sex-matched controls (0.76 ÷ 1.32 = 0.576).

Dan will benefit from lower-extremity conditioning exercises and attention strategies to improve gait velocity and stride length. Using an assist device can improve stability, confidence, and stride length, and ultimately improve gait velocity.

- Improve gait velocity from 77% to 90% of age- and sex-matched normal gait speed. (To calculate the percentage of the patient's current speed to his or her norms, divide the patient's speed by the norm speed and multiply by 100.)
- Improve the patient's ability to ambulate in the home by improving gait velocity from 0.3 m/s to 0.5 m/s with a two-wheeled walker and supervision.

Summary

1. Interventions should focus on lower-extremity gait deviations to minimize fall risk and maximize gait velocity.
2. Gait is no longer an automatic activity for people with PD. Greater mental concentration is required to optimize parameters and reduce risk of falls.
3. Patients who exhibit gait deterioration with dual tasking should be educated about how dual tasking can undermine balance, and they should be advised about how to compensate.

4. People with PD tend to have slower gait velocity than their age-matched norms, resulting primarily from reduced stride length.
5. Gait velocity norms can be used for goal setting.

chapter 13

Compensatory Strategies for Gait Interventions

Because the primary neuropathology of PD cannot be directly treated or rehabilitated, interventions are compensatory in nature. Compensatory strategies are used to maximize function when recovery is not expected. Here are two categories of compensatory strategies:

• The first type of compensatory strategy attempts to use alternate neuronal pathways to facilitate optimal movement. This goal can be accomplished through rhythmic auditory stimulation, attentional strategies, or visual cues. A systematic review examined the effectiveness of various compensatory strategies to improve gait parameters in people with PD. Rhythmical auditory cueing had the strongest evidence for improving gait parameters in this population. Improvement in stride length, which secondarily improved walking speed, was a common denominator of the RAS studies reviewed. Visual and somatosensory cues had insufficient evidence concerning their effects (Lim et al., 2005).

• The second type of compensatory strategy addresses extrinsic factors to improve stability such as ambulating with an assistive device or changing footwear (see chapter 16, "Walkers, Canes, and Footwear"). Gait parameters can also be affected by range of motion or strength impairments. Therapy interventions to address these deficits are rehabilitative in nature (see chapter 3, "Exercise and Rehabilitation Considerations").

This chapter reviews compensatory strategies that take advantage of alternate neuronal pathways to optimize movements.

Rhythmic Auditory Stimulation

Rhythmic auditory stimulation (RAS) uses rhythmical sounds to facilitate motor movement. RAS is primarily used in gait training because gait is by nature a rhythmical activity. Rhythmical sounds can be produced with a metronome or by using music with a simple structure and a strong 2/4 or 4/4 beat. Music is superior therapeutically. Walking to music results in greater improvements in rhythmicity of gait and facilitates greater motor synchronization in response to a beat than does walking to a metronome (Thaut et al., 1997).

Benefits

RAS has been shown to be effective in improving gait parameters in people with PD up to and including Hoehn and Yahr stage 4 (McIntosh et al., 1997). An underlying mechanism that can cause difficulty with gait in people with PD compared with healthy age-matched adults is the lack of rhythmicity, reduced symmetry, and impaired timing of muscle activation patterns relative to the gait cycle. The ability to normalize these impairments has been demonstrated in a study using RAS in a 3 wk walking program. Results exhibited improved rhythmicity, enhanced symmetry of gait, and normalization of EMG patterns in the lower-extremity muscles during the gait cycle (see figure 13.1; Miller et al., 1996).

Gait training with RAS offers superior gains over a walking program without cues. A study compared the effectiveness of a 3 wk walking program using RAS (instrumental music with accentuated rhythm in 2/4 or 4/4 time) to a walking program without RAS. One-third of the group did not participate in a specific walking program. They were asked only to continue their usual daily activities. The RAS group demonstrated an improvement in gait velocity by 24.1%. The walking group without RAS improved by 7.4%. Improvement in gait velocity in the RAS group was primarily attributed to improvement in stride length. The group who continued their normal activities and did not actively participate in any gait training had a 7% reduction in their gait velocity. The results of this study demonstrate additional benefits from a walking program with RAS as well as the negative effects of not actively walking on a regular basis (Thaut et al., 1996).

More modest improvements were found in another study that also examined the benefits of a 3 wk program of rhythmical stimulation. Gait velocity improved 0.05 m/s. The intensity and frequency of training in this study were lower than those of the previously mentioned study. Of significance, a reduction of freezing by 5.5% was noted among freezers (Nieuwboer et al., 2007).

When RAS is initially introduced therapeutically, the clinician may occasionally observe additional subtle changes in patients while walking. These changes may include a relatively more erect posture or spontaneous improvements in arm swing. A more obvious improvement is greater endurance or the motivation to walk more. These changes may be due to greater neuronal involvement of the reticular activating system in response to auditory stimuli (Thaut et al., 1999). The inherent function of the reticular activating system is for fight or flight reactions that stimulate postural and movement responses (Skinner et al., 2004).

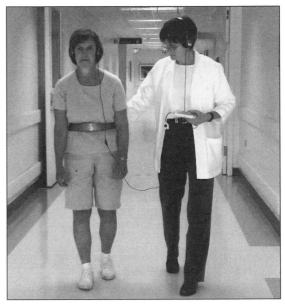

Figure 13.1 Gait training with RAS. The clinician and patient are wearing headsets connected to the same CD player. The patient is listening and walking to the beat of the music. The clinician is observing the patient's response to the music to ensure that she is walking to the beat and effectively showing improvements in gait deficiencies. The clinician may additionally cue the patient if needed to facilitate optimal gait patterns.

RAS has also been shown to deter gait deterioration while dual tasking (Rochester et al., 2005), which is important in fall prevention, but more research is necessary. Clinically, the ability to entrain to the rhythm and improve gait parameters with RAS has been observed in people with various levels of dementia. These changes typically occur with minimal cuing from the therapist.

Benefits Specific to Freezers

People who experience gait deviations such as freezing of gait (FOG) or gait festination are yet more arrhythmic, asymmetrical, and asynchronous than their counterparts who do not freeze or festinate. A lack of muscular synchronization can further weaken strength or power and secondarily impair forward progression. These deficits become even more exaggerated just before a freeze or at the onset of festination (Hausdorff et al., 2003; Nieuwboer et al., 2004a). Freezing is often described as a stutter stepping when lateral weight shift is rapid but forward progress tends to halt. Festination is an involuntary speeding up of gait with progressively smaller step lengths.

Using rhythmical sounds to improve impairments caused by a lack of rhythm or synchronization is a logical approach. The varying responses of freezers and nonfreezers to RAS should be a consideration in clinical interventions. A study of subjects with PD (Hoehn and Yahr stages ranging from 1.5 to 4) compared freezers to nonfreezers in response to different cueing frequencies. At baseline preferred walking speed under noncued conditions, the groups exhibited similar cadences. Freezers, however, demonstrated slower gait velocities because of shorter stride length. Both groups walked under five cuing frequencies relative to their baseline preferred walking cadence: –20%, –10%, baseline, +10%, and +20%. At 10% above baseline cadence, gait velocity improved in both groups, but the freezers exhibited reduced stride length. Nonfreezers demonstrated improved stride length. Freezers showed optimal gains in stride length when auditory cues were 10% below baseline cadence (Willems et al., 2006).

Another study demonstrated optimal entrainment for freezers at baseline cadence (Nieuwboer et al., 2004b). When establishing optimal walking cadences for freezers, the frequency of the rhythm needs to be adjusted to optimize both entrainment and stride length. Because stride length is generally more deficient than cadence in PD gait patterns, therapeutic interventions should focus on increasing stride length instead of cadence. An intervention that causes increased gait velocity coupled with smaller stride length can place the patient at greater risk of falls, especially one who freezes or festinates and is unable to control the forward momentum of the body coupled with an undersized step.

Immediate and Long-Term Benefits

People with PD who exhibit motor fluctuations demonstrate immediate improvement in stride length, cadence, and gait velocity with RAS in both their "on" and "off" states. Although gait velocity is slower during "off" states primarily because of reduced stride length, the relative percentages of improvements were similar in both "on" and "off" groups. Improvement in gait velocity was primarily due to improvement in stride length. See table 13.1 for changes in gait parameters (McIntosh et al., 1997).

Responses to RAS can be immediate, but for long-term carryover a gait training program with RAS is necessary. A study looked at the long-term effects of a 3 wk training program using RAS with people who have PD. The most substantial benefits lasted approximately 3 wk (McIntosh et al., 1998). See table 13.2. The results of this study can be used to educate patients about the need to initiate a daily walking program with RAS for 3 wk to improve

Table 13.1 Immediate Responses From RAS on Gait Parameters: Velocity, Cadence, and Stride Length

	Baseline	Improvements in gait parameters from baseline					
	Maximum gait velocity	Cadence	Stride length	Gait velocity	Cadence	Stride length
Controls (healthy older adults)	1.24 m/s	111 steps/min	134 cm	+14.9% 1.42 m/s	+10.8% 123 steps per min	+3.7% 139 cm
"On" PD	0.70 m/s	98 steps/min	86 cm	+36% 0.95 m/s	+10.8% 108 steps per min	+18.6% 102 cm
"Off" PD	0.56 m/s	91 steps/min	74 cm	+25% 0.70 m/s	+9.9% 100 steps per min	+18.9% 88 cm

Data from G.C. McIntosh et al., 1997, "Rhythmic auditory-motor facilitation of gait patterns in patients with Parkinson's disease," *Journal of Neurology, Neurosurgery, and Psychiatry* 62(1): 22-26.

Table 13.2 Long-Term Effects From RAS Walking Program on PD Subjects*

3 wk walking program with RAS	Pre-rehab	Post-3 wk rehab program	1 wk post-rehab	2 wk post-rehab	3 wk post-rehab	4 wk post-rehab	5 wk post-rehab
Gait velocity in m/min	56.6 m/min	64.5 m/min	61.9 m/min	63.5 m/min	62.6 m/min	58.9 m/min	56.9 m/min
Gait velocity in m/s	0.943 m/s	1.075 m/s	1.032 m/s	1.058 m/s	1.043 m/s	0.982 m/s	0.948 m/s
Percent improvement	Baseline	13.96%	9.38%	12.19%	10.60%	4.06%	0.53%

*Gait velocities rounded to the nearest .001; percentages rounded to the nearest .01%.

Data from G.C. McIntosh, C.P. Hurt, and M.H. Thaut, 1998, "Long-term training effects of rhythmic auditory stimulation on gait in patients with Parkinson's disease," *Movement Disorders* 13(2): 212.

gait parameters. Equally important, patients should be aware of its long-term limitations and establish a maintenance walking program with RAS. In general, people need to walk daily for at least 30 min to prevent deconditioning, regardless of whether the walking is done with or without RAS.

RAS-Based Gait Interventions

The treatment of gait with RAS is fun and uncomplicated. The idea with RAS is to channel the movements of the body to specific time frequencies. Better control of acceleration and velocity as well as smoother movement will result (Thaut et al., 1999). Patients may make

> ### Calculations to Determine Percentage of Gait Velocity Improvement:
>
> 1. Gait velocity after rehab minus baseline gait velocity = X
> 2. X divided by the baseline gait velocity = Y
> 3. Y multiplied by 100 = percentage improvement
>
> #### Sample calculations
>
> Looking at table 13.2, determine the percentage of gait velocity improvement immediately after a walking program with RAS.
>
> 1. 64.5 m/min minus 56.6 m/min = 7.9 m/min
> 2. 7.9 m/min divided by 56.6 m/min = 0.1396
> 3. 0.1396 multiplied by 100 = 13.96% improvement in gait velocity

stepping adjustments in their walking when listening to music to synchronize to the beat (synchronization strategies). When listening to music with a predictable rhythm, people anticipate the upcoming beats, so you may see the step precede the beat of the music. This action is fine as long as the steps are synchronized with the music.

The time difference between step duration and the duration of the rhythmic interval is period error. The occurrence of the step just before a predictable rhythm is considered the dominant rhythmic strategy. You may also see patients adjust their steps in response to the music—they hear the beat and then take a step. The time difference from the sound of the beat to the step is called phase error. When step corrections are necessary for synchronization, period errors are corrected first (making a step in anticipation of the sound). If further synchronization is necessary, a gradual correction of phase errors (stepping after the sound is heard) will occur (Thaut et al., 1999).

How does this apply clinically? Be aware that synchronization strategies exist. Patients should be allowed the time they need to synchronize to the beat before cueing because they may self-correct. If the patient is exhibiting poor synchronization, one of two things may be required: The patient may need more cueing to get started, or you may need to change the number of beats per minute of the music.

Preliminary Considerations

When gait training with RAS, a balance of intensity, safety, and the elicitation of optimal gait parameters should be considered. Because most of the PD population is older, close attention to intensity is necessary. Monitoring RPE and vital signs will guide intensity levels. Gait training with RAS is individualized, so group gait training is not feasible.

The ability of a patient to walk to the beat of the music depends on how well the beat is matched to the patient's walking rhythm or cadence. Patients can more easily lock into the rhythm of the beat if the music is appropriately matched. The ability to lock into the beat of the music is called entrainment. When the patient entrains to the beat, good synchronization between the beat of the music and the person's stepping rhythm can be observed. The methodologies of some RAS studies have resulted in less than optimal outcomes because of mismatching the rhythm to the patient. Optimally, RAS should closely match the person's natural cadence (ranging from 10% below to 10% above the patient's baseline cadence at a preferred walking velocity), which allows optimal stride length and ability to entrain to the beat. One study looked at changes in gait parameters when subjects with PD walked to rhythms 25% greater than their cadences (Suteerawattananon et al., 2004) The lack of improvement in stride length in this study was likely due to the imposed time limitations between each beat and therefore preventing an optimally sized step.

Steps to Effective RAS Gait Training

Follow these basic procedures to create an effective RAS gait training session for your patients:

1. Assess resting blood pressure and heart rate before starting initial training. The patient must be sitting for 5 min to be considered at rest. The feet should be on the floor, and the arm should be at heart level.

2. Measuring cadence is necessary to get started with RAS. Cadence is the number of steps taken per unit of time, typically measured in steps per minute. Count the number of steps in 30 s and multiply by two to find steps per minute (see figure 13.2 and "Calculating Cadence"). Closely match the rhythm of the music (beats per minute) to the patient's cadence (steps per minute) to produce optimal improvement in gait parameters. The rhythm may need to be adjusted up or down for optimal rhythmical entrainment or reduced to allow time for a longer step. Assessing cadence is usually straightforward, but a handheld metronome may be necessary to assess the cadence of people whose gait is variable, arrhythmical, and asymmetrical. While the patient is walking, adjust the beats per minute (BPM) on the metronome until you find optimal entrainment. Set the metronome or select music that closely matches the person's cadence.

3. Before having the patient ambulate to the music, it may be helpful to advise the patient about the parameters to work on while walking to the beat. After the patient is walking, additional cues can help with entrainment: "Step, step, step . . . or left, right, left." If the patient has difficulty improving stride length, the beats per minute can be reduced by five to allow time to take a longer step.

4. To establish baseline endurance with ambulation, monitor either ambulation distance or time while gait training. This can be a starting point for a home walking program with RAS.

5. When the patient becomes proficient with her or his baseline BPM or simply becomes more conditioned, cadence can be increased by 5 to 10 BPM (only if needed) depending on entrainment and ability to maintain optimal stride length. Some patients who already exhibit normal cadence may not need to increase their beats per minute but need to focus

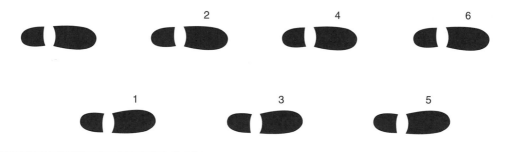

Figure 13.2 To establish cadence (steps per minute), count each step of uninterrupted walking.

> ### Calculating Cadence
>
> Cadence = steps per minute. To calculate cadence:
>
> 1. The patient walks at her or his comfortable pace for 30 s while you count the steps.
> 2. Multiply the number of steps taken in 30 s by 2 to find steps per minute.
>
> Sample problem: Donna took 50 steps in 30 s; 50 steps × 2 = 100 steps per minute.
>
> Cadence norms are 117 steps per minute for women and 111 steps per minute for men (Perry, 1992).

on improving other gait deviations in response to the music. Patients who freeze optimally entrain at baseline cadence (Nieuwboer et al., 2004b); however, individual responses should be your guide.

6. When you have observed good entrainment and optimal stride length to the beat, turn off the metronome or music and have the patient replicate what he or she was doing with the metronome or music. Advise the patient to think about the beat while walking. This approach is called fading because you fade away the auditory cue for carryover.

7. Reassess blood pressure and heart rate. Obtain rate of perceived exertion because various cardiac and blood pressure medications may blunt blood pressure and heart rate responses. When in doubt about your patient's vitals, call your patient's cardiologist or internist.

8. Set up a home RAS program based on responses in therapy.

Optimizing RAS Interventions

M.H. Thaut (2005) offers the following tips for ensuring that your patients receive the best results possible from your RAS gait training efforts.

- Focus on increasing stride length and ground clearance.
- You may observe spontaneous improvement in heel strike with increased stride length. To improve heel strike further, offer additional cues such as "step with your heel down first, to the beat."
- Stop-and-go exercises improve control with starting or stopping during ambulation. Have the patient stop every time you turn off the metronome or music without warning. Similarly, the patient starts walking when you turn the metronome or music back on. The patient should practice stopping with one foot ahead of the other for stability. When starting, the patient may need to emphasize lateral weight shift to allow off loading of the initial step leg.
- Turning: Have the patient practice pacing back and forth, varying the turns from wide to narrow and left to right. The patient should also practice turns in open environments and restricted areas. Encourage your patient to perform turns to the beat.
- Thresholds: The patient can walk through doorways while keeping to the beat of the music.

> ### Posture and RAS
>
> Posture tends to be resistant to all forms of therapy. Attempts to optimize it are frustrating to both the patient and the clinician. Worsening of posture can be multifactorial, including progression of PD, osteoporosis, arthritis, or just being deconditioned. Any improvement in a patient's posture seems to be related to the improvement of general physical fitness.
>
> Because of the energizing component of RAS, some spontaneous improvement in posture may be noted. Improvement in posture is relative, and even minimal improvement is positive. Occasional gentle reminders for postural corrections can be helpful. Unrealistic expectations, however, can harm the patient psychologically. Therapy should emphasize the more treatable components of gait.

- Progress the walking CD to higher BPM (typically by 5 BPM at a time) to improve cadence if deficient. Cadence should not be increased at the sacrifice of stride length. Typically, stride length and ground clearance will be the focus.

- Arm swing and trunk rotation: These parameters are not as critical as gait deviations, which carry a higher fall risk.

- Some people with PD Hoehn and Yahr stage 1 may have only unilateral upper-extremity involvement. People in this category can work on arm swing without sacrificing lower-extremity gait parameters.

- Some patients with PD Hoehn and Yahr stage 1 may show a drag-to type of gait in which one foot lags behind or has a consistently shorter stride length than the other. Focus should be on stepping to the music with the deficient leg. Asymmetry may continue even as the disease progresses to bilateral involvement. Typically, the initial side of involvement continues to be deficient in comparison. You may need to focus on the more deficient leg as in stage 1, but this condition depends on the individual.

Equipment Needs

Here is what you need to get started with an RAS gait intervention program:

- **Music**. Walking CDs with specific beats per minute are needed (beats per minute can be used interchangeably with steps per minute). Music needs to have a simple composition with a strong, easily identifiable 2/4 or 4/4 beat. A selection of music at increments of 5 BPM (or steps per minute) is required to match or adjust to motor responses. Commonly used frequencies are the following: 90 BPM, 95 BPM, 100 BPM, 105 BPM, 110 BPM, 115 BPM, and 120 BPM. On rare occasions frequencies below 90 BPM may be needed, typically because of various comorbidities.

- **Technical equipment**. The necessary equipment items are
  - a portable CD player;
  - two headsets and a dual headphone adaptor, or splitter, so that both the patient and the therapist can listen to the music to confirm appropriate synchronization of the steps to the beat of the music; and
  - a portable metronome (figure 13.3).

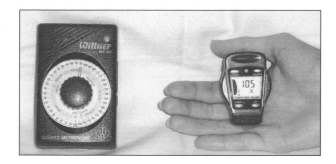

Figure 13.3 Metronomes. The smaller metronome frees up the clinician's hands because it can be clipped to the patient. This unit has greater customization capabilities, such as volume and modifications of the accent beat. Accentuating every second or fourth beat can facilitate movements targeted for one limb.

Resources for BPM-Calibrated Music

Finding music that has a particular number of beats per minute can be time consuming. The following resources can save you significant time and energy.

- The Center for Biomedical Research in Music (CBRM) offers a set of walking CDs at increments of 5 BPM to facilitate treatment of patients at various levels of involvement. These CDs have been composed to optimize therapeutic results by accentuating the beat and minimizing instrumental distractions. Visit www.colostate.edu/depts/cbrm to obtain the CDs.

- Patients who show mild gait deviations and have a walking cadence of 108 or greater can try commercial CDs at www.workoutmusicvideo.com. Before recommending commercial music, however, the clinician should acquire some commercial CDs for clinic use to see whether the patient is able to entrain to music with more distractions and less-pronounced rhythms.

- Those who can follow more complex musical compositions can download music that they enjoy, but they need to know which songs are available at their BPM. The Web site www.BPMlist.com sells a catalogue that offers a variety of songs categorized by BPM. This catalogue can serve as a reference in the clinic. The therapist can make a CD with songs at various BPMs to use in the clinic to test the capability of the patient to entrain to these more complex compositions. The therapist can then make recommendations based on responses.

Guidelines for a Home Walking Program With RAS

As the literature has indicated, 3 wk of RAS improves gait parameters in people with PD and has good carryover for 3 wk. Emphasize to patients that the carryover is limited to 3 wk and that they should periodically reinstitute the walking program with RAS when they experience any decline in their initial gains.

When the appropriate physiological responses to walking with RAS has been confirmed by monitoring blood pressure, heart rate, and rate of perceived exertion, the patient can begin the home program with RAS. The primary goal of RAS is to improve stride length and secondarily gait velocity for functional ambulation but also to reduce other gait deviations. The ultimate goal is to enable the patient to walk 30 min a day to prevent deconditioning and maintain fitness and independence (*Physical activity and health: A report of the surgeon general*, 1996; Coleman, 1999; Sabate et al., 1996). Most patients do not have that kind of endurance, but they can work up to it. The following guidelines will help patients follow a daily walking regimen.

- Start by having the patient walk the same distance that she or he could in therapy.
- If the patient is deconditioned and can perform only 5 min of ambulation, then he or she should walk 5 min two to three times a day and gradually increase the time to build up endurance. From there, the patient can walk 15 min two times a day. The goal is 30 minutes a day, whether it is 5 min × 6, 10 min × 3, or 30 min at one time.
- Issue a walking CD or advise the patient where to buy appropriate music (see "Resources for BPM-Calibrated Music").
- Patients need to have their own portable music player and headset.
- In writing, advise the patient how often and how long to walk initially and how to progress. Establish these guidelines by observing walking endurance in the clinic.
- Part of the walking program involves walking without the music but thinking about the beat. For example, a patient can walk for 20 min with the music and then walk the last 10 min without the music but keeping the same rhythm by thinking about the music.
- People who freeze can practice walking to the music in their homes while going through doorways, turning, and maneuvering in close quarters.

Attention Strategies

What are attention strategies? The basal ganglia are responsible for automatic and sequential movements. When the automaticity of walking is lost, patients need to convert to manual mode by increasing their concentration on walking. Deficient gait parameters can improve if the patient pays attention to walking. The opposite also holds true. If the patient diverts attention from walking such as by dual tasking, gait deviations may worsen (see chapter 12, "Gait Deviations and Instability"). Secondarily, dual tasking can increase the risk of falls in people with movement disorders. Attention strategies involve self-cuing with various phrases to improve gait parameters or redirecting attention to lower-extremity movements when dual tasking.

Benefits and Limitations

The benefits of this compensatory strategy depend on the capability of the patient to stay focused on walking. Cognitive impairments limit the effectiveness of this strategy.

The effectiveness of attention strategies has been demonstrated in subjects with mild PD during their "on" state by Lehman et al. (2005). The focus was to take long steps. Subjects underwent initial training for 10 d during which time they were instructed to take long steps at the onset of session. They were cued again after every two steps. The total distance walked during daily training sessions was 1,800 ft (550 m). Improved gait parameters were noted for as long as 4 wk. Another study looked at the effects of focusing on arm swing versus concentrating on taking larger steps. Step length improved by 18% when the attention focus was to swing the arms deliberately. But if participants were instructed to focus on large steps, step length improvement ranged from 38% to 47% (Behrman et al., 1998).

Patients often voice concerns about improving arm swing during gait. Patients should be advised of the importance of focusing on their feet to optimize stride length and prevent falls. Attention strategies are more effective and more practical than visual cues for gait.

Interventions

When using attention strategies to improve gait deviations we need to be selective about which deviation receives the most attention. Focus should be on the feet to minimize fall risk. My experience is that paying attention to one deviation is much easier (and more effective) than dividing attention among many deviations. Patients agree that working on only one gait deviation is optimal. Walking can be mentally draining when a patient has to focus on taking each step. By mentally repeating a phrase instead of focusing specifically on each step, patients seem to have less difficulty maintaining improved parameters. By focusing on one deviation (by using attentional phrases), an additional deviation may secondarily improve. For example, using the attentional phrase "take long steps" can simultaneously improve stride length and heel strike.

Here is an effective treatment protocol for attention strategies for people with mild PD:

- While the patient is walking, select a phrase or attention strategy to test its effectiveness (see the following options).
- You may initially repeat the phrase aloud to get the patient started and then say it intermittently as needed.
- Encourage the patient to think repeatedly of the phrase while walking. Repeating the phrase mentally helps establish a rhythm while walking.
- Continue to test various phrases or attention strategies using the preceding procedure.
- Select the phrase or attention strategy that produces optimal results and advise the patient to use that option when walking.
- Recommend a walking program that uses the optimal attention strategy.

The following options can be reviewed with patients. This information can also be issued as a handout to promote practice and review (see appendix D for a patient handout about gait attention strategies).

Option #1. Count the number of steps it takes to reach a destination. For example, if you are walking from the kitchen to the living room, count the number of steps it takes to travel that distance. For longer distances, count to a certain number, say 30. When you hit 30 start over with 1 and repeat.

- If only one foot is giving you a problem, then count only the steps you take with that foot. For example, let's say that your left foot is the uncooperative foot:
- The left foot takes a step, and you count "1." The right foot takes a step, and you don't count. The left foot takes a step, and you count "2." The right foot takes a step, and you don't count. Continue counting in this way.

- If both feet are giving you a problem, then count every time you take a step. For example, the left foot takes a step, and you count "1." The right foot takes a step, and you count "2." The left foot takes a step, and you count "3," and so on.

Option #2. Take long steps. Attempt to establish a rhythm while walking by repeatedly thinking "take long steps."

Option #3. Place your heel down first. Using the phrase "heel down first" may help you improve stride length.

Option #4. Attempt to shift your weight more to the left and right as you walk, like a penguin. This option is not applicable to most but may be helpful for someone who exhibits significant freezing.

Patients may sometimes say that they cannot walk as well when they are tired. Maintaining attention is more difficult when tired, and lack of automaticity in gait becomes more apparent. At times, the deterioration of gait when tired can be alarming to patients because they associate it with disease progression. Depending on the symptomology, this may or may not be the case. We can, however, help them put their minds at ease by explaining the connection of mental fatigue with increased difficulty during ambulation.

Case Example: Gait Training for Reduced Stride Length

John is 66 yr old. He has PD Hoehn and Yahr stage 2 and is generally healthy.

Subjective Evaluation

John reports that he enjoys walking but believes that his steps are becoming shorter even though he walks 2 mi (3 km) daily. Walking seems more difficult in the evenings.

Objective Evaluation

John demonstrates good strength and flexibility overall. His balance is good. John completed the 10 m walk in 11 s, so his gait velocity is 0.90 m/s (10 divided by 11 = 0.90). According to the table in appendix B, Male Walking Velocity Norms by Age, the normal gait velocity for men between the ages of 65 and 69 is 1.59 m/s. The following calculation is performed to establish how John's gait velocity compares with healthy age- and sex-matched norms:

$$0.90 \text{ m/s} \div 1.59 \text{ m/s} \times 100 = 56\%$$

John's gait velocity is 56% of his age- and sex-matched norms.

Goal

The single goal established for John is to improve gait velocity from 0.90 m/s to 1.05 m/s to optimize functional ambulation.

Therapeutic Interventions

Through patient education and gait training interventions, John will have a better understanding of his symptoms and how to improve and maintain his abilities.

(continued)

Case Example   *(continued)*

John is taught that walking is not as automatic as it was now that he has PD. With PD, he must devote greater attention to walking. Therefore, if he becomes tired his walking may not be as good. He is advised to continue his daily walks to prevent deconditioning and optimize his ability. John is informed of the efficacy of attention strategies and RAS.

Various gait interventions are instituted. Attention strategies are tested. "Take long steps" offers the greatest improvement in stride length compared with the other attentional strategies tried, and therefore it is recommended. John's cadence is calculated at 105 steps per minute. Resting vital signs are taken. John is advised to walk to the beat of music, focusing on taking longer steps. He is informed that if he has difficulty keeping time with the music (too fast or too slow), the therapist is responsible for changing the music so that it matches him, not the other way around. As John walks to the music he finds that it is too slow. The BPM is increased from 105 to 110. John then demonstrates good entrainment with improved stride length. John's vitals are taken after walking 0.25 mi (0.4 km) with RAS. Normal cardiovascular responses are noted. RPE was "somewhat hard" or "moderate." John is advised of the long-term benefits of RAS and the need for tune-ups when benefits wane. A sample of commercial music is tested for John's ability to entrain. He does well and is given information on commercial music within his BPM range.

Outcomes

After walking 3 wk on a regular basis, improved stride length and secondarily improved velocity can be expected. John's gait velocity was reassessed with the 10 m walk, which demonstrated that he met his goal.

Visual Cues

The goal of using visual cues is to capitalize on alternate neuronal pathways to facilitate improvements in motor responses. Visual cueing is any marking on the floor that the patient can see and step over safely. Studies have shown that visual cues improve stride length and gait velocity (Azulay et al., 1999; Suteerawattananon et al., 2004). These studies have demonstrated the efficacy of increasing stride length by placing a series of parallel lines at equal distance on the floor and having the patient step over the lines. This method may be helpful for household ambulators but would not be practical for community ambulators. The benefits of visual cues are primarily seen when used for freezing, especially start hesitation (when the patient has difficulty initiating the first step) (Kemoun & Defebvre, 2001). Visual cues are more effective than auditory cues during gait initiation. Visual cues improve timing and the magnitude of weight shifting before a person takes the first step (Jiang & Norman, 2006).

A few walkers and canes on the market have lasers. These devices display a laser line on the floor for the patient to step over. Visual cueing ambulatory assist devices have reportedly been ineffective for "on" freezing (Kompoliti et al., 2000). Because the benefits of laser ambulatory assist devices vary by individual, evaluating the effects may aid in making appropriate recommendations. Educating patients about when specific compensatory strategies are most effective can help them self-manage issues as they arise and reduce their anxiety when compensatory strategies are not effective. This guidance will also help patients be educated consumers as new devices enter the market. Patients should be advised to use visual cues primarily for difficulties with start hesitation and for "off" freezing. See chapter 14, "Freezing," for information about the use of visual cues and treatment strategies.

Summary

1. The three types of neurologically based compensatory strategies are rhythmical auditory stimulation (RAS), attention strategies, and visual cues.
2. RAS is the most effective treatment for improving stride length and secondarily improving gait velocity and symmetry and reducing gait variability.
3. RAS is effective in treating people with PD from Hoehn and Yahr stages 1 through 4.
4. Cadence (steps per minute) tends to be more preserved in people with PD than are other gait parameters, but nonetheless cadence needs to be assessed for the implementation of therapeutic intervention with RAS.
5. Therapists need to monitor heart rate, blood pressure responses, and RPE when gait training with RAS.
6. Attention strategies are helpful in modifying gait parameters in people who have mild PD. The focus should be on lower-extremity deviations.
7. Visual cues are most beneficial for start hesitation in freezing.

14

Freezing

*F*reezing is a term commonly used with people who have PD to describe the inability to take steps while walking or when attempting to start walking. Freezing gives the appearance that the feet are glued to the floor. It occurs suddenly and lasts for brief periods, typically less than 10 s, but it can last as long as a minute (Schaafsma et al., 2003). After the freezing episode passes, the patient can resume ambulation until the next episode occurs.

During freezing, lateral weight shifting is rapid and insufficient in magnitude. This circumstance gives the appearance of stuttering feet and interferes with the ability to unload one foot long enough to take a step. Freezing of gait can result in gait instability or falls, especially when coupled with a loss of postural reflexes or a festinating gait (Michalowska et al., 2005). Freezing may occur more frequently with longer periods of disruption as PD progresses. The incidence of freezing in people with mild PD is approximately 7% (Giladi et al., 2001). As PD progresses the incidence of freezing increases to approximately 50%.

Freezing is not exclusive to PD. The incidence of freezing in other movement disorders is 57% in vascular Parkinsonism; 56% in normal pressure hydrocephalus; and 45% in progressive supranuclear palsy, multiple system atrophy, and corticobasal ganglionic degeneration (Giladi et al., 1997). Freezing can be extremely frustrating to patients and disruptive to their functional gait. Unfortunately, medical management such as medications or deep brain stimulation (DBS) is not effective in treating "on" freezing (Davis et al., 2005). Although freezing can affect speech and upper-extremity movements, freezing is discussed here only in its relationship to gait.

General Issues in Freezing

Before we address the evaluation of and interventions for freezing, you should become familiar with terminology, precipitating factors, and theories about why freezing occurs.

Terminology Related to Freezing of Gait

Terminology related to freezing can be confusing because of the use of different words for the same phenomenon. Freezing has been described by various researchers as motor blocks (Giladi et al., 1992), akinesia, or gait ignition failure. The following terms are directly or indirectly related to freezing.

Akinesia is the inability to initiate movement because of severe bradykinesia (slowness of movement and difficulty initiating movement) and hypokinesia (decreased amplitude of movement and progressive lessening of amplitude with each movement) (Fahn, 1995). Akinesia is likely to be associated with the assumption of fixed postures and can last from seconds to hours. Because no strong evidence associates bradykinesia or rigidity with freezing, the terms *akinesia* and *freezing* should not be used interchangeably (Fahn, 1995; Giladi et al., 2001; Hausdorff et al., 2003).

A person who is akinetic can appear to be not even attempting to move, which can be frustrating to the patient and observers. The therapist needs to be sensitive to reports of akinetic states from their patients. Educating the patient and family members can increase awareness of its characteristics and improve understanding. Advice on strategies to reduce time stuck in an akinetic state can reduce frustrations. These strategies are similar to the ones used to improve the control of freezing but are not necessarily as effective. Fixed postures can occur in any position or in transition from one position to another.

In my experience, prolonged akinetic states have not commonly occurred in the clinic, but patients have reported being stuck in one position from 2 to 3 h in their homes. In one case, a person with PD was attempting to get up from the floor and was unable to move from the all-fours position for 3 h. Another patient with PD was stuck in the standing position for 2 h in his bathroom. His feet were not stuttering as would be seen in freezing; they appeared to be bolted to the floor. When akinetic states occur in the clinic, tactile or visual cues (stepping over a pen for gait initiation) or assisted weight shift can facilitate movement.

Freezing is the inability to take steps while walking or when attempting to start walking. Attempted movement is visible (stutter stepping) but nonproductive. *Freezing of gait (FOG)* is the term most commonly seen in literature. The term only specifies when freezing occurs (any time during gait) and does not say anything about what triggers freezing or when freezing occurs during gait.

"Off" freezing is responsive to dopaminergic medications. "Off" freezing occurs when the dopamine levels in the brain are low. This circumstance may occur in a person with PD who has not yet started taking dopaminergic medications or in a person who is taking L-dopa but for some reason has suboptimal dopamine levels. For those who take L-dopa, low dopamine levels may occur in several situations:

- Before taking the first dose of the day because typically L-dopa is not taken at night
- When the benefits of medications wear off prematurely before the next dose
- If the patient forgets to take the medication
- When the progression of PD increases the difficulty of normalizing dopamine levels with medications, causing "off" states to occur more erratically

"On" freezing occurs when dopamine is at the optimal level with dopaminergic medications. The patient is considered "on" when the ability to move improves in response to medications. The cause of "on" freezing is not fully understood because "on" freezing is not responsive to L-dopa (Kompoliti et al., 2000).

Start hesitation is freezing that occurs when a person attempts to initiate the first step to start walking. This hesitation to start walking often happens when a person first gets out of a chair or starts to walk from a static standing position.

Gait ignition failure is an isolated gait disorder that is observed in vascular pseudo-Parkinsonism. The incidence of vascular pseudo-Parkinsonism is approximately 3% to 5%

of all cases of Parkinsonism (Sibon & Tison, 2004). *Gait ignition failure* is a term used for freezing in a person who does not have all the stereotypical gait patterns seen in people with PD. Other than freezing, a person with vascular Parkinsonism exhibits an upright posture with good stride length and good arm swing (Atchison et al., 1993). When describing gait deviations such as difficulties with initiating gait because of freezing, the term *start hesitation* is most commonly used.

Destination hesitation is freezing that occurs when a person with PD approaches an object or intended destination. For example, when someone wants to sit down and is approaching a chair, freezing may occur as the person comes close to the chair. Aggravating factors with destination hesitation are premature reaching for the chair, difficulty with turns, and rushing. Premature reaching may be the patient's attempt to stabilize.

Precipitating Factors of Freezing

Freezing can be triggered by various activities, environmental factors, or psychological factors. Even factors that commonly disrupt gait should be evaluated on an individual basis. In general, freezing occurs more frequently when people with PD are in their "off" state (Schaafsma et al., 2003).

Common freezing triggers are start hesitation, turning, and walking in narrow spaces (Giladi et al., 1992; Schaafsma et al., 2003). Some people have few triggers, whereas others have many. Knowing when freezing occurs will help focus therapeutic interventions. Duplicating activities that cause freezing can help the clinician further evaluate motor dysfunctions and make modifications to minimize freezing episodes. The following is a list of freezing triggers.

- Start hesitation (hesitation when initiating walking)
- Turning (worst with 360° turns) (Schaafsma et al., 2003)
- Walking through narrow spaces
- Destination hesitation (hesitating when approaching a destination)
- Thresholds
- Posture (a forward-flexed posture can create an anterior instability and secondarily trigger a freeze)
- Rushing
- Psychological factors: anxiety, stress, or attention (Fahn, 1995)

Freezing Theories

A number of studies have been done to explore why freezing occurs. Although much remains to be learned, some factors are understood, and some theories have been formulated about the etiology of various types of freezing. Here is some of what we know or can at least suggest with some confidence about start hesitation and freezing of gait.

- **Start hesitation**. Gait initiation deals with the transition of making the proper postural adjustments from static standing to initiating the first step. The difficulty with step initiation appears to be multifactorial. People with PD exhibit decreased force production of their leg muscles, which is necessary for forward propulsion and performance of a normal initial step length (Burleigh-Jacobs et al., 1997; Gantchev et al., 1996). The forward-leaning Parkinsonian posture may at times cause shortening of the initial step (Halliday et al., 1998).

> ### See For Yourself
>
> To see how lack of lateral weight shift can impair a person's ability to take a step, stand with your right side against the wall (close enough to limit lateral weight shift). Now try to start walking with your left foot first (Shumway-Cook & Woollacott, 2001).

As postural control becomes more impaired (as seen with disease progression with PD), the COM (center of mass) and the COP (center of pressure) tend to be more closely coupled (Gantchev et al., 1996; Halliday et al., 1998; Hass et al., 2005). This circumstance reduces weight-shifting forces both anteriorly–posteriorly and laterally along the horizontal axis. If weight shifting is of insufficient magnitude the patient will use a stutter type of stepping and will not be able to unload the potential swing leg long enough to take a step. Generally, people with PD also require more time to make the necessary postural adjustments before taking their first step, which is an additional contributing factor in the delay of gait initiation (Burleigh-Jacobs et al., 1997; Gantchev et al., 1996). These factors are further exacerbated when the patient is "off."

- **Freezing of gait (FOG).** Several factors have been examined in connection with FOG.
  - EMG: FOG studies have investigated the EMG activity of the anterior tibialis and gastrocnemius muscles before freezing. Patients with freezing demonstrated premature timing and reduced amplitude of both muscle groups. The freezing group showed a relative exaggeration of the anterior tibialis muscle when compared with the gastrocnemius, which was postulated to be an attempt to pull the leg forward in compensation for lack of pushoff. Ultimately, insufficient force is present for forward progression or stopping (Albani et al., 2003; Nieuwboer et al., 2004).
  - Rhythmicity: People with PD who exhibit "on" or "off" freezing are yet more arrhythmic or dysrhythmic in their gait patterns than their counterparts who do not freeze. This holds true even when they are not experiencing a freezing episode (Hausdorff et al., 2003). The disruption of the rhythmicity of gait in people with PD is even greater just before a freezing episode (Nieuwboer et al., 2001).
  - Gait asymmetry: People who freeze demonstrate greater asymmetry of gait and reduced rhythmicity from one leg to the other than do those who do not freeze (Plotnik et al., 2005).
  - Stride length: With "off" freezing a progressive loss of stride length occurs because of the inability to generate force coupled with the inability to control the rhythmicity of gait (Nieuwboer et al., 2001).

Evaluating Freezing

Generally, freezing patterns are primarily established through the patient's reports and through observation of activities in the clinic. Seventy-five percent of the people with PD who experience freezing of gait report that their worst freezing occurs in the home and the least in the neurologist's office (Nieuwboer et al., 1998). This finding only accentuates the need for a thorough subjective evaluation. A helpful tool that can lend some objectivity to freezing is the Freezing of Gait Questionnaire (see appendix A), which was developed to assess the severity of freezing of gait (FOG) unrelated to falls (Giladi et al., 2000).

Here are some general guidelines to remember when evaluating for freezing:

Subjective Evaluation

See "Subjective Evaluation," appendix C. In addition, do the following:

• **Define the term freezing**. Before asking any questions about freezing, explain the definition of freezing and demonstrate if necessary to ensure that the patient understands what is being asked. Commonly used descriptors for freezing are "feet glued to the floor" and "stutter stepping."

• **Ask if freezing occurs**. If the answer is no, you are done with the freezing part of the evaluation. If the answer is yes, you need to know the precipitating factors.

• **Ask when freezing occurs**. Sometimes the patient will be unable to remember all aggravating factors. Reviewing a list of freezing triggers with the patient can often save time. The patient can then report more easily which of the potential triggers are problematic. Here is a list of potential triggers and conditions:

- Start hesitation: when attempting to start walking
- Turning
- Walking through narrow spaces
- Destination hesitation: when reaching a destination
- Thresholds (doorways)
- Change in floor surface
- Posture (throws balance forward) or when the walker moves too far ahead of the patient
- Rushing
- When "on" (if applicable)
- When "off" (if applicable)
- Freezing of gait: freezing while walking with no other known precipitating factors; may be secondary to festination

Objective Evaluation

Observations for freezing can start when the patient gets out of the chair in the waiting room, continue during the gait evaluation, and end when the person sits back down. Note when freezing occurs. See figure 14.1 for the freezing evaluation process.

Freezing Interventions

Combinations of interrelated factors contribute to freezing episodes. First, impaired synchronous muscle activation patterns can affect force production and secondarily lateral weight shift and forward propulsion. Second, a lack of symmetry and rhythmicity of gait is more accentuated in those who freeze. So, treatment interventions should focus on facilitating force production and weight shifting, and improving rhythmicity and symmetry of gait.

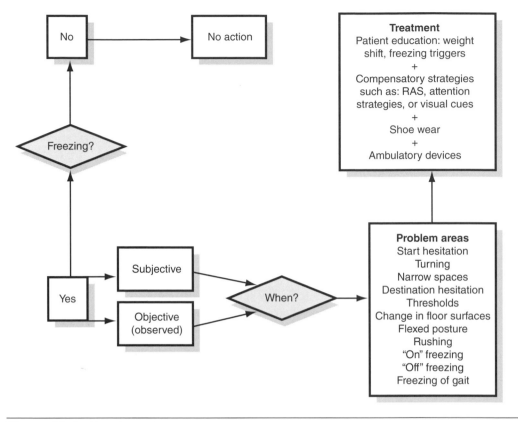

Figure 14.1 Freezing evaluation process.

Treatment strategies for freezing encompass compensatory strategies similar to those used in gait training.

Freezing compensatory strategies, which capitalize on the use of alternate neuronal networks or modification of extrinsic factors, are as follows:

- Rhythmic auditory stimulation to improve gait rhythmicity
- Attention strategies to improve lateral weight shift to unlock or prevent a freeze
- Visual cues for start hesitation
- Use of an assistive ambulatory device if needed
- Modification of footwear

Freezing that occurs from forward bent postures, rushing, or psychological factors requires interventions that focus on patient education. Patients need to be made aware of how postures or behaviors can trigger a freeze. They will then have the tools to troubleshoot and modify their behaviors accordingly.

General Interventions

A common denominator in interventions for freezing is improving lateral weight shifting either indirectly with rhythmic auditory stimulation (RAS) or more directly with additional maneuvers that have been reported by patients to be helpful.

Improving Rhythmicity and Force Production

Various studies have looked at the effects of RAS on gait for people with PD. One study noted that one patient demonstrated immediate improvement in freezing during turns with RAS but experienced no carryover (McIntosh et al., 1997). Another study found a 5.5% reduction in freezing after a 3 wk walking program with rhythmical stimulation (Nieuwboer et al., 2007).

My experience with using RAS to reduce freezing has demonstrated positive results. Patients who have been compliant with a 3 wk walking program (5 d a week) using RAS have reported a reduction in the severity and frequency of freezing. Walking to RAS has been shown to improve rhythmicity and symmetry of gait (del Olmo & Cudeiro, 2005; Thaut et al., 1999). Treatment with RAS has demonstrated improved symmetry of muscle activation of the anterior tibialis and gastrocnemius confirmed with EMGs (Thaut et al., 1999). Listening to rhythmical music also has an energizing effect on the reticular activating system (Thaut et al., 1999), which can enhance force production and secondarily improve weight shifting.

Refer to chapter 13, "Compensatory Strategies for Gait Interventions," for treatment procedures with RAS. Because people with PD who freeze have greater impairments in rhythmicity, muscle synchronization, and symmetry than their nonfreezing counterparts, those who freeze require a more regimented program for maintenance than do those who do not freeze.

Patient-Reported Strategies

Other maneuvers reported by patients have been helpful in breaking a freezing episode. Note that the effectiveness of these maneuvers varies from one person to the next. Testing each maneuver for its effectiveness can help with recommendations. From the following list, the maneuver of taking a step backward before starting to walk forward has been notably more effective than the others. In more severe cases or during "off" freezing, stepping over something offers good results. Patients can further practice the maneuvers at home to see which are most effective in breaking their freeze.

- Take a step backward before starting to walk forward.
- March in place.
- Take a step sideways before stepping forward.
- Step over an object or over someone else's foot placed perpendicular to the patient's foot.
- Imagine stepping over a line.

Interventions for Specific Issues

At times specific problems with freezing require more individual attention and may require a modification or combination of interventions to optimize outcomes (see table 14.1).

Start Hesitation

Using attention strategies to promote lateral weight shift as well as maintaining this weight shift toward the stance leg can help control freezing with start hesitation. Increasing the excursion and duration of a lateral weight shift allows more time to take a longer initial step. Encouraging lateral weight shift can be difficult if a forward-leaning posture is

Table 14.1   Freezing Interventions

Freezing triggers	Treatment suggestions	Goals
Feet catching on floor surfaces	Recommend footwear with smooth low-friction soles or resurfacing of existing shoes (see chapter 16). Avoid soles with ridges and soft rubber.	Reduce severity (duration and frequency) of freezing for fall prevention demonstrated by improvement on Freezing of Gait Questionnaire score (see appendix A). Reduce reported frequency of tripping or risk of falls caused by improper footwear.
1. Start hesitation 2. "On" freezing 3. Thresholds	Use an attention strategy to focus on accentuating and prolonging timing of lateral weight shift to optimize stride length of initial step. Attempt taking a step backward before stepping forward. Use rhythmical auditory stimulation (RAS).	
Freezing when turning	Improve foot placement and advancement (see chapter 15) and avoid rushing. Use RAS.	Improve stability or reduce loss of balance during turns.
Freezing of gait	Use rhythmic auditory stimulation during gait activities and home walking program. Use attention strategies to facilitate stride length and lateral weight shift. Use ambulatory device if needed.	Increase patient awareness of the effects of posture on freezing.
Forward-flexed posture	Educate patient on the effects of posture on freezing. Use attention strategy to optimize posture during freezing episode.	
"Off" freezing	Use visual cues, such as an object to step over or floor marking. Increase lighting.	
Rushing	Educate patient concerning the effects of rushing on freezing and allowing more time for activities. Practice gait activities without rushing.	
Freezing in narrow spaces	Practice ambulation in tight areas. Based on observations, make recommendations on foot placement and weight shifting.	

propelling the patient's balance forward. Attempting to minimize this postural deviation first and then following up with the lateral weight shift will result in a more stable and more effective initial step (see the patient handout on freezing in appendix D).

At times the patient's base of support may be so narrow that any effective lateral weight shift can be destabilizing. My experience in attempting to increase patients' natural narrow base of support has demonstrated that they are resistant to any carryover. These people may need to rely on an ambulatory assist device to widen their base of support and allow an effective lateral weight shift to unload the stepping limb without jeopardizing stability. Visual cues have been shown to facilitate greater force production and lateral weight shift than immediate responses to auditory cues for gait initiation (Jiang & Norman, 2006). A practical use of laser ambulatory devices is to facilitate the initiation of gait. As previously mentioned, Nieuwboer and colleagues (2007) noted improvements of freezing after 3 wk exposure to RAS. My observation is that freezing is more resistant than stride length to achieving long-term improvements from RAS (see chapter 13, "Compensatory Strategies for Gait Intervention"). Optimal improvements in stride length can be appreciated for approximately 3 wk after an RAS program (McIntosh et al., 1998). Depending on freezing severity, I have observed that long-term improvements of freezing persist for about 1 wk, thus indicating the need for long-term exposure to an RAS program.

Turning

Frequently, freezing during turns is aggravated by rushing or improper foot placement. While turning, the outside foot, which has to cover the greatest distance in the turn, lags behind. For example, when making a left turn the right foot (the foot on the outside of the circle) needs to take a bigger step than the inside foot, but it does not. As the turn proceeds, the outside foot lags further behind, resulting in instability and freezing. See chapter 15 for turning strategies.

Negotiating Doorways, Thresholds, or Floor Surface Changes

Doorways, thresholds, or simply a change in floor surface can cause freezing. If the patient perceives thresholds or floor surfaces as a balance threat, the increased anxiety can trigger a freeze. Repeated exposure to such triggers using compensatory strategies can improve confidence or self-management (figure 14.2).

Compensatory strategies may include rhythmic auditory stimulation or attention strategies to emphasize a lateral and prolonged weight shift. Taking a step back before proceeding forward is often effective. Severe freezers may benefit from visualization to accentuate lateral weight shifting by thinking of word phrases such as "walking like a duck," "like a penguin," or "waddling." Patients may respond differently to various phrases. A trial of walking to the various phrases may be necessary to establish optimal lateral weight shift responses. Some patients with dementia can identify with word phrases. When walking through thresholds while using RAS, minimization of verbal cues can allow the patient to hook into (entrain) the beat more spontaneously (see chapter 13, "Compensatory Strategies for Gait Interventions").

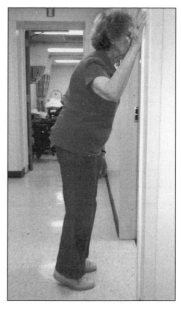

"On" Versus "Off" Freezing

Generally, "off" freezing tends to be responsive to visual cues. Patients often complain of problems with freezing when first getting out of bed and attempting their first step. Placing an object on the floor parallel to the bed such as a sock that has a contrasting color to the floor has reportedly been helpful (see chapter 4, "Equipping Caregivers," figure 4.3). The patient steps over the sock to break the freeze. Some patients may need the initial visual object for only a few days. After it is removed, they can imagine stepping over the object.

Figure 14.2 Reaching for the doorframe is a typical balance strategy when freezing in a doorway. The feet are incapable of assisting in balance recovery during a freeze.

Forward Bent Posture

Patients should attempt to correct their posture only if it is causing an imbalance or freeze. A forward-flexed posture is resistant to any form of medical or physical intervention and is difficult to correct for any length of time. Patients should be made aware of how their posture can affect freezing as well as therapeutic limitations concerning improving postural deviations. If able, the patient should stand as erect as possible before lateral weight shifting to attempt to regain control over a freezing episode. Ambulatory assistive devices may or may not be beneficial for freezing that is exacerbated with forward-flexed postures. Their use should be evaluated on an individual basis.

Rushing

For some patients rushing is the main freezing trigger. Rushing is one of the most difficult freezing triggers to treat because it seems to be more of a personality trait or lifelong habit. When such people freeze, they want to rush out of their freeze, which is yet more destabilizing. Rushing also increases fall risk because movements are quick and the ability to respond effectively is hampered.

People who freeze primarily from rushing can eliminate many of their freezing episodes if they slow down. This outcome can be observed in the clinic. As the patient walks at a more normal cadence and avoids rushing, freezing episodes melt away. But during the next therapy visit, the person may report no changes in freezing at home. Continued patient education is often necessary to reinforce the fact that rushing aggravates freezing and increases the risk of falls. Unless the behavior of rushing is modified, freezing will continue to occur. Patients can be advised that by not rushing they can get from point A to point B quicker because freezing will be reduced.

Anxiety

Freezing that occurs from anxiety is often associated with fear of falling. Patients who freeze often report feeling anxious in crowded areas because of the possibility of being bumped off balance or because they do not want to slow down other people. Patients can become more anxious if they *feel* rushed (not actually rushing, as noted above). For example, a person can be walking fine but start freezing after discovering that someone is walking behind her or him. Patients often state, "I don't want to slow anyone down." Patients often compensate and simply stop walking until the person behind them has passed.

A family member may need to be taught how to assist a patient with prolonged lateral weight shifting. To enhance feelings of security and stability, the patient should lean in the direction of the assisting person. In some patients, using an ambulatory assist device can enhance feelings of stability and profoundly improve freezing episodes. For general anxiety, antianxiety drugs can be considered. But these should be discussed only as a last resort if anxiety is interfering with mobility because this class of drugs (benzodiazepines, discussed in chapter 8) can also increase fall risk. The risk–benefit ratio, of course, is the key to the decision.

Equipment-Related Interventions

Various types of canes, walking sticks, and walkers may help or hinder, depending on how they are used.

• **Canes and walking sticks**. Ambulatory assist devices such as an inverted cane or a laser cane are not effective for most "on" freezing. Such ambulatory assist devices often fail to help control freezing episodes (Kompoliti et al., 2000). The inverted walking stick has been found to worsen freezing (Dietz et al., 1990), and in my opinion it is a safety hazard

Lee has PD Hoehn and Yahr stage 3 and is cognitively intact.

Subjective Evaluation

Lee reports that she has fallen many times because of freezing. When she starts to walk, just touching something seems to help. She does not use an ambulatory assistive device. Richard (Lee's husband) states that in the morning, before Lee takes her L-dopa medications and freezing is worst, he helps Lee with walking. He does this by standing in front of her and walking backward while holding her hands. In her "off" state, Lee's gait is more narrowly based and freezing occurs more frequently while ambulating. Lee's triggers for freezing are start hesitation and turns. Doorways seem to be a trigger only with "off" freezing. Her score on the Freezing of Gait Questionnaire is 14. If time constraints are a problem during the initial evaluation, the questionnaire can be given to the patient to complete at home or administered on the next visit before implementing freezing interventions. My experience, however, is that subjective reports without the questionnaire can offer significant insight into interventions.

Objective Evaluation

Lee is in her "on" state during the evaluation. Lee is observed to freeze during turns and with start hesitation. Turning observations reveal reduced advancement of the outside foot, rushing, and instability caused by pivots. Other than instability during turns, gait is steady without an assist device. No freezing is noted with linear ambulation, and no narrowness of her base is noted.

Goals

The following goals were established for Lee:

- She will report improved control of freezing episodes during start hesitation, turns, and while ambulating in the "off" state to improve stability (this can be reassessed purely on the patient's feelings of improved control or through an improved score on the Freezing of Gait Questionnaire).
- Her caregiver (Richard) will demonstrate proper technique in assisting the patient while walking to minimize strain and optimize safety.
- Lee will demonstrate proper use of the walker.
- Lee will also demonstrate proper turning technique to improve stability (improved advancement of outside foot, avoidance of rushing or pivoting).

Therapeutic Interventions

Patient education and caregiver involvement should be an integral part of therapeutic interventions to reduce stress and strain. The biomechanics or kinematics of freezing and turning instability is explained. Patient educational handouts are issued regarding these areas (see appendix D). Richard is informed that his current method of helping Lee with walking is suboptimal because it can create greater anterior instability, further exacerbate freezing, and jeopardize his ability to support Lee in the event

(continued)

Case Example *(continued)*

of a loss of balance. Lee is informed about how a walker can improve freezing and stability while walking in her "off" state. She is advised that visual cueing can help with start hesitation in her "off" state. When attempting her first step, she can step over a visual cue such as a sock on the floor or her husband's foot placed perpendicular to her own foot (see figure 14.3, *a* and *b*).

Proper body mechanics regarding freezing and turns are reviewed and practiced. Richard is instructed about how to assist Lee with lateral weight shift by standing at her side. For gait training, a two-wheeled walker is recommended. Because Lee is reluctant to use a walker, she is advised to borrow one from a lending closet. Walking regularly with RAS is recommended.

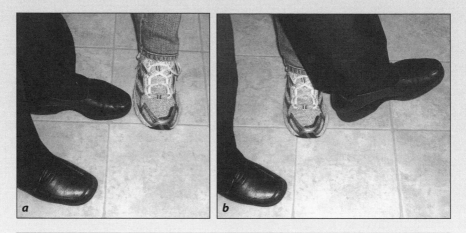

Figure 14.3 Visual cue for start hesitation. When freezing occurs the caregiver can *(a)* place one foot in front of the person who is frozen and *(b)* have the person step over it.

Outcomes

Lee's ability to reduce freezing will depend on attention strategies to improve lateral weight shifting while "on" and using a walker when "off" to allow lateral weight shift in the presence of a narrow base of support. If Lee continues to resist using a walker for "off" states, Richard will be able to assist her more effectively and safely. Improving turning stability will require Lee to modify habitual behaviors (such as rushing or pivoting) and use attention strategies to improve advancement of the outside foot.

because it may cause tripping (figure 14.4*a*). Some patients have reported improvement with the laser cane, which produces a visible laser beam on the floor that the patient attempts to step over. This option is much safer because it does not create an obstacle (figure 14.4*b*). My observation is that visual cues are most effectively used for start hesitation and "off" freezing.

• **Walkers**. For some people, the main trigger for a freeze may be allowing the walker to get too far ahead. Therapists and health professionals are probably more familiar than they would like to be with the phrase "get closer to the walker!" After repeated reminders these words lose their effectiveness. When the walker is too far ahead the elbows are typically fully extended and the patient is leaning forward. Instruction to relax the elbows can facilitate elbow flexion during walking and secondarily bring the patient closer to the walker. This suggestion can be reinforced with tactile cues. The patient can be told, "When we are walking, every time I tap the front side of your elbow I want you to relax your elbows and try to keep them relaxed." Instructing a family member or caregiver

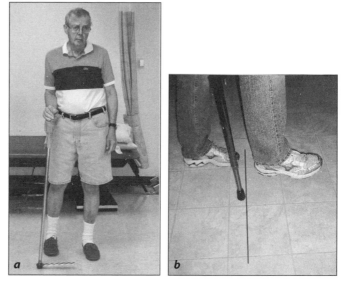

Figure 14.4 Instep mobility products: *(a)* inverted walking stick; *(b)* laser cane.

will help with consistency. If this technique is ineffective and serious freezing persists because the walker is too far forward, then using a walker with fewer wheels may be necessary for safety. On rare occasions, a pickup walker may be needed for control and stability.

Freezing can still occur when the patient is walking within the walker boundaries. Using handbrakes effectively during a freeze can be critical to stability or fall prevention. Patients who freeze may either delay the use of their handbrakes or make no attempt to use them. The saying "squeeze when you freeze" will alert the patient to do just that. Practice is typically necessary to ensure understanding. Stop-and-go drills are helpful. The patient is told to make a sudden stop. When doing so, the emphasis is on squeezing the handbrakes first and secondarily stopping walking.

Summary

1. Not all people with PD have freezing.
2. Freezing can occur in people with other movement disorders, and they can benefit from similar interventions.
3. The severity, frequency, and aggravating factors of freezing vary from one person to the next.
4. Visual cues are most effective for "off" freezing.
5. Therapeutic interventions can improve control of freezing episodes but do not resolve freezing problems.
6. Exaggerated lateral weight shift and prolonged timing of the weight shift is necessary to control freezing.
7. Rhythmical auditory stimulation can be effective in reducing freezing.
8. Therapeutic interventions should address patient-specific freezing triggers.

15

Turning While Ambulating

Making turns while ambulating can be one of the more destabilizing aspects of walk-ing for people with Parkinson's (Willemsen et al., 2000). Alterations in turning ability during gait occur in people with PD as early as Hoehn and Yahr stages 1 and 2, even before changes in linear walking emerge (Ferrarin et al., 2006). Common turning strate-gies seen in people with PD are wider turns, reduced stride length, and increased stepping variability (Huxham et al., 2008). Before entering a turn, people with PD also tend to slow down and take more steps (Crenna et al., 2007).

These turning adaptations in people with PD may result from basal ganglia dysfunction in combination with attempting to stabilize turns. Patients who fall as the result of turning are generally not sensitive to strategies that may offer greater stabilization. For example, instead of entering the turn slowly and making a wide turn, they rush and then pivot. The activity of turning can be compared to the dynamics of turning a car. Slow turns are easily controlled in a vehicle. All four wheels remain on the ground, and passengers remain in place in their seats. But if the driver turns quickly to the left, passengers slide toward the right. During a quick turn the initial forward momentum of the car pulls the car and the passengers to the side. The effect of high-momentum forces has been demonstrated with linear walking in which greater velocity has the potential to cause greater instability (Pai et al., 2000).

Making turns requires greater lateral center of mass (COM) control than does linear walking, which may contribute to the lateral instability observed (see figure 15.1). Stack et al. (2006) found that people with PD who reported difficulties with turning experienced frequent freezing or falls.

Factors Contributing to Turning Instability

Previous chapters have pointed out that people with PD exhibit greater difficulty with lateral stability than do people without PD. This effect becomes more pronounced with increased disease severity because of their narrow base of support coupled with postural instability and limited trunk mobility (Dimitrova et al., 2004). Turning is one of the most common aggravating factors of freezing, which itself can be destabilizing (Bloem et al., 2004). Insta-bility is further compounded with hip abductor strength deficiencies, which are unrelated to PD and are associated with aging and deconditioning (Rogers & Mille, 2003).

Even when a person is mildly affected, asymmetry of foot advancement during turns can play havoc with balance. Although patients voice difficulty with turns, they often do not

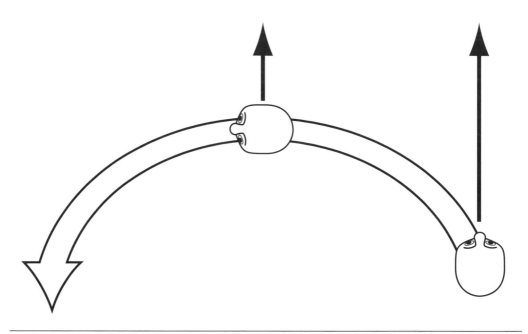

Figure 15.1 Anterior forces with linear ambulation become destabilizing lateral forces during turns.

understand why they are unsteady. Turning instability is often (but not always) the result of underscaled stepping of the outside foot or an impairment of lateral weight-shifting capability. The outside foot tends to lag progressively farther behind as the inside foot forges ahead with its turn. When this occurs, the base of support narrows, creating progressive instability in the presence of continued lateral forces. For example, when making a left turn, the right foot (the foot on the outside of the circle) lags behind. Normally, the outside foot should be taking a larger step than the inside foot because it needs to cover more distance to complete the turn (see figure 15.2). Some people take a backward step with the inside foot during a turn. This maneuver may be compensating for difficulties with advancement of the outside foot. Patients who have pronounced unilateral symptoms typically have problems when turning away from their affected side. Greater concentration (attention strategies) may be needed to bring the more involved foot around, and prolonging weight shifting may be required to offer more time for the involved foot to take a longer step.

Evaluating Turns

Although turning asymmetries can be observed even when a patient is in an "on" state, obtaining the patient's reports on turning difficulties remains important for making appropriate interventions.

• **Subjective evaluation**. Patients should be asked whether they have difficulty with turning. People who report difficulty with turning frequently have problems with freezing (Stack et al., 2006). If they do, freezing should also be addressed. See "Subjective Evaluation" in appendix D for further questioning about freezing triggers.

• **Objective evaluation**. The objective evaluation of turns is purely observational. I have found that if the patient is asked to pace back and forth (making 180° turns) for a

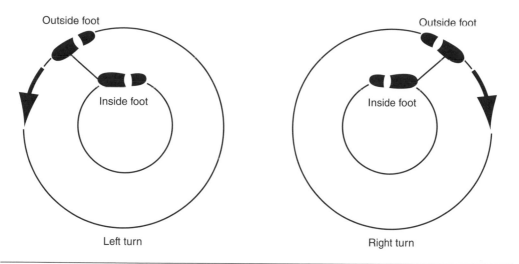

Figure 15.2 These demonstrate the foot positioning of the outside foot to enhance stability during turns. Some overlap offers greater stability.

distance of approximately 15 to 20 ft (4.5 to 6 m), he or she tends to concentrate more on the linear gait than turning. This activity can expose natural turning habits. Because PD typically affects one side more than the other, turns in one direction may be more difficult. Patients tend naturally to turn in the direction in which they feel more steady or comfortable. Observing both left and right turns can bring out those differences. Make note of deviations. Also, observe sharper turns or turns with a smaller turning radius because those tend to be truer to life and more difficult. Appendix C, "Objective Evaluation," item 5 (page 241) provides a useful checklist for noting the patient's turning strategies. These items include the following:

- Normal
- Multistep
- Pivotal
- Freezing
- Narrow based
- Guarded
- Right turn with reduced advancement of the left foot
- Left turn with reduced advancement of the right foot
- Rushing
- Unstable

Interventions to Improve Turns

Other than addressing musculoskeletal impairments that contribute to turning instability, modification of turning habits is the primary focus. Educating patients about the causes of turning difficulties and their effects on stability can facilitate learning of new strategies. But certain strategies are not possible with some patients because of intrinsic factors that are resistant to physical interventions. For example, a very narrow-based gait is difficult to treat (see chapter 8, "Balance Evaluation," for information about treatable and difficult-to-treat intrinsic factors). In addition, impaired cognition can prevent learning of new strategies. In such cases, an assistive device (cane or walker) may be needed before optimal turning strategies can be implemented. The following interventions can be useful in the treatment of turns.

General Strategies

Some patients may require only a few of the listed interventions to improve turning ability. Others will require intensive practice with turns using various compensatory strategies as well as conditioning and flexibility exercises. The following interventions are useful for improving turning ability:

- **Strength and ROM training**. Target musculoskeletal impairments that may affect turning stability. These impairments are often, but not always, hip abductor weakness and limited axial flexibility.

- **Rhythmical auditory stimulation (RAS)**. Rhythmical auditory stimulation has been shown to reduce variability of step timing during turns in both freezers and nonfreezers (Willems et al., 2007). See chapter 13, "Compensatory Strategies for Gait Interventions," for a thorough discussion of RAS.

- **Modifying speed**. Educate the patient to avoid rushing or abrupt, fast turning movements.

- **Reducing turning degree**. One study compared the turning dynamics of a subject with PD Hoehn and Yahr stage 3 with an older adult subject. The subject with PD demonstrated a tendency to turn more sharply as the turning arc increased (Morris et al., 2001). I have observed this tendency clinically. Turning through a greater turning arc often leads to more pivotal types of turns, especially in smaller spaces. Turns of 360° are reportedly more precipitous of freezing than 180° turns (Schaafsma et al., 2003). I have found, especially with people who freeze, that a 180° turn is also more precipitous of freezing and destabilizing than a 90° turn. People often perform 180° turns during daily activities such as approaching a chair. By approaching the chair from the side, the turn can be reduced to 90°. Reviewing side approaches can functionally reduce difficulties by minimizing the arc of the turn. See chapter 9, "Chair Transfers," for interventions (pages 118–119).

- **Step length training**. Review proper turning to increase step length of the outside foot (see appendix D for a patient handout about turns). The patient may need to use attention strategies because turning may not be as automatic as it was in the past. Step length adjustments of the outside foot may be needed. Patients initially tend to overstep with the outside foot, which can be equally destabilizing. Some patients have great difficulty understanding the mechanics of performing 180° turns. Visual cues can be used as a training tool to help these patients improve their turning capability. The following strategy may be needed to enhance step length training:
  - Colored floor discs can be used as stepping pads.
  - Arrange three discs in an equilateral triangle, placed about one of your patient's step lengths apart. For training purposes, the peak of the triangle can be referred to as the nose and the base of the triangle can be the eyes.
  - Place a mirror image of the three discs approximately 10 ft (3 m) away. (If the triangles are too close together, the patient is likely to become dizzy because of having to enter another turn too soon.)

- The patient walks back and forth, alternating left and right turns while stepping on the discs. The pivoting foot stays on the nose disc as the outer foot steps from one disc (eye) to the next. The stepping sequence is pivot, step, pivot, step. The pivot occurs before the outside foot steps to the next disc. Fine-tuning adjustments for foot placement are often necessary (see figure 15.3, *a–f*).

- If a patient demonstrates difficulties with turns in only one direction, interventions should focus on that direction.

Case Example: Difficulty With Turns While Ambulating

Gary is 60 yr old and has PD Hoehn and Yahr stage 3. Parkinsonian symptoms are greater on his right side.

Subjective Evaluation

Gary is an active person who walks and exercises regularly. His chief complaint is difficulty with turns that on occasion has caused loss of balance. He denies having fallen, but he freezes with turns and start hesitation.

Objective Evaluation

Gary is asked to pace back and forth initially without further instructions. Gary is observed to turn only to the right when making 180° turns. He is then asked to continue pacing but to perform left turns. While making 180° left turns Gary demonstrates reduced advancement of his right foot, mild freezing, and instability. Mild freezing is also noted when he gets out of a chair and attempts to start walking.

Goals

Two goals are established for Gary:

- To improve stability with left turns
- To reduce freezing with left turns

Therapeutic Interventions

Patient education and body mechanics training helps Gary to self-analyze and manage difficulties with turns.

• Gary is informed that because his symptoms are worse on his right side, he has greater difficulty taking a larger step with the right foot to make left turns. Therefore, when making left turns he needs to pay more attention to the right foot and, if necessary, make a right turn if he finds himself in an unstable situation.

• Turning with emphasis on advancement of the outside foot is reviewed and practiced. Gary is issued a patient handout on turns (see appendix D) for future self-management. Although freezing was mild, antifreezing strategies are reviewed.

Outcomes

Attention strategies are commonly needed to improve turns. With a little practice Gary improved turning stability simply by increasing the step length of his outside foot. Secondarily, he was able to reduce freezing.

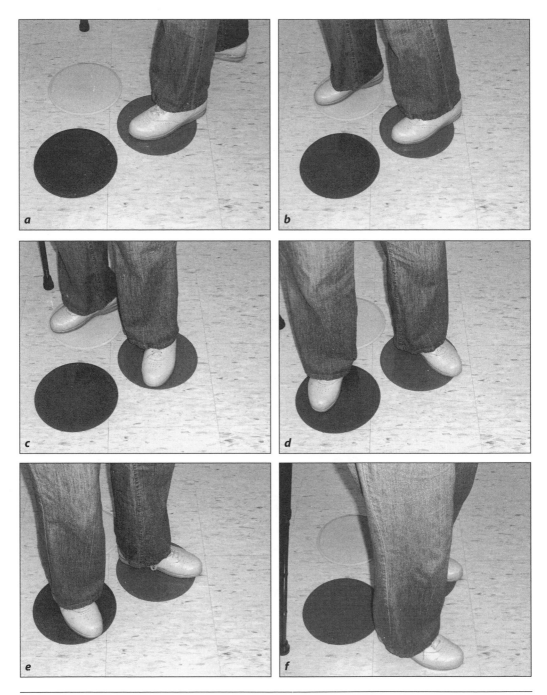

Figure 15.3 *(a–f)* These images demonstrate pivot–step sequence training facilitated with visual attention strategies to improve advancement of the outside foot during turns.

Specific Situations and Conditions

Depending on the severity of turning difficulties, additional educational and physical interventions may be necessary.

- **Turning radius**. Narrow spaces may trigger freezing when a person attempts to turn. Patients should practice narrow and wide turns using the concept of increasing the advancement of the outside foot. Making wider turns can improve stability but is not practical in smaller spaces. The goal is to train for turning adaptability given the environmental demands.

- **Recovering after a fall**. If someone has difficulty with turns and falls, the caregiver can place a chair at the head end and the foot end to reduce the difficulty of getting up for both the patient and the caregiver. The patient can more easily stand up by using the chair placed at the head end. After the person is standing, the caregiver can pull up the other chair so that the patient can sit down without needing to turn.

- **People who freeze**. Those who freeze may need to focus on increasing the excursion of lateral weight shifting and prolonging the timing of the lateral weight shift to free up the outside foot long enough to take a longer step (see chapter 14, "Freezing"). Reducing the degree of the turn may be needed as well.

- **Patients with a narrow base**. Although a person with PD may demonstrate a normal-width base of support during gait, the base of support tends to narrow during a turn (Morris et al., 2001). People with PD Hoehn and Yahr stages 1 through 3 can modify the base of support during turns with practice if the base of support with linear ambulation is not too narrow and cognition allows carryover. But if a person with PD already has a very narrow base of support with linear ambulation or if cognition prevents modifications during turns, then an assist device may be needed for additional lateral stability.

- **Dual tasking**. On occasion I have discovered from patients' reports and later observed that when dual tasking patients tend to rotate the trunk without any attempt to move the feet, causing immediate imbalance. This pattern seems to be most commonly triggered when a person in the kitchen or a closet picks up an object and immediately performs a turn. Patient education to promote awareness and caution can help with prevention. Redirecting attention to the feet instead of what is being carried can help with moving the feet sooner rather than later.

Summary

1. Instability during turns is multifactorial.

2. Rushing is often destabilizing when turning.

3. Attention strategies may be necessary to improve turns.

4. Stability with turns can significantly improve by improving foot advancement of the outside foot and accentuating lateral weight shift.

5. An ambulatory assist device may be necessary for stability if the patient's base of support is naturally too narrow.

6. Turns of 90° are easier to perform than turns of 180°. Patients should try to approach chairs and other destinations from the side.

7. Rhythmical auditory stimulation can help improve turning strategies by reducing variability of step duration.

16

Walkers, Canes, and Footwear

As mentioned in chapter 8, "Balance Evaluation," intrinsic factors (factors related to the patient) increase the risk of falls. Some of these factors are modifiable, such as strength, flexibility, and to some extent balance (see chapter 3, "Exercise and Rehabilitation Considerations"). Some patients can improve sufficiently from therapy to progress from using a cane to using no assistive device. Even with the best efforts to improve these areas, however, a person can continue to be unsteady and unsafe. At this point we need to look at modifying extrinsic factors (factors related to the environment) to reduce the risk of falls.

Modification of extrinsic factors should involve a comprehensive approach with occupational therapy (OT) and physical therapy (PT). Occupational therapy addresses home environmental modifications and the needs of activities of daily living (ADL), which would include the use of a cane or walker during ADL. Physical therapy can focus on safe ambulation using ambulatory assist devices or changes in footwear. This chapter discusses extrinsic factors relative to gait to improve safety and function. The guidelines and recommendations offered here are based almost solely on my clinical experience. Over the years, I have made recommendations in over 350 individual cases regarding walker needs.

Matching Walkers to Patients

Matching the walker to patient needs can be a challenge. Many types of walkers are on the market. Options and styles change over the years. Recommending the best walker requires consideration of many variables. Our job is to find the best match and to prioritize features for safety and mobility.

The topic of using a walker can be a sensitive issue for many patients. A walker is often viewed as a sign of going downhill. From the patient's perspective, the onset of unsteadiness was not sudden, as seen with a stroke, but its potential progressive nature can cause apprehension. Over time the patient has made adaptations in response to unsteadiness. Usually a person who is less steady or has a fear of falling tends to limit activities to avoid falls or loss of balance. When a patient voices concerns about an assist device being an indicator of going downhill, the therapist should clear up the misconception. Becoming deconditioned by limiting activities only accelerates impairments, resulting in greater disability. If a patient is able to become more active, safely, then deconditioning can be prevented or reversed. This point should be made clear to the patient.

On the other hand, the patient may not be psychologically ready to discuss the possible need for an assist device. In such a case the discussion may need to wait, but the need for it should not be forgotten. Establishing rapport with the patient and working on other fall prevention issues can help pave the way for later acceptance and compliance.

Having various types of walkers in the clinic for the patient to "test drive" helps in the selection of the safest and most practical walker. I have often found that patients have never tried to use a walker and truly do not know how much a walker can improve their mobility. A casual approach can help relieve some anxiety about using a walker. The therapist may say, "Let's just go for a walk with this walker and let me know what you think."

Patients should be made aware of the pros and cons of various walkers so that they can be educated consumers when buying one. An open dialogue between the patient and therapist can help ensure understanding of walker options. Giving the patient a list of reputable vendors will pave the road to making this a more pleasant process. Patients should contact their insurers and affiliated dealers to understand the level of coverage. The clinician should give the patient a written summary of walker recommendations such as walker height, type, seat, and wheels. Providing specifications minimizes confusion with the vendor and ensures the right fit for the patient. After the patient buys the walker, the therapist should review features for optimal safety and ensure proper height adjustment.

Walker Features

Many walker characteristics are involved in establishing the best fit for the patient (table 16.1). Larger wheels roll better on a variety of surfaces and facilitate outdoor ambulation. The weight of the walker is a consideration for portability. What type of braking mechanism does the walker have? The ability to stop the walker and control its velocity is critical for safe ambulation. Various seats are available to meet the needs of the patient. Walker height is a routine consideration for physical therapists, but not all walkers come in your patient's size. If you are recommending a particular brand of walker, make sure that it can be adjusted to your patient's height. See chapter 5, "Postural Variations and Dystonia," for exceptions to walker height adjustments. Consider the following features when making recommendations about walkers.

Wheels

Many questions must be answered about the most suitable type of wheels for a given patient. The issues to address are wheel size, number, and whether the wheels are swivel or stationary.

Size

The basic principle to keep in mind here is that the larger the wheels are, the better they roll. Here are the specifics:

- **Three-inch (7.6 cm) wheels (two-wheeled walkers).** Consider this size for indoor ambulators who have thin carpeting. These wheels are too small to push easily on thicker carpeting.
- **Five-inch (12.7 cm) wheels (two-wheeled walkers).** Recommend this size for those who are primarily indoor ambulators. This size moves more easily on thicker carpeting and can be used for short distances outdoors, but uneven terrain can easily catch the back legs. Glides are made of plastic and do not endure outdoor surfaces.
- **Six-inch wheels (15.2 cm) (four-wheeled walkers).** This size functions well for indoor ambulation. This size of wheel can also be used for outdoor ambulation on a limited

Table 16.1 Walker Criteria Considerations

Walker type	Wheel size	Portability	Brake system	Seat
Two-wheeled Lightest walker (approx. 5 to 6 lb, or 2.3 to 2.7 kg)	5 in. (12.7 cm) better than 3 in. (7.6 cm) for indoor use	Easily portable	None needed	Typically has no seat but some have seat capability
Four-wheeled (approx. 11 to 16 lb, or 5 to 7.3 kg)	5 in. (12.7 cm)—indoors 6 in. (15.2 cm)—limited outdoor use 8 in. (20.3 cm) or larger—regular outdoor use	Portability needs to be evaluated depending on patient abilities or family or caregiver support. Walker weight can affect portability Backrests: Strap backrest or bar backrest models are available. Strap backrest models are more portable than bar backrest models	Handbrakes: Four-wheeled walkers should have handbrakes for safety Slowdown brakes: This additional feature facilitates greater control of walker speed	Stationary seat: Most common. It offers a deeper seat than the flip-up seat Flip-up seat: More functional for ambulation and standing activities. Allows more room to walk inside the walker and permits easier access to counter or tabletops
Weighted walker (approx. 19 lb or more, or 8.6 kg or more)	Consider wheel size and compliance of floor surface	Most difficult to transport because of weight	Handbrakes: Some have additional slowdown brakes Few have reverse brakes	Stationary or flip-up seat that allows access to basket

basis. Wheels of this size are not able to handle uneven terrain consistently. Handbrakes are necessary.

- **Eight-inch wheels (20.3 cm) or larger (four-wheeled walkers).** This size of wheel is ideal for outdoor use because the walker can roll efficiently over uneven terrain. Handbrakes are necessary.

Number

Walkers may have from zero to four wheels.

- **Pickup walker.** Rarely is a pickup walker recommended. Pickup walkers significantly reduce gait velocity, but they may be necessary for safety. This type of walker is indicated for people who are unable to control the velocity of any rolling walker, such as those who have severe freezing or festination and whose feet cannot keep up with the velocity of the walker. The gap between a rolling walker and the patient can widen quickly, resulting in a fall.

- **Two-wheeled walker.** This is the typical hospital-issue collapsible folding walker with glides on the back. It is practical for people walking indoors. This walker is the lightest of all rolling walkers and therefore the easiest to transport. Because it does not require handbrakes, it is simple to use, an added benefit for those who are cognitively impaired. The two-wheeled walker may be a better option than the four-wheeled walker for people who have difficulty controlling walker velocity or keeping the walker close enough for balance control. People with a festinating gait may need this type of walker, but they should be assessed individually.

- **Three-wheeled walker.** This type of walker can be helpful in stabilizing gait but is not as stable as the four-wheeled walker. Three-wheeled walkers may be lighter than their four-wheeled counterparts, but they lack a seat, which may be important when the patient is fatigued or experiencing "on" or "off" motor fluctuations.

- **Four-wheeled walker.** This type is the most versatile. It is good for indoors or outdoors depending on wheel size. A seat is standard. Walker weight varies, and options vary.

Swivel versus stationary

Stationary wheels do not swivel. The choices affect maneuverability and stability.

- **Swivel wheels.** Any walker with three or more wheels has swivel wheels and turns well. Turning can be problematic for people with PD (see chapter 15, "Turning While Ambulating"). Swivels are beneficial and generally recommended, although swivel wheels on a two-wheeled walker hamper control of walker movement with linear ambulation.

- **Stationary wheels.** Stationary wheels (which do not swivel) are recommended only for two-wheeled walkers. Although turning with stationary wheels can be cumbersome, linear ambulation is more stable or controlled.

Weight

Walker weight can be critical for portability. Two questions need to be asked: Who will be lifting the walker into and out of the car, and how capable is the designated lifter? The answers may determine the type of walker selected. If a patient lives in assisted living, does not drive, and has grown children who will lift the walker into and out of the car, then walker weight may not be an issue. But for a frail older patient who still drives, walker weight will play a significant role. Before buying a walker, the patient or designated lifter should attempt to load and unload it from the car. If a similar walker is available in the clinic, loading and unloading capability can be assessed and practiced there.

Here are the walker options in terms of weight:

- **Pickup walker.** This is the lightest of all walkers, weighing approximately 5 to 6 lb (2.3 to 2.7 kg).

- **Two-wheeled walker.** This is also a light walker, ranging from 6 to 7 lb (2.7 to 3.2 kg). The rear legs have glides to allow easy pushing.

- **Lightweight four-wheeled walker.** This kind of walker weighs approximately 11 to 13 lb (5.0 to 5.9 kg) and has 5 or 6 in. (12.7 to 15.2 cm) wheels.

- **Standard four-wheeled walker.** This walker weighs approximately 14 to 16 lb (6.4 to 7.3 kg).

- **Weighted walker.** Weighing approximately 19 lb (8.6 kg) or more, this type of walker is recommended when extra stability is needed to maintain balance. It is suitable for either backward fallers or people who continue to fall or remain unsteady with their current walker. If independent ambulation is a goal, this type of walker may be needed. The main drawback of a weighted walker is that it is difficult to lift into and out of a car.

Braking Mechanisms

The ability to control the velocity of the walker is necessary for safety. Various types of braking mechanisms are available to address this potential problem:

- **Standard handbrake.** This handbrake must be squeezed to slow down or stop the walker. This type of braking system is standard. Patients with cognitive impairments may not be able to use this type of brake effectively, although this may not be an issue if ambulation is closely supervised.

- **Reverse handbrake.** This handbrake must be released to activate the braking mechanism. In other words, the person must squeeze the handbrake to allow the walker to move during ambulation. If the patient releases or forgets to squeeze the handbrake, the walker stops. This safety feature is useful for those with cognitive impairments or those who have difficulties with dual tasking.

- **Slowdown brakes.** A mechanism located on the back wheels of the walker offers continual resistance to the wheels to help control the walker velocity. The resistance is adjusted initially and then only as needed. Slowdown brakes can be beneficial for people who tend to festinate or have difficulty controlling walker velocity (see figures 16.1 and 16.2). I have observed that patients initially rely on this mechanism and later wean themselves. I am not sure whether this device initially works as a training tool or the added resistance makes ambulation fatiguing. Perhaps by becoming more conditioned, patients may improve stability and control and no longer need the device.

Seat

Each of the two types of seat options offers advantages and disadvantages:

- **Flip-up seat.** A flip-up seat can be swiveled up and out of the way while standing or ambulating (see figure 16.3). The disadvantage is that the flip-up seat is not as deep as a stationary seat. The flip-up seat offers several advantages:

  - Turns in smaller spaces are possible because the patient can be inside the walker during the turn.

- The patient can stand farther inside the walker and thus more easily reach items on a counter.
- The seat offers greater clearance when tipping the walker back to go up curbs.
- The walker can be closer to the curb when the patient steps down.
- The patient can walk farther inside the walker, which can improve control of walker velocity.

• **Standard, or stationary, seat.** This type of seat is much deeper than the flip-up seat, which makes it more comfortable. The seat folds up only when folding the entire walker for transporting it. More seats are being made with padding for extra comfort. The disadvantages of this kind of seat are the following:

- Increased turning clearance is needed.
- The seat interferes with reaching over a counter.
- The seat presents interference when tipping the walker backward to go up a curb.
- When going down a curb the walker needs to be positioned farther from the curb to allow room for the feet to step down.
- The seat may impede the ability to walk close to the walker.

These disadvantages may not be a problem if the patient lives in a home with plentiful space, never goes up or down curbs, and is able to stay close to the walker.

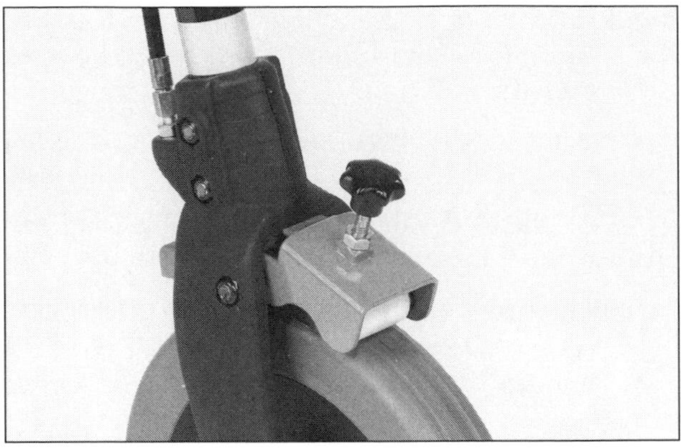

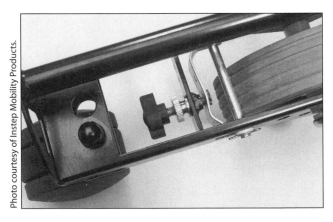

Photo courtesy of Clarke Health Care.

Figure 16.1 Dolomite slowdown brakes.

Photo courtesy of Instep Mobility Products.

Figure 16.2 U-step slowdown brakes.

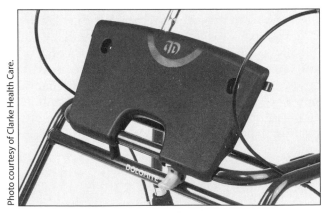

Photo courtesy of Clarke Health Care.

Figure 16.3 Flip-up walker seat.

Back Support

Generally speaking, people with PD do not require much support when sitting. The level of support from either a back strap or bar is sufficient. The strap conforms better to the person's back than the bar does. Some strap lengths are adjustable to accommodate various posture and body types. The type of back support typically is not an issue for trunk stability, but it can be a factor in portability.

- **Back strap:** The strap makes the walker much less bulky and easier to transport, which makes this feature superior to the padded bar support.
- **Padded bar:** The bar feature is more common than the back strap but bulkier. Some bars are removable to reduce bulkiness for transporting.

Relevant Patient Characteristics

Cognitive function, presence of motor fluctuations, direction of instability, and the patient's endurance can dictate the type of walker needed. Cognition and the presence of motor fluctuations are two nonmodifiable variables for the rehab professional. Improvements in stability are possible depending on pathology or impairments. Endurance is the most rehabilitatable variable, and improvement should occur easily with the appropriate walker. For example, a four-wheeled walker with 8 in. (20.3 cm) wheels allows easy outdoor ambulation, and a two-wheeled walker can be sufficient for indoor ambulation.

Cognitive Impairment

Cognitive deficits may affect the type of walker needed to ensure safety.

- A simpler walker design may be necessary for people with dementia.
- Handbrakes can be a safety issue if the patient is unable to use them effectively. Few walkers have the reverse handbrake feature described earlier. Two-wheeled walkers do not require additional braking mechanisms for safety and are therefore easier to use by those with cognitive impairments.
- If assistance or supervision of another person is required for safe ambulation regardless of the assistive device used, then walker versatility become important to optimize mobility and minimize caregiver strain. For example, if the patient enjoys outdoor ambulation and a caregiver can control walker velocity, a four-wheeled walker may be an option.

Motor Fluctuations

Predictability or unpredictability of motor fluctuations can dictate walker needs:

- "Wearing off" symptoms are predictable episodes of potential instability when at end dose of L-dopa. The patient may need to use the walker only for predictable "off" states.
- Diurnal "off" states can be significant. Some patients may need to use their walker only when they first get up in the morning before their first dose of PD medications becomes effective. A walker may also be needed in the evening when the daily dosing of L-dopa may start to wear off. In addition, patients become tired and do not walk as well. Using a walker on an as-needed basis can be sufficient for fall prevention and is usually more palatable to the patient.
- Some people with PD experience abrupt "on-off" episodes and unpredictable periods of impaired mobility. When patients exhibit these symptoms they are advised to use their

walker at all times. A walker with a seat may alleviate the apprehension of not having a place to sit during an abrupt "off" period. Patients who experience "on-off" episodes tend to be reluctant to use the walker at all times because during their "on" time they can be quite independent with ambulation.

Direction of Instability

Walkers can improve general stability. Backward instability can increase the challenge of walker selection.

• **Forward and lateral instability**. Depending on other variables, any walker is helpful in preventing forward falls or a lateral loss of balance because the walker increases the base of support anteriorly and laterally.

• **Backward instability**. Because a walker does not increase the base of posterior support, a weighted walker provides a more effective counterbalance of forces. The U-step has a base that extends farther posteriorly than conventional walkers do, a feature that improves backward stability, especially during static standing. On occasion, adjusting the height of a conventional walker to a lower level than is customary can alleviate some posterior instability.

Endurance

Endurance should always be considered in selecting a walker so that the device does not deter the patient from walking to his or her potential.

• **Community ambulator**. A four-wheeled walker with 8 in. (20.3 cm) wheels may be appropriate for an active community ambulator.

• **Household ambulator**. A two-wheeled or four-wheeled walker with 5 in. (12.7 cm) wheels may be sufficient for a household ambulator who has limited potential to become a community ambulator.

Environmental Factors

Ground or floor surfaces should be considered when determining wheel size.

• Plush carpeting can cause difficulty when pushing a walker with 3 in. (7.6 cm) wheels. Larger wheels (5 in., or 12.7 cm, or greater) may be necessary.

• The uneven surfaces often encountered while walking outside require wheels 8 in. (20.3 cm) or more in diameter. Thus, if a patient prefers walking outside the walker must meet that specification.

Stairs are the most common environmental barrier when it comes to walkers. Curbs can also be problematic, but at least there are methods to overcome this barrier with the walker.

Stairs

When a person lives in a house with stairs the ideal situation is to have a walker on each level. Financially, having more than one walker may not be possible. Whether the person lives alone or not, an occupational therapist should make a home visit to assess all possible alternatives for safe solutions not only with the stairs but with all ADLs including walker modifications (e.g., adding a pouch or tray to help carry items).

A lightweight two-wheeled walker or pickup walker would be the lightest to carry up and down the stairs. Having the patient practice carrying a walker up and down the stairs in therapy can confirm whether this option is feasible. If the patient does not live alone, a family member could carry the walker to the next level. The capability of that family member should be assessed to see whether this option is viable.

The patient may need to move to an environment with fewer barriers to optimize safety and independence, such as a retirement community or assisted living. This option can be an emotional decision fueled by financial concerns. A team approach from the patient's physician, social services, occupational therapy, and physical therapy may be necessary for such a transition. Additional in-home service is another option. Social services can help the patient sort out options based on the patient's level of function, support systems, and finances.

Curbs

Maneuvering safely up and down curbs with a walker requires practice. Because the sequence of manipulating the walker can be involved, the patient must use the proper technique regularly to avoid forgetting it. Fortunately, sidewalk ramps at street intersections have significantly diminished the need for being able to go up and down curbs. But barriers at home residences persist. These barriers require maneuverability similar to that needed to go up or down a curb. Going up and down a curb is easier when using a walker with a flip-up seat when compared with using a walker with a stationary seat. Some patients may not be able to follow these instructions because of cognitive impairments. Involving a family member with the procedures can reduce difficulties for both the patient and the family member.

Technique for Going Up Curbs

The steps for going up curbs with a walker follow. For an illustration of this technique, see figure 16.4, *a–d*.

1. Roll the front wheels of the walker against the curb (figure 16.4*a*).
2. Step back but do not move the walker. Keep brakes on or squeezed while tilting the walker onto the back wheels. When the front wheels are above curb level and the weight of the walker is on the back wheels, release the brakes and roll the walker so that the back wheels are against the curb and the front wheels are on the curb (figure 16.4*b*).
3. Simply roll the back wheels up the curb (figure 16.4*c*).
4. Before stepping up on the curb, make sure that enough clearance is available for your feet and that the brakes are on (figure 16.4*d*).

Technique for Going Down Curbs

The steps for going down curbs with a walker follow. For an illustration of these steps, see figure 16.5, *a–c*.

1. Walk to the edge of the curb with the walker.
2. Roll the front wheels off the curb and then use the brakes as you step closer to the walker.
3. Roll the back wheels off the curb and use the brakes as you step to the edge of the curb.
4. Allow room to step down while keeping the brakes on.

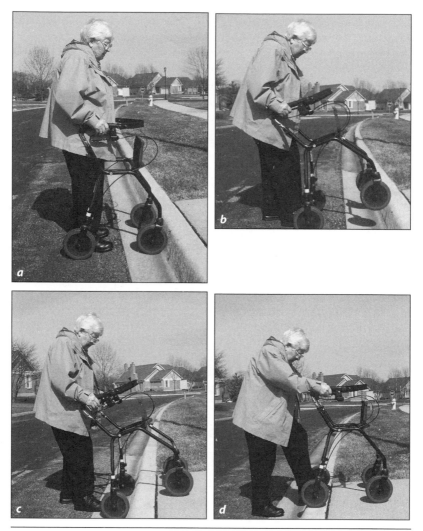

Figure 16.4 *(a)* Roll the front wheels against the curb; *(b)* squeeze the brakes and tilt the walker; roll the walker on the back wheels to the curb; *(c)* roll the back wheels onto the curb; *(d)* squeeze the brakes while stepping up on the curb.

Manufacturers

All walkers have pros and cons. The key is to determine the characteristics necessary for optimal safety and mobility of each patient, because every person with PD is unique. Regardless of walker brand, gait training strategies with walkers remain similar. See Appendix D "Gait Training Strategies when Using a Walker". The following manufacturers are only a few of many, but the walkers mentioned here have features that make them more suitable than many others for the PD population. All three manufacturers offer walkers in a wide range of heights. See table 16.2 for walker brands and features.

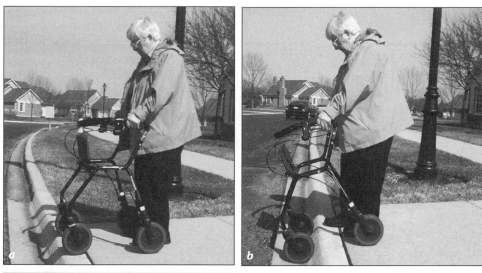

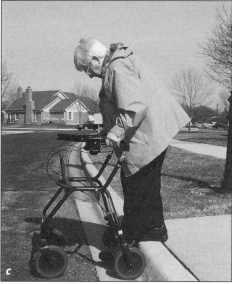

Figure 16.5 *(a)* Step close to the walker before descending the curb; *(b)* roll the front wheels and then the back wheels over the curb; squeeze the brakes when stepping closer to the curb; *(c)* squeeze the brakes while stepping down.

• Invacare carries a variety of walkers. The strap backrest makes them more portable than walkers with stiff backrests. This manufacturer makes one of the few two-wheeled walkers available with a flip-up seat (figure 16.6a). Invacare also makes a four-wheeled walker with a flip-up seat (figure 16.6b).

• The U-step walker offers more stability for those who are less steady (see figure 16.7). A unique feature of this walker is the reverse hand-braking system, which tends to be safer for those who are cognitively impaired. The unique frame offers good support for people who lose their balance backward. The U-step walker also has the slowdown brake feature. The weight of this walker makes it more difficult to transport, which may be a consideration.

• Dolomite walkers also have the strap backrest. The Dolomite Legacy has a flip-up seat and 8 in. (20.3 cm) wheels (see figure 16.8). Optional slowdown brakes are available for this model.

Table 16.2 Walker Brands and Features

Brand	Walker name	Walker weight	Wheel size	Number of wheels	Seat	Slowdown brakes
Made by many manufacturers	Standard two-wheeled walker	Approximately 6 lb (2.7 kg)	5 in. (12.7 cm) fixed	2 wheels and 2 glides	No seat	No
Invacare	Walklite	11 lb (5.0 kg)	5 in. (12.7 cm) fixed	2 wheels and 2 glides	Flip-up for more walking room	No
Invacare	Rollite Rollator	16.5 lb (7.5 kg)	8 in. (20.3 cm)	4 wheels	Flip-up for more walking room	No
Dolomite	Legacy	15 lb (6.8 kg)	8 in. (20.3 cm)	4 wheels	Flip-up for more walking room	Yes
Instep Mobility	U-step	19 lb (8.6 kg)	Two side wheels are 5.5 in. (14.0 cm). Five additional wheels are 3 in. (7.6 cm)	7 wheels	Flip-up for access to basket. Patient is able to walk inside walker without seat flipping up because of walker base configuration	Yes

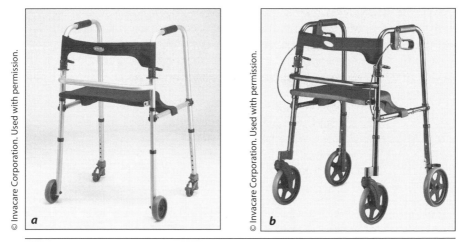

© Invacare Corporation. Used with permission.

Figure 16.6 *(a)* Invacare Walklite; *(b)* Invacare Rollite Rollator.

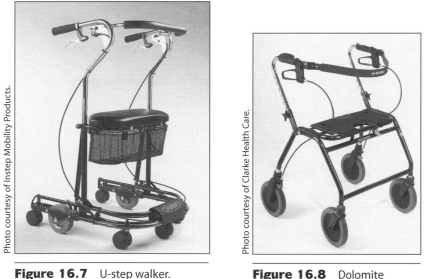

Photo courtesy of Instep Mobility Products.

Photo courtesy of Clarke Health Care.

Figure 16.7 U-step walker.

Figure 16.8 Dolomite Legacy walker.

Canes

As with walkers, the need for a cane should be evaluated on an individual basis. Patients in the earlier stages of PD, Hoehn and Yahr stages 1 and 2 (postural reflexes intact), may benefit from a cane. A cane offers improved lateral stability for a narrowly based gait. It can also improve lateral weight shift in people whose posture exhibits significant scoliosis, which can adversely affect weight-shifting capability to one side.

However, even at the earlier stages, if a patient exhibits significant freezing with momentous anterior instability, a cane may not offer enough support to prevent an anterior loss of balance. Canes can potentially cause greater instability because of their dual tasking effect. Using a cane has been shown to inhibit grasping as a strategy for balance recovery (Bateni et al., 2004). Some people with PD have great difficulty keeping the cane out to the side, thus creating a tripping hazard. Quad canes in general tend to be a greater tripping hazard and should be avoided. Some people with PD who have motor fluctuations may be steady with a cane during their "on" state and need a walker during their "off" state.

Footwear

People with PD who exhibit reduced ground clearance during the swing phase of gait are at risk of tripping. In addition, deviations from normal foot-loading patterns have been noted during the stance phases of gait in people with PD. Reduced impact occurs at heel strike, and forefoot loading is higher than normal (Kimmeskamp & Hennig, 2001). This loading pattern in combination with reduced ground clearance can cause the forefoot to catch on the ground surface. The greater the friction between the sole of the forefoot and the ground surface, the greater the likelihood that the foot will be caught. From a therapeutic standpoint this problem can be reduced by altering shoe choices.

Addressing Footwear With the Patient

When a patient reports problems with the feet catching or sticking to various floor surfaces and causing imbalance, evaluation of the patient's current footwear is warranted. Descriptors such as catching or sticking should be distinguished from problems such as tripping on uneven surfaces. Although both problems result from reduced ground clearance, the latter may not necessitate a change in footwear. People with gait deviations such as freezing or festination should be advised about specific footwear that minimizes sticking. Soles with a lower friction coefficient can significantly reduce catching.

Not surprisingly, however, simply advising your patient to change footwear does not always translate into action. People can be attached to their current footwear or be financially unable to manage expensive footwear. One study examined the attitudes of older people toward sturdy footwear. The researchers interviewed 652 people over the age of 64. Twenty-six percent of the people interviewed wore sturdy shoes, and approximately 66% had worn sturdy shoes at some time. Participants did not change their footwear in response to a fall. Barriers to wearing sturdy shoes included foot problems, difficulty donning the shoes, expense, style, and lack of knowledge about the importance of wearing sturdy shoes (Dunne et al., 1993).

Fortunately, all these issues can be addressed through a combination of patient education and guiding the patient toward choosing appropriate footwear. Moreover, commercial footwear continues to become more sophisticated. Some styles are available for people who have claw toes. Some are made deeper to accommodate a shoe insert or ankle–foot orthosis (AFO). Donning and doffing is facilitated by the use of Velcro closures or long-handled shoehorns.

Footwear Recommendations

Proper footwear recommendations begin with advising patients what not to wear. They then need to be shown why they should wear something else. Finally, they need to be guided in what they should wear.

Crucial Shoe Characteristics

Following these shoe guidelines can reduce the risk of falls:

- Avoid ridged soles. Ridges catch more easily on carpeting.
- Crepe soles and soles with a soft rubbery material as seen in running shoes should be avoided (Warshaw, 1999).
- Soles need to have a sufficiently large surface area for an optimal base of support.
- Lower-heeled shoes can reduce forward imbalance problems caused by a forward-flexed posture or postural instability (Tencer et al., 2004).
- Well-fitting shoes with sufficient toe room and a supportive heel counter offer both comfort and stability. Loose-fitting footwear such as sandals should be avoided.
- Soles that are worn can cause imbalance or undue stress on the foot. Shoes should be resoled or replaced.

Patient Education

As noted earlier, persuading patients to buy different shoes is not always easy. Simply telling them that their current footwear is dangerous is not always sufficient. Information and demonstration are often needed.

When you advise patients to buy shoes with firm low-friction soles, they tend to be more concerned about slipping than they are about tripping. This priority is understandable because recovering from a slip is more difficult and may be more injurious. But the concern about slipping with a low-friction sole is more of a perceptual issue than an actual threat. Patients should be informed that catching their feet presents the main fall risk and reassured that the level of friction of their new shoes will not cause slips.

Patients who are reluctant to change their footwear are often convinced by experiencing a temporary trial of friction reduction of their current soles. This can be done by wrapping the shoe in a pillowcase (see figures 16.9, *a* and *b*). Before wrapping the shoe, the person should first walk a sufficient distance to observe catching or sticking. The more problematic foot is then wrapped with a pillowcase, which is anchored by strong adhesive tape. The end product looks like a pillowcase moccasin. The sole area needs to be wrinkle free and taut (see figure 16.9*c*). The patient then walks with the pillowcase-wrapped shoe. Immediate gait improvement should be noted and pointed out to the patient.

So how does the patient check for low friction when buying new shoes? Sliding a hand along the bottom of the shoe and checking for tackiness or a feeling of the skin dragging on the sole indicates excessive friction. This method may need to be demonstrated using the patient's current footwear. Patients should "test drive" potential new footwear in the store on carpeted and tile surfaces to evaluate whether their feet are catching less. Proper footwear can be verified with a confirmed reduction in catching of the feet.

Recommended Shoe Brands

PW Minor and SAS are shoe manufacturers who offer shoes that reduce the catching experienced with a Parkinsonian gait. Some styles of these supportive shoes have sufficient depth to accommodate orthotics or an AFO (ankle–foot orthosis). Both manufacturers carry styles that come in either a tie lace or Velcro closure. Recommended PW Minor styles are Canfield Leisure and Canfield Pleasure. SAS also offers a variety of styles. Recommended SAS styles

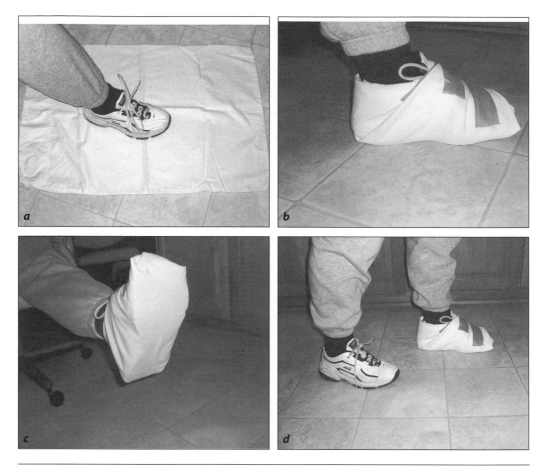

Figure 16.9 *(a)* For smaller feet, the pillowcase can be folded in half; *(b)* the foot is wrapped in a pillowcase that is anchored with tape; *(c)* the sole area should be wrinkle free and taut; *(d)* a trial walk in the pillowcase-wrapped shoe allows the patient to experience the benefits of a lower-friction sole.

are Free Time and Me Too for women, and Time Out and VTO for men. These brands and styles meet the necessary sole requirements. Looking at the soles of some of these models can give a baseline for comparison for recommending additional brands. Web sites to refer to are www.pwminor.com and www.arthritis.com.

Modifying Old Shoes

Shoe repair shops can resurface many shoes. The forefoot of the sole is removed and replaced with a low-friction material, typically leather and is typically called a leather half sole. The resurfaced area should include the area of the metatarsal heads. Not all shoe soles can be resurfaced, but the shoe repair person should make this judgment. Resurfacing is an economical option. People who are fond of their current shoes appreciate having this option (figure 16.10).

Tina is 78 and has PD Hoehn and Yahr stage 4.

Subjective Evaluation

Tina lives with her husband, George, in a one-level home that requires only one step to enter. She states that going up and down that one step is becoming more difficult. She no longer drives, but her husband does. She is ambulatory with a two-wheeled walker that she uses at all times but complains it is hard to manage. She received this walker from a friend. She denies experiencing any falls, but states that her foot catches at times. Ambulation is primarily indoors, except when she goes out to visit family. She bought running shoes a few months ago because she thought that they would offer more stability. She states that she does not exercise and has not been on the floor in years. Therefore, she does not know whether she would be able to get up if she fell.

Objective Evaluation

Tina comes to therapy with her two-wheeled walker, which is visibly hard for her to push and is adjusted too high. She walks far behind the walker, causing her to walk on her toes occasionally. The walker has 3 in. (7.6 cm) wheels, and the glides on the back legs have worn through to the rubber tips, causing the walker to drag. Tina's gait presents with short shuffling steps. Notably, her feet frequently catch on the tile flooring. She is wearing running shoes with ridged soles. She is generally deconditioned, and her ROM is generally limited.

Goals

Several goals were established for Tina:

- Become independent with HEP for general conditioning and flexibility to optimize mobility
- Be able to verbalize understanding of proper footwear for fall prevention
- Demonstrate proper use of the walker for fall prevention
- Demonstrate proper body mechanics with going up and down curbs while using her walker
- Demonstrate floor transfers with minimal assistance and use of furniture for support

Therapeutic Interventions

The need for increasing ambulation and exercise to improve abilities and reverse deconditioning is explained. The patient is advised that footwear with soft rubbery soles and ridges can cause her feet to catch and result in a loss of balance. Recommendations are offered regarding alternative footwear. The following physical interventions are made:

- **Walker**: Glide caps are applied, and walker height is adjusted. If the walker is still difficult to push after making these modifications, she may need 5 in.

(continued)

Case Example *(continued)*

(12.7 cm) wheels. Because of her limited outdoor ambulation and the capability of her husband (marginally steady with a cane), a four-wheeled walker is not pursued. Transporting her lightweight two-wheeled walker will be less difficult than moving a heavier four-wheeled walker.

- **Exercise**: Tina is instructed in a HEP that addresses impairments.
- **Gait and transfers training**: Gait training is done with the walker on level surfaces and up and down curbs. Tina and her husband practice floor transfers.

Outcomes

With a comprehensive exercise program, increased ambulation with a properly fitted and properly working walker, and appropriate footwear, Tina can be expected to achieve her goals.

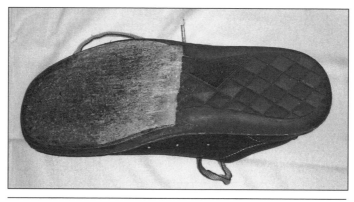

Figure 16.10 Sole of resurfaced shoe.

Summary

1. Matching a walker to the patient requires knowledge of walker features, patient needs, and environmental factors.

2. Having various types of trial walkers in the clinic can facilitate assessment of patient ability to maneuver the walker safely and ensure appropriate walker selection.

3. Steadiness should be confirmed with the recommended assist device. This task is accomplished with external perturbations in various directions during static standing and while ambulating with that particular device.

4. The patient's ability to control the speed of the walker is a primary safety consideration.

5. Patients should be educated about the pros and cons of various walkers so that they can participate in the walker selection process.

6. Issuing written information on individual walker requirements, including walker height, will help avoid confusion with the vendor when the patient is purchasing a walker.

7. If appropriate, the patient or caregiver should try loading the recommended walker in the car before buying.

8. The patient should follow up with the therapist after buying the walker to ensure understanding of all features, to make sure that height is adjusted correctly, and to ensure proper use of the walker.

9. Canes can help or hinder balance and need to be evaluated on an individual basis.

10. Indications to address footwear are the feet being caught on floor surfaces, creating instability. This can be due to reduced ground clearance while walking, freezing, or gait festination.

11. Firm low-friction soles reduce the chances that the feet will catch.

12. Patient education on proper footwear is often necessary to improve awareness and ensure compliance with recommendations.

13. Shoe resurfacing is an economical way to achieve a reduction of sole friction and thus reduce the risk of falls.

A

Rating Scales
and Questionnaires

CONTENTS

Rating Scales

Rating scales constructed for people with PD are intended to standardize criteria and methodology in establishing disease severity and dysfunction or disability. They are primarily used by physicians to determine the effectiveness of medications or surgical interventions. They are also used to determine the effectiveness of new drugs or other new therapeutic interventions. Some scales can be brief and determine only the stage of disease progression such as the Hoehn and Yahr Clinical Staging Scale (Hoehn & Yahr, 1967), one of the oldest and most widely used scales. The scale was developed before L-dopa became available and therefore does not account for motor fluctuations. Because of its limitations, the Hoehn and Yahr scale is typically used in combination with other scales. A scale that focuses more on functional abilities is the Schwab and England Activities of Daily Living Scale (Schwab and England, 1969). A more recently developed scale, the Unified Parkinson's Disease Rating Scale, is the most comprehensive scale and most widely used scale to date (Fahn et al., 1987).

An awareness of these scales can help with the understanding of research implications for physical management. For example, some of the physical interventions may be effective for people with PD Hoehn and Yahr stages 1 and 2 but not for Hoehn and Yahr stages 3 and 4. Other interventions may be effective for Hoehn and Yahr stages 1 through 4. Interventions for stage 5 are primarily directly to caregivers. Therapists also use scales for research. Many scales are used for Parkinson's. Only the three most commonly used scales have been listed here.

Hoehn and Yahr Staging of Parkinson's Progression

Stage 1 = Unilateral disease

Stage 2 = Bilateral disease, balance intact

Stage 3 = Mild to moderate bilateral disease; some postural instability; physically independent

Stage 4 = Severe disability; still able to walk or stand unassisted

Stage 5 = Wheelchair bound or bedridden unless aided

Modified Hoehn and Yahr Staging of Parkinson's Progression

Stage 1 = Unilateral disease

Stage 1.5 = Unilateral and axial involvement

Stage 2 = Bilateral disease, balance intact

Stage 2.5 = Mild bilateral disease with recovery on pull test

Stage 3 = Mild to moderate bilateral disease; some postural instability; physically independent

Stage 4 = Severe disability; still able to walk or stand unassisted

Stage 5 = Wheelchair bound or bedridden unless aided

Schwab and England Activities of Daily Living Scale

100% = Completely independent. Able to do all chores without slowness, difficulty, or impairment. Essentially normal. Unaware of any difficulty.

90% = Completely independent. Able to do all chores with some degree of slowness, difficulty, and impairment. Might take twice as long. Beginning to be aware of difficulty.

80% = Completely independent in most chores. Take twice as long. Conscious of difficulty and slowness.

70% = Not completely independent. More difficulty with some chores. Some take three to four times as long. Must spend a large part of the day with chores.

60% = Some dependency. Can do most chores, but with much difficulty and effort. Errors occur; some chores impossible.

- 50% = More dependent. Help needed with half, slower, and so on. Difficulty with everything.
- 40% = Very dependent. Can assist with all chores, but few alone.
- 30% = With effort, now and then does a few chores alone or begins alone. Much help needed.
- 20% = Nothing alone. Can be a slight help with some chores. Severe invalid.
- 10% = Totally dependent, helpless, complete invalid.
- 0% = Vegetative functions such as swallowing, bladder functions, and bowel functions are not operating. Bedridden.

Reprinted, by permission, from R.S. Schwab and A.C. England, Jr., 1960, "Projection technique for evaluating surgery in Parkinson's Disease," *Journal of Nerve and Mental Disorders* 130: 556-566.

Unified Parkinson's Disease Rating Scale (UPDRS)

This scale is the most comprehensive and widely used. Longitudinally, patients are reassessed with this tool to follow the progression of Parkinson's or, in some fortunate cases, lack of progression. This rating scale is divided into four sections. Section I addresses mentation, behavior, and mood. Section II addresses activities of daily living (ADLs) during "on" and "off" periods. Section III addresses motor function during "on" periods. Section IV addresses motor complications from medications. The higher the score, the greater the disability. A score of zero indicates no disability.

Section I—Mentation, Behavior, and Mood

1. Intellectual impairment

   0 = None.

   1 = Mild. Consistent forgetfulness with partial recollection of events and no other difficulties.

   2 = Moderate memory loss, with disorientation and moderate difficulty handling complex problems. Mild but definite impairment of function at home with need of occasional prompting.

   3 = Severe memory loss with disorientation for time and often to place. Severe impairment in handling problems.

   4 = Severe memory loss with orientation preserved to person only. Unable to make judgments or solve problems. Requires much help with personal care. Cannot be left alone at all.

2. Thought disorder (because of dementia or drug intoxication)

   0 = None.

   1 = Vivid dreaming.

   2 = Benign hallucinations with insight retained.

   3 = Occasional to frequent hallucinations or delusions; without insight; could interfere with daily activities.

4 = Persistent hallucinations, delusions, or florid psychosis. Not able to care for self.

3. Depression

    0 = None.

    1 = Periods of sadness or guilt greater than normal, never sustained for days or weeks.

    2 = Sustained depression (1 wk or more).

    3 = Sustained depression with vegetative symptoms (insomnia, anorexia, weight loss, loss of interest).

    4 = Sustained depression with vegetative symptoms and suicidal thoughts or intent.

4. Motivation and initiative

    0 = Normal.

    1 = Less assertive than usual; more passive.

    2 = Loss of initiative or disinterest in elective (nonroutine) activities.

    3 = Loss of initiative or disinterest in day-to-day (routine) activities.

    4 = Withdrawn, complete loss of motivation.

Section II—Activities of Daily Living (for Both "On" and "Off")

5. Speech

    0 = Normal.

    1 = Mildly affected. No difficulty being understood.

    2 = Moderately affected. Sometimes asked to repeat statements.

    3 = Severely affected. Frequently asked to repeat statements.

    4 = Unintelligible most of the time.

6. Salivation

    0 = Normal.

    1 = Slight but definite excess of saliva in mouth; may have nighttime drooling.

    2 = Moderately excessive saliva; may have minimal drooling.

    3 = Marked excess of saliva with some drooling.

    4 = Marked drooling, requires constant tissue or handkerchief.

7. Swallowing

    0 = Normal.

    1 = Rare choking.

    2 = Occasional choking.

    3 = Requires soft food.

    4 = Requires NG tube or gastrostomy feeding.

8. Handwriting

    0 = Normal.

    1 = Slightly slow or small.

    2 = Moderately slow or small; all words are legible.

3 = Severely affected; not all words are legible.

4 = Most words are not legible.

9. Cutting food and handling utensils

0 = Normal.

1 = Somewhat slow and clumsy, but no help needed.

2 = Can cut most foods, although clumsy and slow; some help needed.

3 = Food must be cut by someone, but can still feed slowly.

4 = Needs to be fed.

10. Dressing

0 = Normal.

1 = Somewhat slow, but no help needed.

2 = Occasional assistance with buttoning, getting arms in sleeves.

3 = Considerable help required, but can do some things alone.

4 = Helpless.

11. Hygiene

0 = Normal.

1 = Somewhat slow, but no help needed.

2 = Needs help to shower or bathe, or very slow in hygienic care.

3 = Requires assistance for washing, brushing teeth, combing hair, going to bathroom.

4 = Foley catheter or other mechanical aids.

12. Turning in bed and adjusting bed clothes

0 = Normal.

1 = Somewhat slow and clumsy, but no help needed.

2 = Can turn alone or adjust sheets, but with great difficulty.

3 = Can initiate, but not turn or adjust sheets alone.

4 = Helpless.

13. Falling (unrelated to freezing)

0 = None.

1 = Rare falling.

2 = Occasionally falls, less than once per day.

3 = Falls an average of once daily.

4 = Falls more than once daily.

14. Freezing when walking

0 = None.

1 = Rare freezing when walking; may have start hesitation.

2 = Occasional freezing when walking.

3 = Frequent freezing; occasionally falls from freezing.

4 = Frequent falls from freezing.

15. Walking

    0 = Normal.

    1 = Mild difficulty. May not swing arms or may tend to drag leg.

    2 = Moderate difficulty, but requires little or no assistance.

    3 = Severe disturbance of walking; requires assistance.

    4 = Cannot walk at all, even with assistance.

16. Tremor (symptomatic complaint of tremor in any part of the body)

    0 = Absent.

    1 = Slight and infrequently present.

    2 = Moderate; bothersome to patient.

    3 = Severe; interferes with many activities.

    4 = Marked; interferes with most activities.

17. Sensory complaints related to Parkinsonism

    0 = None.

    1 = Occasionally has numbness, tingling, or mild aching.

    2 = Frequently has numbness, tingling, or aching; not distressing.

    3 = Frequent painful sensations.

    4 = Excruciating pain.

Section III—Motor Examination

18. Speech

    0 = Normal.

    1 = Slight loss of expression, diction, or volume.

    2 = Monotone, slurred but understandable; moderately impaired.

    3 = Marked impairment, difficult to understand.

    4 = Unintelligible.

19. Facial expression

    0 = Normal.

    1 = Minimal hypomimia, could be normal poker face.

    2 = Slight but definitely abnormal diminution of facial expression.

    3 = Moderate hypomimia; lips parted some of the time.

    4 = Masked or fixed facies with severe or complete loss of facial expression; lips parted 0.25 in. (0.6 cm) or more.

20. Tremor at rest (head, upper and lower extremities)

    0 = Absent.

    1 = Slight and infrequently present.

    2 = Mild in amplitude and persistent, or moderate in amplitude but only intermittently present.

    3 = Moderate in amplitude and present most of the time.

    4 = Marked in amplitude; interferes with eating.

21. Action or postural tremor of hands

    0 = Absent.

    1 = Slight; present with action.

    2 = Moderate in amplitude; present with action.

    3 = Moderate in amplitude with postural holding as well as action.

    4 = Marked in amplitude; interferes with feeding.

22. Rigidity (judged on passive movement of major joints with patient relaxed in sitting position; cogwheel ignored)

    0 = Absent.

    1 = Slight or detectable only when activated by mirror or other movements.

    2 = Mild to moderate.

    3 = Marked, but full range of motion easily achieved.

    4 = Severe; range of motion achieved with difficulty.

23. Finger taps (tapping thumb with index finger in rapid succession)

    0 = Normal.

    1 = Mild slowing or reduction in amplitude.

    2 = Moderately impaired. Definite and early fatiguing. May have occasional arrests in movement.

    3 = Severely impaired. Frequent hesitation in initiating movements or arrests in ongoing movement.

    4 = Can barely perform the task.

24. Hand movements (opening and closing hands in rapid succession)

    0 = Normal.

    1 = Mild slowing or reduction in amplitude.

    2 = Moderately impaired. Definite and early fatiguing. May have occasional arrests in movement.

    3 = Severely impaired. Frequent hesitation in initiating movements or arrests in ongoing movement.

    4 = Can barely perform the task.

25. Rapid alternating hand movements (pronation and supination movements of hands, vertically and horizontally, with as large an amplitude as possible, both hands simultaneously)

    0 = Normal.

    1 = Mild slowing or reduction in amplitude.

    2 = Moderate impairment. Definite and early fatiguing. May have occasional arrests in movement.

    3 = Severely impaired. Frequent hesitation in initiating movements or arrests in ongoing movement.

    4 = Can barely perform the task.

26. Leg agility (tapping heel on the ground in rapid succession, picking up entire leg; amplitude at least 3 in., or 7.6 cm)

0 = Normal.

1 = Mild slowing or reduction in amplitude.

2 = Moderately impaired. Definite and early fatiguing. May have occasional arrests in movement.

3 = Severely impaired. Frequent hesitation in initiating movements or arrests in ongoing movement.

4 = Can barely perform the task.

27. Rising from chair (attempting to rise from a straight-backed chair with arms folded across chest)

0 = Normal.

1 = Slow or may need more than one attempt.

2 = Pushes self up from arms of seat.

3 = Tends to fall back and may have to try more than one time but can get up without help.

4 = Unable to rise without help.

28. Posture

0 = Normal erect.

1 = Not quite erect, slightly stooped posture; could be normal for older person.

2 = Moderately stooped posture, definitely abnormal; can be slightly leaning to one side.

3 = Severely stooped posture with kyphosis; can be moderately leaning to one side.

4 = Marked flexion with extreme abnormality of posture.

29. Gait

0 = Normal.

1 = Walks slowly, may shuffle with short steps but no festination (hastening steps) or propulsion.

2 = Walks with difficulty but requires little or no assistance; may have some festination, short steps, or propulsion.

3 = Severely stooped posture with kyphosis; can be moderately leaning to one side.

4 = Cannot walk at all, even with assistance.

30. Postural stability

0 = Normal.

1 = Retropulsion but recovers unaided.

2 = Absence of postural response; would fall if not caught by examiner.

3 = Very unstable, tends to lose balance spontaneously.

4 = Unable to stand without assistance.

31. Body bradykinesia and hypokinesia (combining slowness, hesitancy, decreased arm swing, small amplitude, and poverty of movement in general)

0 = None.

1 = Minimal slowness, giving movement a deliberate character; could be normal for some persons. Possibly reduced amplitude.

2 = Mild degree of slowness and poverty of movement that is definitely abnormal. Alternatively, some reduced amplitude.

3 = Moderate slowness, poverty, or small amplitude of movement.

4 = Marked slowness, poverty, or small amplitude of movement.

Section IV—Complications of Therapy (in the Past Week)

A. Dyskinesias

32. Duration: In what proportion of the waking day are dyskinesias present? (Historical information.)

0 = None

1 = 1–25% of the day

2 = 26–50% of the day

3 = 51–75% of the day

4 = 76–100% of the day

33. Disability: How disabling are the dyskinesias? (Historical information; may be modified by office examination.)

0 = Not disabling

1 = Mildly disabling

2 = Moderately disabling

3 = Severely disabling

4 = Completely disabling

34. Painful dyskinesias: How painful are the dyskinesias?

0 = No painful dyskinesias

1 = Slight

2 = Moderate

3 = Severe

4 = Marked

35. Presence of early morning dystonia (historical information)

0 = No

1 = Yes

B. Clinical Fluctuations

36. Are "off" periods predictable?

0 = No

1 = Yes

37. Are "off" periods unpredictable?

    0 = No

    1 = Yes

38. Do "off" periods come on suddenly, within a few seconds?

    0 = No

    1 = Yes

39. What proportion of the day is the patient "off" on average?

    0 = None

    1 = 1–25% of the day

    2 = 26–50% of the day

    3 = 51–75% of the day

    4 = 76–100% of the day

C. Other Complications

40. Does the patient have anorexia, nausea, or vomiting?

    0 = No

    1 = Yes

41. Are any sleep disturbances present, such as insomnia or hypersomnolence?

    0 = No

    1 = Yes

42. Does the patient have symptomatic orthostasis? (Record the patient's blood pressure, height, and weight on the scoring form.)

    0 = No

    1 = Yes

Questionnaires

Like scales, questionnaires help determine the effectiveness of interventions and are often used to determine research outcomes. Although they rely on the patient's or caregiver's subjective reports, questionnaires help make outcomes more objective. The accuracy of reporting, however, depends on cognitive integrity, which should be a consideration when administering a questionnaire. The Freezing of Gait Questionnaire is a brief questionnaire that is a practical tool for the clinician to use in goal setting and objectifying outcomes related to freezing interventions. The Parkinson's Disease Quality of Life Questionnaire, often used in PD research, is also included (Jenkinson et al., 1997). The patient can complete it at home. This questionnaire is not critical to establish outcomes because physical therapists commonly use other tools to establish the effectiveness of their interventions (see appendix B).

Freezing of Gait Questionnaire

This questionnaire was developed to assess the severity of freezing of gait (FOG) unrelated to falls. Typically, patients freeze more at home than when in the clinic. Therefore, the severity of freezing is established more from the patient's report than from clinical observation. This questionnaire is highly reliable and moderately correlated with the ADL and motor components of the Unified Parkinson's Disease Rating Scale (Giladi et al., 2000).

1. During your worst state, how do you walk?

   0 = Normally

   1= Almost normally, somewhat slowly

   2 = Slowly but fully independent

   3 = Need assistance or walking aid

   4 = Unable to walk

2. Are your gait difficulties affecting your daily activities and independence?

   0 = Not at all

   1 = Mildly

   2 = Moderately

   3 = Severely

   4 = Unable to walk

3. Do you feel that your feet become glued to the floor while walking, making a turn, or when trying to initiate walking (freezing)?

   0 = Never

   1 = Very rarely—about once a month

   2 = Rarely—about once a week

   3 = Often—about once a day

   4 = Always—whenever walking

4. How long is your longest freezing episode?

   0 = Never happened

   1 = 1–2 seconds

   2 = 3–10 seconds

   3 = 11–30 seconds

   4 = Unable to walk for more than 30 seconds

5. How long is your typical start hesitation episode (freezing when initiating the first step)?

   0 = None

   1 = Takes longer than 1 second to start walking

   2 = Takes longer than 3 seconds to start walking

   3 = Takes longer than 10 seconds to start walking

   4 = Takes longer than 30 seconds to start walking

6. How long is your typical turning hesitation (freezing when turning)?

   0 = None

   1 = Resume turning in 1 to 2 seconds

   2 = Resume turning in 3 to 10 seconds

   3 = Resume turning in 11 to 30 seconds

   4 = Unable to resume turning for more than 30 seconds

Reprinted from *Parkinsonism and Related Disorders,* Volume 6, N. Giladi, H. Shabtai, E.S. Simon, S. Biran, J. Tal, & A.D. Korczyn, "Construction of freezing of gait questionnaire for patients with Parkinsonism," pg 6, © 2000, with permission from Elsevier.

PDQ-39

Parkinson's Disease
Quality of Life Questionnaire

and

scoring system

HEALTH SERVICES RESEARCH UNIT
DEPARTMENT OF PUBLIC HEALTH
UNIVERSITY OF OXFORD

Version 1.1

DUE TO HAVING PARKINSON'S DISEASE, how often have you experienced the following, <u>during the last month</u>?

Due to having Parkinson's disease, how often <u>during the last month</u> have you . . ..

*Please tick **one box** for each question*

	Never	Occasionally	Sometimes	Often	Always
1. Had difficulty doing the leisure activities which you would like to do?	☐	☐	☐	☐	☐
2. Had difficulty looking after your home, e.g. DIY, housework, cooking?	☐	☐	☐	☐	☐
3. Had difficulty carrying bags of shopping?	☐	☐	☐	☐	☐
4. Had problems walking half a mile?	☐	☐	☐	☐	☐
5. Had problems walking 100 yards?	☐	☐	☐	☐	☐
6. Had problems getting around the house as easily as you would like?	☐	☐	☐	☐	☐
7. Had difficulty getting around in public?	☐	☐	☐	☐	☐
8. Needed someone else to accompany you when you went out?	☐	☐	☐	☐	☐
9. Felt frightened or worried about falling over in public?	☐	☐	☐	☐	☐
10. Been confined to the house more than you would like?	☐	☐	☐	☐	☐
11. Had difficulty washing yourself?	☐	☐	☐	☐	☐
12. Had difficulty dressing yourself?	☐	☐	☐	☐	☐
13. Had problems doing up buttons or shoe laces?	☐	☐	☐	☐	☐
14. Had problems writing clearly?	☐	☐	☐	☐	☐
15. Had difficulty cutting up your food?	☐	☐	☐	☐	☐
16. Had difficulty holding a drink without spilling it?	☐	☐	☐	☐	☐
17. Felt depressed?	☐	☐	☐	☐	☐
18. Felt isolated and lonely?	☐	☐	☐	☐	☐
19. Felt weepy or tearful?	☐	☐	☐	☐	☐
20. Felt angry or bitter?	☐	☐	☐	☐	☐

*Please check that you have ticked **<u>one box for each question</u>**
before going on to the next page*

Due to having Parkinson's disease, how often <u>during the last month</u> have you . . ..

Please tick **one box** for each question

	Never	Occasionally	Sometimes	Often	Always
21. Felt anxious?	☐	☐	☐	☐	☐
22. Felt worried about your future?	☐	☐	☐	☐	☐
23. Felt you had to conceal your Parkinson's from people?	☐	☐	☐	☐	☐
24. Avoided situations which involve eating or drinking in public?	☐	☐	☐	☐	☐
25. Felt embarrassed in public due to having Parkinson's disease?	☐	☐	☐	☐	☐
26. Felt worried by other people's reaction to you?	☐	☐	☐	☐	☐
27. Had problems with your close personal relationships?	☐	☐	☐	☐	☐
28. Lacked support in the ways you need from your spouse or partner? *If you do not have a spouse or partner, please tick here* ☐	☐	☐	☐	☐	☐
29. Lacked support in the ways you need from your family or close friends?	☐	☐	☐	☐	☐
30. Unexpectedly fallen asleep during the day?	☐	☐	☐	☐	☐
31. Had problems with your concentration, e.g. when reading or watching TV?	☐	☐	☐	☐	☐
32. Felt your memory was bad?	☐	☐	☐	☐	☐
33. Had distressing dreams or hallucinations?	☐	☐	☐	☐	☐
34. Had difficulty with your speech?	☐	☐	☐	☐	☐
35. Felt unable to communicate with people properly	☐	☐	☐	☐	☐
36. Felt ignored by people?	☐	☐	☐	☐	☐
37. Had painful muscle cramps or spasms?	☐	☐	☐	☐	☐
38. Had aches and pains in your joints or body?	☐	☐	☐	☐	☐
39. Felt unpleasantly hot or cold?	☐	☐	☐	☐	☐

*Please check that you have ticked <u>**one box for each question**</u> before going on to the next page*

Coding system for questions

All questions on the PDQ-39 are coded in the same way. We recommend that data is entered using the following codes.

- 0 = Never
- 1 = Occasionally
- 2 = Sometimes
- 3 = Often
- 4 = Always (or cannot do at all, if applicable)

Dimensions and their questions

Mobility

10 questions, nos. 1 to 10

Activities of daily living (ADL)

6 questions, nos. 11 to 16

Emotional well being

6 questions, nos. 17 to 22

Stigma

4 questions, nos. 23 to 26

Social support

3 questions, nos. 27 to 29

Cognitive impairment (Cognitions)

4 questions, nos. 30 to 33

Communication

3 questions, nos. 34 to 36

Bodily discomfort

3 questions, nos. 37 to 39

Scoring for each dimension

Each dimension is calculated as a scale from 0 to 100
0 = no problem at all; 100 = maximum level of problem

If the response to a question is missing, no scale score
is calculated for that individual for that dimension

Formula for scoring each dimension

$$\frac{\text{sum of scores of each question in dimension}}{4 \text{ (max. score per question)} \times \text{nos. questions in dimension}} \times 100$$

Mobility

(scores of questions 1+2+3+4+5+6+7+8+9+10) / (4 × 10) × 100

Activities of daily living

(scores of questions 11+12+13+14+15+16) / 4 × 6) × 100

Emotional well being

(scores of questions 17+18+19+20+21+22) / 4 × 6) × 100

Stigma

(scores of questions 23+24+25+26) / 4 × 4) × 100

Social support

(scores of questions 27+28+29) / 4 × 3) × 100

note: if respondents indicate that they do not have a spouse or partner on question 28 then social support can be calculated as follows:

Social support = (scores of questions 27+29) / (4 × 2) × 100

Cognitions

(scores of questions 30+31+32+33) / (4 × 4) × 100

Communication

(scores of questions 34+35+36) / (4 × 3) × 100

Bodily discomfort

(scores of questions 37+38+39) / (4 × 3) × 100

No changes may be made to the questionnaire without written permission.

The Health Services Research Unit is a non-profit making organisation which is part of the University of Oxford. The Parkinson's Disease Society of Great Britain is a charitable organisation.

For further information, please contact
Crispin Jenkinson
Health Services Research Unit
Department of Public Health
University of Oxford
Old Road Campus
Headington, Oxford, OX3 7LF, UK
Tel: (01865) 289441
Email:
CRISPIN.JENKINSON@DPHPC.OX.AC.UK
http://www.publichealth.ox.ac.uk/units/hsru/PDQ/
Fax: (01865) 226711

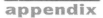

appendix

B

Tests

CONTENTS

Testing is the backbone for establishing baselines and measuring progress. Following established procedural protocol in testing is essential for accurate and comparable results. Balance, leg strength and endurance, and gait velocity are measurable contributors to functional abilities.

Balance

Procedures for these balance tests are described. The Berg balance test has proved to be a good measure of functional performance in people with PD Hoehn and Yahr stage 2 (bilateral involvement with postural reflexes intact). The TUG is a highly reliable test that can detect performance improvements resulting from therapy in people with PD. The functional reach, while not a sensitive tool to predict fall risk, can be used to measure anterior stability. Tests to measure postural stability (the pull test or the push and release test) are reviewed in chapter 7, "Postural Instability."

Leg strength is important for mobility and balance. The chair stand test (see figure on page 232) can measure deficits. The patient's test results can be compared to norms for goal setting and monitoring progress. See table B.1, Norms for Chair Stand Test by Age and Sex.

Optimization of gait velocity is needed for functional ambulation in the community. To establish baseline gait velocity, see chapter 12, "Gait Deviations and Instability." For goal setting and monitoring progress, you can compare your patient's gait velocity with norms (see table B.2, Female Walking Velocity Norms by Age, and table B.3, Male Walking Velocity Norms by Age).

Berg Balance Test

Patient criteria: This test cannot be performed with an assist device.

Item description	Score (0–4)
1. Sitting to standing	_____
2. Standing unsupported	_____
3. Sitting unsupported	_____
4. Standing to sitting	_____
5. Transfers	_____
6. Standing with eyes closed	_____
7. Standing with feet together	_____
8. Reaching forward with outstretched arm	_____
9. Retrieving object from floor	_____
10. Turning to look behind	_____
11. Turning 360°	_____
12. Placing alternate foot on stool	_____
13. Standing with one foot in front	_____
14. Standing on one leg	_____
Total	_____

General Instructions

Demonstrate each task or give instructions as written. When scoring, record the lowest response category that applies for each item.

In most items, the subject is asked to maintain a given position for a specific time. Progressively more points are deducted if the time or distance requirements are not met, if the subject's performance warrants supervision, or if the subject touches an external support or receives assistance from the examiner. Subjects should understand that they must maintain their balance while attempting the tasks. The choice of which leg to stand on or how far to reach is left to the subject. Poor judgment will adversely influence the performance and the scoring.

Equipment required for testing are a stopwatch or watch with a second hand and a ruler or other indicator of 2, 5, and 10 in. (5, 12.5, and 25 cm). Chairs used during testing should be of reasonable height. Either a step or a stool (of average step height) may be used for item #12.

1. Sitting to standing

Instructions: Please stand up. Try not to use your hands for support.

☐ 4 Able to stand without using hands and stabilize independently

☐ 3 Able to stand independently using hands

☐ 2 Able to stand using hands after several tries

- ☐ 1   Needs minimal aid to stand or to stabilize
- ☐ 0   Needs moderate or maximal assist to stand

2. Standing unsupported

    Instructions: Please stand for 2 min without holding onto anything.

    - ☐ 4   Able to stand safely for 2 min
    - ☐ 3   Able to stand for 2 min with supervision
    - ☐ 2   Able to stand for 30 s unsupported
    - ☐ 1   Needs several tries to stand for 30 s unsupported
    - ☐ 0   Unable to stand for 30 s unassisted

    If a subject is able to stand for 2 min unsupported, score full points for sitting unsupported. Proceed to item #4.

3. Sitting with back unsupported but feet supported on floor or on a stool

    Instructions: Please sit with arms folded for 2 min.

    - ☐ 4   Able to sit safely and securely for 2 min
    - ☐ 3   Able to sit for 2 min under supervision
    - ☐ 2   Able to sit for 30 s
    - ☐ 1   Able to sit for 10 s
    - ☐ 0   Unable to sit without support for 10 s

4. Standing to sitting

    Instructions: Please sit down.

    - ☐ 4   Sits safely with minimal use of hands
    - ☐ 3   Controls descent by using hands
    - ☐ 2   Uses back of legs against chair to control descent
    - ☐ 1   Sits independently but has uncontrolled descent
    - ☐ 0   Needs assistance to sit

5. Transfers

    Instructions: Arrange a chair or chairs for a pivot transfer. Ask the subject to transfer one way toward a seat with armrests and one way toward a seat without armrests. You may use two chairs (one with and one without armrests) or a bed and a chair.

    - ☐ 4   Able to transfer safely with minor use of hands
    - ☐ 3   Able to transfer safely but has definite need of hands
    - ☐ 2   Able to transfer with verbal cueing or supervision
    - ☐ 1   Needs one person to assist
    - ☐ 0   Needs two people to assist or supervise to be safe

6. Standing unsupported with eyes closed

   Instructions: Please close your eyes and stand still for 10 s.

   - ☐ 4   Able to stand for 10 s safely
   - ☐ 3   Able to stand for 10 s with supervision
   - ☐ 2   Able to stand for 3 s
   - ☐ 1   Unable to keep eyes closed for 3 s but stays steady
   - ☐ 0   Needs help to keep from falling

7. Standing unsupported with feet together

   Instructions: Place your feet together and stand without holding.

   - ☐ 4   Able to place feet together independently and stand for 1 min safely
   - ☐ 3   Able to place feet together independently and stand for 1 min with supervision
   - ☐ 2   Able to place feet together independently and hold for 30 s
   - ☐ 1   Needs help to attain position but able to stand for 15 s feet together
   - ☐ 0   Needs help to attain position and unable to hold for 15 s

8. Reaching forward with outstretched arm while standing

   Instructions: Lift your arm to 90°. Stretch out your fingers and reach forward as far as you can. (The examiner places a ruler at the end of the fingertips when the arm is at 90°. The fingers should not touch the ruler while reaching forward. The recorded measure is the distance forward that the fingers reach while the subject is in the most forward-leaning position. When possible, ask the subject to use both arms when reaching to avoid rotating the trunk.)

   - ☐ 4   Can reach forward confidently more than 25 cm (10 in.)
   - ☐ 3   Can reach forward more than 12.5 cm (5 in.) safely
   - ☐ 2   Can reach forward more than 5 cm (2 in.) safely
   - ☐ 1   Reaches forward but needs supervision
   - ☐ 0   Loses balance while trying to reach; requires external support

9. Picking up object from the floor from a standing position

   Instructions: Pick up the shoe or slipper placed in front of your feet.

   - ☐ 4   Able to pick up slipper safely and easily
   - ☐ 3   Able to pick up slipper but needs supervision
   - ☐ 2   Unable to pick up slipper but reaches 2 to 5 cm (1 to 2 in.) from slipper and keeps balance independently
   - ☐ 1   Unable to pick up slipper and needs supervision while trying
   - ☐ 0   Unable to try or needs assist to keep from losing balance or falling

10. Turning to look behind over left and right shoulders while standing

Instructions: Turn to look directly behind you over toward your left shoulder. Repeat to the right. (To encourage a better twist turn, the examiner may pick an object directly behind the subject for him or her to look at.)

☐ 4 Looks behind from both sides and weight shifts well
☐ 3 Looks behind one side only; other side shows less weight shift
☐ 2 Turns sideways only but maintains balance
☐ 1 Needs supervision when turning
☐ 0 Needs assist to keep from losing balance or falling

11. Turning 360°

Instructions: Turn completely around in a full circle. Pause. Then turn a full circle in the other direction.

☐ 4 Able to turn 360° safely in 4 s or less
☐ 3 Able to turn 360° safely one side only in 4 s or less
☐ 2 Able to turn 360° safely but slowly
☐ 1 Needs close supervision or verbal cueing
☐ 0 Needs assistance while turning

12. Placing alternate foot on step or stool while standing unsupported

Instructions: Place each foot alternately on the step or stool. Continue until each foot has touched the step or stool four times.

☐ 4 Able to stand independently and safely and complete eight steps in 20 s
☐ 3 Able to stand independently and complete eight steps in more than 20 s
☐ 2 Able to complete four steps without aid but with supervision
☐ 1 Able to complete more than two steps but needs minimal assist
☐ 0 Needs assistance to keep from falling or is unable to try

13. Standing unsupported with one foot in front

Instructions (demonstrate to subject): Place one foot directly in front of the other. If you feel that you cannot place your foot directly in front, try to step far enough ahead so that the heel of your forward foot is ahead of the toes of the other foot. (To score 3 points, the length of the step should exceed the length of the other foot and the width of the stance should approximate the subject's normal stride width.)

☐ 4 Able to place foot tandem independently and hold for 30 s
☐ 3 Able to place foot ahead of the other independently and hold for 30 s

□ 2   Able to take small step independently and for hold 30 s

□ 1   Needs help to step but can hold for 15 s

□ 0   Loses balance while stepping or standing

14. Standing on one leg

Instructions: Stand on one leg as long as you can without holding.

□ 4   Able to lift leg independently and hold for more than 10 s

□ 3   Able to lift leg independently and hold for 5 to 10 s

□ 2   Able to lift leg independently and hold for 3 s or longer

□ 1   Tries to lift leg, is unable to hold for 3 s, but remains standing independently

□ 0   Unable to try or needs assist to prevent fall

□   Total score (maximum = 56)

Reprinted, by permission, from Katherine Berg.

Timed Up and Go

This quick screening test was established to detect balance and mobility problems in older people (Podsiadlo & Richardson, 1991).

Setup: Mark a 3 m (10 ft) distance from a chair.

Procedure:

1. The patient should perform the test with her or his usual assistive device.

2. Starting position: The patient is seated.

3. Use this instruction: "Stand up from the chair, walk to the mark, turn at your normal pace, and return to sitting back in the chair."

4. Observe and time the patient while he or she rises from an armchair, walks 3 m, turns, walks back, and sits down again.

5. Allow one practice test and then record the average of three trials (in seconds).

6. The final score is the average of the three trials.

Scoring categories: The scoring categories are not specific to people with Parkinson's or those with movement disorders but can be used as a tool to detect change in performance resulting from therapeutic intervention.

Less than 10 s: indicates independence in balance and mobility

20 s to 29 s: indicates increased fall risk

Greater than 30 s: indicates dependence in most ADLs and mobility

Functional Reach

Although functional reach (Duncan et al., 1990) is not a sensitive instrument in detecting fall risk in the Parkinson's population, it can detect improvement after therapeutic interventions. Functional reach deficits can also help guide HEP needs.

Procedure:

- Place a ruler horizontally at shoulder height.
- Patient position: The feet are shoulder-width apart, the arm is raised to 90°, and the hand is in a fisted position.
- Record the starting position of the third metacarpal to the ruler.
- During the test the upper extremity is not allowed to touch the wall or measuring device.
- Use this instruction: "Reach forward as far as possible without losing your balance or taking a step."
- Record the end position of the third metacarpal to the ruler.
- Measure the difference between the starting and ending positions.

Leg Strength

Leg strength is important for mobility and balance. The chair stand test can measure deficits. The patient's test results can be compared with norms for goal setting and monitoring progress (see table B.1, Norms for Chair Stand Test by Age and Sex).

Chair Stand Test Procedure and Norms

This test is from Rickli & Jones, 2001.

- **Equipment**: Stopwatch and folding chair with a seat height of 17 in. (43 cm). The chair is placed against a wall to prevent tipping.
- **Starting position**: Sitting in the middle of the chair with a straight back, feet on the floor, and arms crossed at the wrist and held against the chest (see figure B.1).
- **Instructions**: On the command "Go," the patient rises to a full stand and then returns to a seated position. The patient should perform one or two practice repetitions to ensure understanding. The patient is encouraged to perform as many repetitions as possible in 30 s but should stop if she or he experiences any pain. Reinforce rising to a full stance and touching the buttocks to the chair before starting another repetition.
- **Scoring**: The score is the total number of stands completed in 30 s. If the person is more than halfway up at the end of 30 s, the movement counts as a full stand.

- **Safety tips**: Brace the chair against a wall; spot for balance problems; immediately stop the test if the patient complains of pain.
- **Adaptations**: If the patient is not able to perform any repetitions, the test score would be 0 repetitions in 30 s. The test could be modified to enable the patient to perform a timed test and establish a baseline.

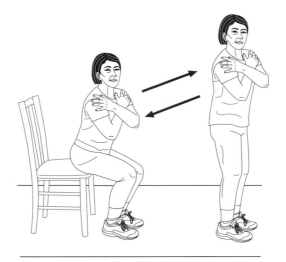

Figure B.1 The chair stand test.

Table B.1 Norms for Chair Stand Test by Age and Sex

Age	Women	Men
60–64	12–17 repetitions	14–19 repetitions
65–69	11–16 repetitions	12–18 repetitions
70–74	10–15 repetitions	12–17 repetitions
75–79	10–15 repetitions	11–17 repetitions
80–84	9 –14 repetitions	10–15 repetitions
85–89	8 –13 repetitions	8–14 repetitions
90–94	4–11 repetitions	7–12 repetitions

Adapted, by permission, from R.E. Rikle and C. Jones, 2001, *Senior fitness test manual* (Champaign, IL: Human Kinetics, 87).

Table B.2 Female Walking Velocity Norms by Age

Age	Meters per second (m/sec)	Meters per minute (m/min)	Miles per hour (mph)*	Kilometers per hour (km/h)*
60–64	1.52 m/sec	91.2 m/min	3.40 mph	5.47 km/h
65–69	1.43 m/sec	85.8 m/min	3.20 mph	5.15 km/h
70–74	1.38 m/sec	82.8 m/min	3.09 mph	4.97 km/h
75–79	1.29 m/sec	77.4 m/min	2.89 mph	4.65 km/h
80–84	1.17 m/sec	70.2 m/min	2.62 mph	4.22 km/h
85–89	1.08 m/sec	64.8 m/min	2.42 mph	3.89 km/h
90–94	0.90 m/sec	54.0 m/min	2.01 mph	3.23 km/h

*Rounded to the nearest hundredth.
Adapted, by permission, from R.E. Rickle and C. Jones, 2001, *Senior fitness test manual* (Champaign, IL: Human Kinetics).

Table B.3 Male Walking Velocity Norms by Age

Age	Meters per second (m/sec)	Meters per minute (m/min)	Miles per hour (mph)*	Kilometers per hour (km/h)*
60–64	1.70 m/sec	102.0 m/min	3.80 mph	6.11 km/h
65–69	1.59 m/sec	95.4 m/min	3.56 mph	5.73 km/h
70–74	1.55 m/sec	93.0 m/min	3.47 mph	5.58 km/h
75–79	1.40 m/sec	84.0 m/min	3.13 mph	5.04 km/h
80–84	1.32 m/sec	79.2 m/min	2.95 mph	4.75 km/h
85–89	1.20 m/sec	72.0 m/min	2.68 mph	4.31 km/h
90–94	1.02 m/sec	61.2 m/min	2.28 mph	3.67 km/h

*Rounded to the nearest hundredth.
Adapted, by permission, from R.E. Rickle and C. Jones, 2001, *Senior fitness test manual* (Champaign, IL: Human Kinetics).

Documentation

CONTENTS

Documentation as a whole, from the time of the evaluation process to the writing of progress notes for follow-up visits, can be challenging when treating specialized populations such as people with PD. The questions asked, the tests given or performed, and the interventions performed often necessitate additional considerations. These considerations address impairments and dysfunction specific to the PD population such as "on" state versus "off" state mobility, dyskinesias, freezing, impairment of postural reflexes, and DBS. All documentation in this appendix is intended to be used as a guide and can be reproduced for the use of those who bought this book. The suggestions in these samples were developed from years of personal experience with the PD population.

Subjective Evaluation

A thorough subjective exam can produce many insights into the causes of imbalance, mobility problems, and caregiver needs. The subjective evaluation for people with PD is unique in that this population may or may not experience motor fluctuations in response to L-dopa medication. If a person with PD is being seen for musculoskeletal problems and heat or electrical modalities are being considered, establish whether the person has an implanted deep brain stimulator. Many of these modalities are either contraindicated or require precautionary considerations. Information provided here in parentheses is intended for instructional or educational purposes for the therapist to facilitate accurate communication or understanding. This portion of the evaluation form is intended to be used as a guide to unveil the unique symptoms of this population.

Pain: Does pain limit you from your activities or sleeping?   ☐ no;   ☐ yes

Patient medical history: _____

Medications: _____

Precautions: _____

Home environment

1. Do you live alone or with others?

   ☐ alone;   ☐ with spouse or significant other;   ☐ family;

   ☐ caregiver: ___ h/d, ___ d/wk

2. What type of home do you live in?

   ☐ single-level home;   ☐ apartment or condominium;

   ☐ multilevel home;   ☐ two-level home;   ☐ basement;

   ☐ other _____

3. Stairs?

   Interior: ___ no; ___ yes

   ☐ no railing;   ☐ railing on one side;   ☐ railing on both sides;

   ☐ elevator

   Exterior: ___ no; ___ yes; number of steps _____

   ☐ no railing;   ☐ railing on one side;   ☐ railing on both sides

Current level of function

1. Do you have difficulties with getting in and out of bed?

   ☐ no;   ☐ yes: ☐ sometimes;   ☐ all the time;

   ☐ no assistance needed;

   ☐ assistance needed: ☐ sometimes;   ☐ always

2. Do you have difficulties with getting in and out of a chair?

☐ no; ☐ yes: ☐ sometimes; ☐ all the time;

☐ no assistance needed;

☐ assistance needed: ☐ sometimes; ☐ always

3. Do you need assistance or use an assist device for walking?

☐ no; ☐ yes: ☐ straight cane; ☐ quad cane; ☐ pickup walker;

☐ two-wheeled walker; ☐ three-wheeled walker;

☐ four-wheeled walker; ☐ weighted walker; ☐ wheelchair;

☐ assistance of another person

4. If the answer to question #3 is yes, when do you need assistance or the use of an assist device?

☐ during "off" times; ☐ at night; ☐ outdoors only;

☐ all the time

5. Do you own any assistive devices?

☐ no; ☐ yes: ☐ straight cane; ☐ quad cane; ☐ pickup walker;

☐ two-wheeled walker; ☐ three-wheeled walker;

☐ four-wheeled walker; ☐ weighted walker; ☐ wheelchair

Subjective information related to balance and falls

1. Do you feel unsteady while standing in one spot? (This may be an indication of postural instability or orthostatic hypotension.)

☐ no; ☐ yes: ☐ rarely; ☐ frequently; ☐ all the time

Onset: ☐ recent; ☐ chronic

2. Do you feel unsteady while walking? (If yes, reasons can be multifactorial.)

☐ no; ☐ yes: ☐ rarely; ☐ frequently; ☐ all the time

Onset: ☐ recent; ☐ chronic

3. Do you have difficulty turning while walking?

☐ no; ☐ occasionally; ☐ frequently

4. Have you had any loss of balance in the past 6 mo? (Describe loss of balance or near fall to the patient and differentiate from an actual fall.)

☐ no; ☐ yes: Frequency _____

Direction of loss of balance:

☐ forward; ☐ backward; ☐ left; ☐ right; ☐ inconsistent

Causes of loss of balance:

☐ tripping; ☐ turning; ☐ rushing; ☐ freezing; ☐ reaching;

☐ when fatigued; ☐ when distracted; ☐ when "on"; ☐ when "off"

5. Have you had any falls in the past 12 mo? (Describe what a fall is. Two or more falls in the past 12 mo indicates an increased risk of falls. See chapter 8, "Balance Evaluation").

☐ no; ☐ yes: Frequency _____

Direction of falls:

☐ forward; ☐ backward; ☐ left; ☐ right; ☐ inconsistent

Causes of falls:

☐ tripping; ☐ turning; ☐ rushing; ☐ freezing; ☐ reaching;

☐ when fatigued; ☐ when distracted; ☐ when "on"; ☐ when "off"

6. Do you need help getting up from the floor (regardless of a fall)?

☐ no; ☐ sometimes; ☐ all the time;

☐ don't know; haven't been on the floor

Subjective information related to Levodopa

1. Are you taking Levodopa (Sinemet, Madopar, Sinemet CR, or Stalevo)?

☐ yes; ☐ no

2. Do you experience "wearing off" symptoms? (Does a predictable gradual worsening of Parkinson's symptoms occur before the next medication dose?)

☐ yes; ☐ no; ☐ NA if not taking L-dopa

3. Do you experience "on-off" symptoms? (Do the effects of Levodopa become more erratic and unrelated to the medication cycle? Is the exacerbation of Parkinsonian symptoms abrupt and unpredictable?)

☐ yes; ☐ no; ☐ NA if not taking L-dopa

4. Do you freeze? (Define freezing to patient and demonstrate if necessary.)

☐ no; ☐ yes: when? _____

☐ start hesitation; ☐ turning; ☐ narrow spaces;

☐ destination hesitation; ☐ thresholds; ☐ rushing; ☐ walking;

☐ "on" freezing; ☐ "off" freezing; ☐ change in floor surfaces

5. During evaluation patient is reportedly

☐ "on"; ☐ "off"

☐ NA if not taking dopamine replacement medication or not experiencing motor fluctuations

Subjective information related to fear of falling

1. Are you concerned about losing your balance or falling?

☐ never; ☐ sometimes; ☐ most of the time; ☐ always

Subjective information related to physical health awareness and maintenance

1. Exercise program

   Stretching?

   ☐ no;   ☐ yes: frequency _____

   Strengthening?

   ☐ no;   ☐ yes: frequency _____

   Walking?

   ☐ no;   ☐ yes: distance _____ or time _____; frequency _____

   Other activities: _____

   Comments: _____

From M. Boelen, 2009, *Health Professionals' Guide to Physical Management of Parkinson's Disease* (Champaign, IL: Human Kinetics).

Objective Evaluation

As with the subjective evaluation, this portion of the evaluation is intended to be used as a guide.

1. **Posture**
   - **Forward head posture:**
     ☐ within normal limits for age; ☐ minimal; ☐ moderate;
     ☐ severe or drop-head posture
   - **Forward trunk leaning:**
     ☐ minimal; ☐ moderate; ☐ severe or camptocormic posture
   - **Thoracic kyphosis:**
     ☐ normal for patient's age; ☐ moderate; ☐ severe
   - **Scoliosis:**
     ☐ mild; ☐ moderate; ☐ severe; ☐ thoracic L/R; ☐ lumbar L/R;
     ☐ S curve; ☐ C curve
   - **Flexed knees:**
     ☐ minimal; ☐ moderate; ☐ severe
   - **Is forward posture compensatory to prevent backward LOB?**
     ☐ yes; ☐ no; ☐ NA; ☐ unable to determine

   Comments_____

   _____

2. **Abnormal tone or movements**
   ☐ **Rigidity:**
     ___ mild; ___ moderate; ___ severe; Location _____
   ☐ **Dyskinetic:**
     ___ mild; ___ moderate; ___ severe; Location _____
   ☐ **Tremor:**
     ___ mild; ___ moderate; ___ severe; Location _____
   ☐ **Dystonia:**
     ___ mild; ___ moderate; ___ severe; Location _____

   Interference with functional activities _____

   _____

3. **Strength deficits** _____

   _____

   _____

4. ROM (only deficits noted)

☐ **Cervical limitations:**
___ rotation L/R;   ___ retraction;   ___ sidebending L/R

☐ **Trunk limitations:**
___ rotation L/R;   ___ lumbar flexion;   ___ extension

☐ **Hip limitations:**
___ extension L/R;   ___ abduction L/R;   ___ flexion L/R

☐ **Ankle limitations:**
___ dorsiflexion L/R;   ___ eversion L/R;   ___ plantarflexion L/R

☐ **Shoulder limitations:**
___ internal rotation L/R;   ___ external rotation L/R;
___ extension L/R;   ___ flexion L/R;   ___ horizontal abduction L/R

Comments_____

_____

5. Bed Mobility

- **Rolling**
  ☐ independent;   ☐ performs with difficulty;   ☐ requires ___ assist
- **Supine to sitting**
  ☐ independent;   ☐ performs with difficulty;   ☐ requires ___ assist
- **Sit to supine**
  ☐ independent;   ☐ performs with difficulty;   ☐ requires ___ assist

Chair transfers

- **Sit to stand**
  ☐ able, uses arms to help;   ☐ requires > 1 attempt;
  ☐ requires ___ assist;   ☐ able, without arms
- **Stand to sit**
  ☐ unsafe (misjudges distance, falls into chair);   ☐ requires ___ assist;
  ☐ uses arms or not a smooth motion;   ☐ safe, smooth motion
- **Immediate standing balance**
  ☐ unsteady _____;   ☐ steady without support;
  ☐ steady with walker
- **Chair stand test**
  Repeated sit to stand without upper-extremity support from seat
  height 17 in. (43 cm): patient is able to perform _____ repetitions
  in 30 s.

  Modifications: _____

  (Refer to appendix B for chair stand test procedure and norms.)

- **Gait**
  - ☐ narrow based; ☐ wide based; ☐ freezing; ☐ festination;
  - ☐ ataxic; ☐ weaving: __ L __ R; ☐ reduced ground clearance: __ L __ R;
  - ☐ reduced stride length; __ L __ R; ☐ reduced trunk rotation;
  - ☐ reduced arm swing: __ L __ R; ☐ reduced heel strike: __ L __ R;
  - ☐ Trendelenburg: pelvis drop: __ L _ R; ☐ other _____
  - Assistive device: _____
  - Gait velocity is ___ m/s or ___ m/min.
  - Gait velocity is ___ % of age- and sex-matched norms.

  (Refer to appendix B for walking velocity norms.)

- **Turning technique during ambulation**
  - ☐ normal; ☐ multistep; ☐ pivotal; ☐ freezing; ☐ narrow based;
  - ☐ guarded; ☐ right turn with reduced advancement of left foot;
  - ☐ left turn with reduced advancement of right foot; ☐ rushing; ☐ unstable

6. Balance

a. Postural reflexes (pull tests need a perturbation of sufficient force to cause loss of balance). See chapter 7, "Postural Instability," for procedure.

1. Unexpected pull test (retropulsive perturbation):
   - ☐ normal, may take two steps to recover;
   - ☐ takes three or more steps, recovers unaided;
   - ☐ would fall if not caught;
   - ☐ spontaneous tendency to fall or unable to stand unaided (test not executable)

   OR
   - ☐ push and release test;
   - ☐ recovers independently with one step of normal length and width;
   - ☐ two to three small steps backward but recovers independently;
   - ☐ four or more steps backward but recovers independently;
   - ☐ steps but needs to be assisted to prevent a fall;
   - ☐ falls without attempting a step or unable to stand without assistance

2. Lateral waist pull:
   - ☐ normal, recovers unaided; ☐ lack of trunk righting;
   - ☐ crossover step; ☐ delay in step initiation;
   - ☐ underscaled step; ☐ no step, needs to be caught

b. Lateral perturbations while walking with or without assist device:
_____

  ☐ steady;   ☐ unsteady but able to self-recover;
  ☐ unsteady, needs assist

c. Select balance tests as appropriate: _____

  ☐ Berg balance score (BBS) _____ /56;
  ☐ timed up and go (TUG) _____ s;
  ☐ functional reach ___ in. or ___ cm;
  ☐ tandem stance ___ s;
  ☐ single-leg stance ___ s;
  ☐ retrowalking: ___ steady; ___ guarded; ___ retropulsion; ___ needs to be caught

Comments _____

From M. Boelen, 2009, *Health Professionals' Guide to Physical Management of Parkinson's Disease* (Champaign, IL: Human Kinetics).

Sample Goals

Circle the numbered goals that apply and check the applicable boxes in that goal.

HEP and Conditioning

1. The patient will demonstrate independence and understanding of a home exercise program (with or without assistance) to improve (independence of a home exercise program is critical for long-term benefits):

    ☐ lower-extremity strength;

    ☐ flexibility: ___ axial; ___ lower extremities; ___ upper extremities;

    ☐ balance;   ☐ flexibility and strength of postural muscles

2. The patient will demonstrate improvement in lower-extremity conditioning and reduced fall risk with improved chair stand test performance from ___ reps in 30 s to ___ reps without upper-extremity support. (The norm for the patient's age- and sex-matched control is ___ reps in 30 s.)

Bed Mobility

1. The patient or caregiver will verbalize or demonstrate decreased difficulty with bed mobility requiring _____ assist:

    ☐ with bed assist rail;   ☐ without bed assist rail

Chair Transfers

1. The patient will demonstrate improved body mechanics to decrease difficulty with sit to stand:

    ☐ able to stand up on first attempt: ___ with arms; ___ without arms

    ☐ able to stand up with ___ minimal; ___ moderate; ___ maximal assist

2. The patient will safely and consistently back up to the chair before sitting to prevent falls.

3. The patient will exhibit improved balance control from stand to sit with or without upper-extremity support (will minimize falling backward into the chair).

Gait

1. The patient will verbalize or demonstrate improved control of freezing with the following triggers to reduce fall risk and improve mobility:

    ☐ start hesitation;   ☐ turning;   ☐ narrow spaces;

    ☐ destination hesitation;   ☐ thresholds;   ☐ rushing;   ☐ walking;

    ☐ "on" freezing;   ☐ "off" freezing;   ☐ change in floor surfaces

2. The patient will improve in the Freezing of Gait Questionnaire from ___ to ___.

3. The patient will improve gait velocity for functional ambulation from ___ m/s to ___ m/s. (The age- and sex-matched norm is ___ m/s.)

4. The patient will improve stability with turns by demonstrating

   ☐ reduced occurrence of pivoting;

   ☐ improved advancement of the left foot with right turns;

   ☐ improved advancement of the right foot with left turns;

   ☐ reduced rushing

5. The patient will demonstrate understanding of how to use the ambulatory assist device properly and safely in the following conditions:

   ☐ turning;   ☐ braking;   ☐ walking within the parameters of the device; ascending and descending curbs;

   ☐ ascending and descending ramps

Floor Transfers

The patient or caregiver will demonstrate understanding of floor transfer technique:

☐ independently;   ☐ with minimal assist;   ☐ with moderate assist;

☐ with maximal assist

Shoes

The patient will verbalize understanding of how footwear can affect balance.

Balance

1. The patient will demonstrate understanding of a staggered stance position to improve stability with static standing.

2. The patient will be able to perform a stepping strategy in response to a loss of balance to reduce the risk of falls.

3. The reduction in fall risk will be demonstrated by improvement in the following balance test performances:

   ☐ Berg balance score (BBS) ___ /56;   ☐ timed up and go (TUG) ___ s;

   ☐ functional reach ___ in. or ___ cm;   ☐ tandem stance ___ s;

   ☐ single-leg stance ___ s

From M. Boelen, 2009, *Health Professionals' Guide to Physical Management of Parkinson's Disease* (Champaign, IL: Human Kinetics).

Sample Progress Note

This abbreviated version of a sample progress note is intended to offer ideas for verbiage of interventions. The form is not all inclusive, but it covers the more common areas unique to the Parkinson's population. The patient's level of function and responses to treatment, although not always mentioned in this sample, should be noted with any intervention. Where appropriate, caregiver involvement should be incorporated (gait or transfers).

Subject: _____

Objective:

Balance and Compensatory Strategies

- Base of support (BOS)—reviewed with the patient how to improve anterior–posterior steadiness with standing activities by increasing the base of support with a staggered foot stance.
- Compensatory stepping strategy
  - Reviewed with the patient a compensatory stepping response in the following directions:
    ☐ posterior;   ☐ anterior;   ☐ lateral
  - Induced stepping responses were
    ☐ effective in balance recovery;   ☐ underscaled or overscaled;
    ☐ inconsistent;   ☐ delayed;
    ☐ ineffective, requiring assist for fall prevention;   ☐ absent

Ambulation

- Attention strategies

  Attention strategies to improve stride length and symmetry of gait were reviewed with the patient. Optimal attention strategy is
    ☐ heel down first;   ☐ taking long steps;   ☐ counting steps;
    ☐ exaggeration of lateral weight shifting;
    ☐ NA if no improvement noted

- Freezing

  Reviewed and practiced with patient antifreezing strategies targeting the following triggers:
    ☐ start hesitation;   ☐ turns;   ☐ narrow spaces;
    ☐ destination hesitation;   ☐ thresholds

- Rhythmic auditory stimulation (RAS)

  Gait training with _____ (assist device) facilitated by rhythmic auditory stimulation at the following beats per minute (BPM) _____ and requiring _____ assist. Optimal entrainment noted at _____ BPM. Endurance _____.

- Vitals
  - Resting blood pressure and heart rate when sitting: _____
  - Blood pressure and heart rate after ambulation: _____
  - Rate of perceived exertion (RPE) after ambulating: _____
- Walker instruction

  Reviewed and practiced proper use of handbrakes for

  □ velocity control;   □ freezing episodes—"squeeze when you freeze";

  □ use of locking mechanism when using walker seat;

  □ ramps and sloped surfaces
- Turns

  Instructed and practiced the patient in proper turning strategies while ambulating with emphasis on

  □ advancement of the outside foot;   □ turning in narrow spaces;

  □ avoidance of pivoting;   □ staying close to the walker during turns;

  □ turning with the walker as a unit (four-wheeled walker);

  □ proper sequencing of the walker and foot placement (two-wheeled or pickup)
- Footwear

  Reviewed with the patient proper shoe wear—a low-friction sole to reduce the possibility of the feet sticking or catching.

Transfer Training

- Chair transfers
  - Sit to stand: Instructed the patient in proper body mechanics to reduce difficulties (scooting to the edge of the chair, foot placement, leaning forward).
  - Stand to sit: Instructed the patient in body mechanics to improve safety and prevent backward loss of balance (reaching for armrests, leaning forward, attempting to sit in the back part of the seat, and relaxing the knees).
  - Chair approach: Reviewed and practiced with the patient various angles of approaching chairs to minimize turns (i.e., approaching a chair directly, requiring a 180° turn, versus approaching from the side, requiring a 90° turn).
- Bed mobility
  - Instructed the patient in log rolling and side lying to sitting.
  - Instructed the patient in using a bed assist rail to facilitate rolling, sitting up, and lying down.
  - Instructed the caregiver in assisting the patient with bed mobility.

- Floor transfers
  - Instructed the patient in floor transfers with and without the support of furniture or external support.
  - Instructed the caregiver in how to assist the patient safely during floor transfers.
  - Advised the patient and caregiver of the benefits of a medical alert system.

Assessment: _____

Plan: _____

From M. Boelen, 2009, *Health Professionals' Guide to Physical Management of Parkinson's Disease* (Champaign, IL: Human Kinetics).

Patient Handouts and Interventions

CONTENTS

This appendix is intended to provide the tools needed for interventions. The patient handouts in this appendix are reproducible. The "Problem-Oriented Treatment Interventions" section offers a quick reference for interventions based on problem areas.

Can Therapy Help Me?

A person with Parkinson's who answers yes to any of these questions should obtain a referral from his or her doctor for the appropriate therapist. The patient should check with the insurance company to ensure coverage and make an appointment with a therapist who is knowledgeable about Parkinson's.

Physical Therapy

- ☐ Do you experience difficulties with moving in bed or getting out of a chair?
- ☐ Do you feel unsteady while standing, walking, or turning?
- ☐ Are you stopping yourself from being more active because you feel unsteady?
- ☐ Is it difficult for you to catch your balance?
- ☐ Have you fallen or have you experienced great difficulty in getting up from the floor?
- ☐ Do your feet tend to stutter or stick to the ground?
- ☐ Do you want to learn how to stay in optimal shape?

Occupational Therapy

- ☐ Are you having problems with your handwriting?
- ☐ Do you have trouble using utensils when eating?
- ☐ Do you have difficulty or require assistance with bathing or dressing?
- ☐ Are you fearful or unsteady when stepping in or out of your tub or getting on or off your toilet?
- ☐ Have you had any falls in your home?
- ☐ Do you have difficulty engaging in your favorite leisure activities or hobbies?

Speech Therapy

- ☐ Have you had recurring pneumonia or chest congestion?
- ☐ Do you cough or clear your throat when you are eating?
- ☐ Do you feel food or pills getting stuck in your throat?
- ☐ Do you have problems with drooling?
- ☐ Do you require extra time to eat, or does food get stuck in your mouth or cheeks?
- ☐ Do people ask you to repeat yourself or speak up?
- ☐ Have you noticed that you are mumbling, have a soft voice, or speak in monotone?
- ☐ Have you noticed problems with your memory?
- ☐ Do you have trouble concentrating?

From M. Boelen, 2009, *Health Professionals' Guide to Physical Management of Parkinson's Disease* (Champaign, IL: Human Kinetics). Reprinted, by permission, from J. Holt.

Freezing

Freezing is often described as the feet sticking to the ground. Its frequency and severity vary from one person to another. Aggravating factors that cause freezing also vary from one person to another.

If you are freezing try the following:

Stop attempting to take any steps.

Lean to one side long enough to allow the opposite foot to take a step and start walking.

If you are freezing because of your posture try the following:

First, correct your posture.

Then lean to one side long enough to allow the opposite foot to take a step and start walking.

Besides the previous recommendations, one of these maneuvers may further help to break a freeze. See which one works best for you.

1. Take one step backward before starting to walk forward.
2. March in place before starting to walk.
3. Take a step sideways before starting to walk forward.
4. Step over a marking on the floor.

Tip: You will be more successful if you do not rush.

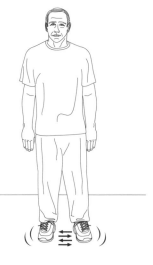

a

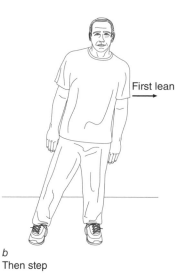

First lean

b
Then step

From M. Boelen, 2009, *Health Professionals' Guide to Physical Management of Parkinson's Disease* (Champaign, IL: Human Kinetics).

Attention Strategies—
Options to Make Walking Less Difficult

Walking can become difficult at times because one foot or both feet are not moving as they should. Walking may not be as automatic as it was in the past, so you need to concentrate on taking larger steps or picking up your feet to avoid tripping. The following options are suggestions to make walking easier and safer. Use the option that works best for you.

Option #1

Count the number of steps that you need to reach a destination. For example, if you are walking from the kitchen to the living room, count the number of steps that it takes to travel that distance. For longer distances count up to a certain number, say 30. When you hit 30, start over with 1.

- If only one foot is giving you a problem, then count only the steps that you take with that foot. For example, suppose that your left foot is the uncooperative foot. Your left foot takes a step, and you count "1." Your right foot takes a step, and you don't count. Your left foot takes a step, and you count "2." Your right foot takes a step, and you don't count, and so on.
- If both feet are giving you a problem, then count every time you take a step. For example, your left foot takes a step, and you count "1." Your right foot takes a step, and you count "2." Your left foot takes a step, and you count "3," and so on.

Option #2

Take long steps. Attempt to establish a rhythm as you are walking by repeatedly thinking "take long steps." Practice this deliberately as an exercise on a daily basis.

Option #3

"Heel down first." At times you may be able to take longer steps and pick up your foot more if you attempt to get your heel down first as you take a step. Mentally repeat this phrase.

Option #4

Attempt to shift your weight more to the left and right as you walk. Walk like a penguin.

Option#5

Walk to music with a rhythm that matches your walking pace.

From M. Boelen, 2009, *Health Professionals' Guide to Physical Management of Parkinson's Disease* (Champaign, IL: Human Kinetics).

Medical Alert Systems

Candidates for medical alert systems:

- A person who lives alone and is at risk of falling
- A person who does not live alone but is at risk of falling and is alone for periods during the day or night
- A person who is unable to get up from the floor even with the assistance of a family member or caregiver

How Does a Medical Alert System Work?

You wear a wristband or a necklace with a push button at all times. The push button device is waterproof so that you can wear it in the shower or while washing dishes. If you fall and are unable to get up from the floor, you push the button. The service will call you on a special phone that also acts as an intercom. The service will talk to you to assess the situation and send help to your home. The system can relieve stress because you know that help is available.

Who Offers Medical Alert Systems?

The following organizations offer these services.

American Red Cross: check local listing
Lifeline: www.LifelineSystems.com, 800-543-3546
Medical Alert: http://medicalalarm.com, 800-588-0200
AlertOne: www.Alert-1.com, 800-882-2280
Lifefone: www.lifefone.com, 800-330-5909

From M. Boelen, 2009, *Health Professionals' Guide to Physical Management of Parkinson's Disease* (Champaign, IL: Human Kinetics).

Recommendations for People With Hypotension

- When first getting out of bed in the morning, change positions slowly because blood pressure can drop significantly at this time.
- If taking medication for hypotension, place it on the nightstand so that you can take it before getting out of bed in the morning.
- Place both feet on the ground when first sitting on the edge of the bed (do not let your feet dangle), perform ankle pumps, and pause before standing up.
- Large meals, especially those high in refined carbohydrates, can cause drops in blood pressure. Therefore, attempt to eat smaller meals that are not rich in refined carbohydrates. Limit activities immediately after a meal.
- Increase fluid intake to avoid dehydration.
- Know what triggers your symptoms and have a plan of action. For example, if you feel lightheaded while standing, sit immediately. If no place to sit is available, squat and press on your abdomen. Lean against a wall for added support.
- Avoid prolonged static standing. Sit when getting dressed, preparing a meal, or ironing. Use a bathtub bench when showering if needed.
- Avoid bending down. Use wheeled laundry baskets that are higher off the ground. When performing yard work have a lawn chair nearby so that you can go from a kneeling position to sitting before standing all the way up.
- Elevate the head of the bed by using either a wedge or leg extensions at the head of the bed.
- Avoid constipation because straining can result in feeling lightheaded.
- Try to stay cool.
  - Take warm showers instead of hot showers.
  - Take advantage of fans or air conditioning during the hot months of the year.

From M. Boelen, 2009, *Health Professionals' Guide to Physical Management of Parkinson's Disease* (Champaign, IL: Human Kinetics).

Staggered Standing

Purpose: To improve steadiness and prevent a loss of balance while standing. You do this by increasing your base of support. The steadiest foot position is with your feet shoulder-width apart and one foot somewhat ahead of the other.

Use option #2 or #3 when

standing and talking to someone,

waiting for an elevator,

opening a door,

picking up something from the floor,

reaching in a cabinet or closet, or

standing in line.

Option #1—not optimal

This foot position is wider than a natural stance position. It will not protect you from losing your balance forward or backward, but it will increase steadiness to the left and right.

Option #2—to prevent forward loss of balance

This foot position is wider than a natural stance position. One foot is somewhat ahead of the other (far enough to feel steady). This position is more stabilizing for people who are unsteady in the forward direction. Some people may be steadier with the right foot forward, and others may be steadier with the left foot forward.

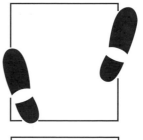

Option #3—to prevent backward loss of balance

This foot position is also wider than a natural stance position. One foot is somewhat ahead of the other (far enough to feel steady). You will have greater stability in the backward direction by placing your feet in a parallel position so that the heels are farther apart.

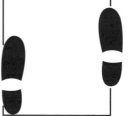

From M. Boelen, 2009, *Health Professionals' Guide to Physical Management of Parkinson's Disease* (Champaign, IL: Human Kinetics).

Standing Up From a Chair

Purpose:

1. To reduce difficulty with getting out of a chair
2. To improve steadiness when initially standing

Positioning:

- First, scoot to the edge of the chair.
- Slide your feet back under your knees (slide one foot farther back to increase steadiness with initial standing).
- Lean forward with your shoulders. Doing so is important and will help your balance.
- Stand up.

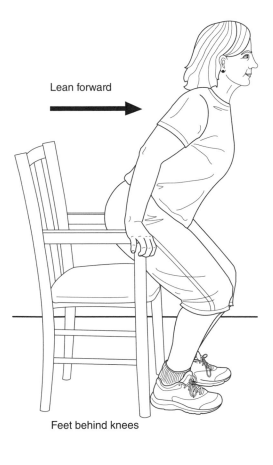

Lean forward

Feet behind knees

From M. Boelen, 2009, *Health Professionals' Guide to Physical Management of Parkinson's Disease* (Champaign, IL: Human Kinetics).

Turning While Walking

At times people become unsteady while turning because the foot on the out-side of the circle tends to lag behind the inside foot. As a result the legs become tangled. A simple rule is to avoid letting the outside foot lag behind. Taking a step that is too large can also cause unsteadiness.

> Left turns: Take a bigger step with your right foot so that it just passes your inside foot.
>
> Right turns: Take a bigger step with your left foot so that it just passes your inside foot.

General tips to be steadier

> Slow down on your turns (as you would when driving a car).
>
> Avoid pivoting.
>
> Try to keep your feet apart.
>
> Make a wider turn if practical.

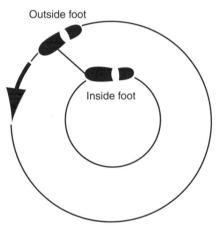

Left turn

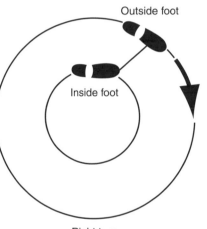

Right turn

From M. Boelen, 2009, *Health Professionals' Guide to Physical Management of Parkinson's Disease* (Champaign, IL: Human Kinetics).

Voluntary Stepping

Purpose: To improve the size and speed of your step so that you do not fall when you lose your balance.

Exercise: Hold on to the kitchen sink or a stable chair.

- Physically and mentally practice taking a quick step in the direction in which you tend to feel unsteady or lose your balance.
- After you have taken a step, shift your weight onto that foot.
- Mentally, you may need to exaggerate your step.
- Practice with one leg until it feels steady and natural. Then repeat with the other leg.
- Step diagonally when focusing on a forward or backward direction. Doing this will make you steadier.

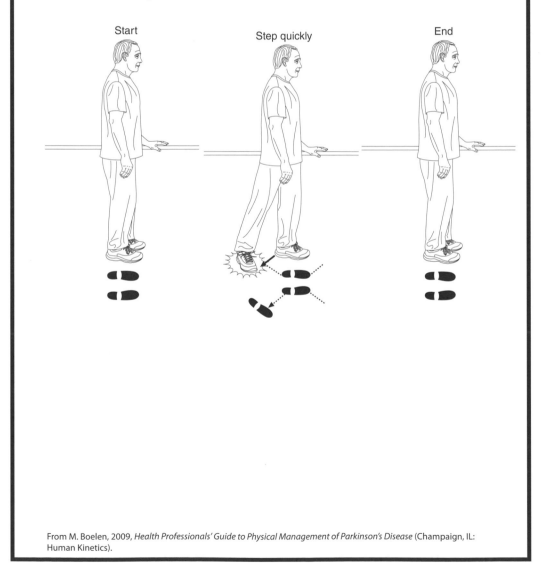

Start   Step quickly   End

From M. Boelen, 2009, *Health Professionals' Guide to Physical Management of Parkinson's Disease* (Champaign, IL: Human Kinetics).

What to Do After a Fall

1. Do not try to get up right away.

2. Before attempting to get up, mentally note whether any areas feel injured. Any suspicion of injury requires medical attention.

3. Attempt to relax for a moment before getting up.

4. If you are in your "off" medication state and not very mobile, wait until medications are working before getting up. If you are not alone, someone can make you comfortable with a pillow in the meantime.

5. Before you attempt to get up, someone should bring a chair close to you so that you can use it for support to get up.

6. An additional chair could be placed behind you before you get up if you have difficulty turning. After you are standing, you can sit on the chair without having to turn.

From M. Boelen, 2009, *Health Professionals' Guide to Physical Management of Parkinson's Disease* (Champaign, IL: Human Kinetics).

Problem-Oriented Treatment Interventions

The following lists address various treatment interventions for specific areas of need. They are a brief synopsis of interventions covered in this book. More detailed information can be obtained by referring to the relevant chapters. Treatment interventions are not all inclusive but encompass those that I have found to be commonly used or effective.

Conditioning and Prevention

Treatment Interventions

Exercises should target impairments or potential impairments (areas of increased rigidity). Minimize the number of exercises by addressing more than one impairment with each exercise.

Functional exercises such as repeated sit to stands can be more rewarding and may increase adherence.

Incorporate speed with lower-extremity exercises for power strength and balance.

Emphasize lifetime conditioning. Maintaining fitness is the patient's responsibility. The target for ambulation is 30 min daily.

Have the patient exercise when Parkinson's medications are working or during the "on" time for optimal results.

Use visual or tactile targets to maximize motion as needed.

Bed Mobility

Treatment Interventions

Review bed mobility with a bed transfer rail to minimize sequential movements and difficulty with rolling and side lying to and from sitting.

An open armchair next to the bed is another option.

Review with the caregiver and patient optimal body mechanics to minimize caregiver back strain.

Suggest that the patient use satin sheets or satin pajamas but not both.

Blanket support or lightweight covers can decrease problems with lower-extremity mobility.

From M. Boelen, 2009, *Health Professionals' Guide to Physical Management of Parkinson's Disease* (Champaign, IL: Human Kinetics).

(continued)

Chair Transfers

Table D.1   Treatment Interventions

Sequence and body mechanics	Review and break down the sequence and body mechanics of the sit-to-stand movement. 1. Scoot to the edge of the chair to allow proper foot placement. 2. Slide feet back (place one foot farther back for greater stability when initially standing). 3. Lean forward before and during the liftoff phase of standing up. Repetition of this activity facilitates learning.
Leaning forward	1. The therapist or caregiver can facilitate the action by placing a hand over the upper back to maintain forward leaning during liftoff or to prevent falling back into the chair when sitting down. 2. Supportive objects (such as a walker) may help with forward leaning because they can increase confidence. 3. Visual triggers (such as a coffee table in front of a couch) may impede leaning forward. Remove the visual trigger.
Seat height	Vary seat height to enable a successful attempt to move from sitting to standing.
Turning arc	When approaching a chair, the patient can reduce the turning arc from 180° to 90° by approaching from the side.
Friction	The patient can change clothing fabric or seat cushion fabric to reduce friction.

From M. Boelen, 2009, *Health Professionals' Guide to Physical Management of Parkinson's Disease* (Champaign, IL: Human Kinetics).

(continued)

Gait

Table D.2 Treatment Interventions

Freezing	Lateral weight shifts need to be accentuated and maintained to allow an effective initial step.
	Have the patient practice antifreezing strategies. Target precipitating factors. Issue the handout on antifreezing strategies.
	Use visual cues for "off" freezing and start hesitation.
	Perform gait training with rhythmic auditory stimulation (RAS) and practice precipitating factors.
Stride length	Use attention strategies to improve stride length for people with mild PD. Issue the handout on optional attention strategies.
	Rhythmic auditory stimulation (RAS) improves stride length and secondarily gait velocity. It is effective for people with PD Hoehn and Yahr stages 1 through 4 and those with cognitive deficits. Issue guidelines about a tailored walking program.
Turning	Use attention strategies when patients practice left and right turns. Patients should go from wide to narrow and take larger steps with the outside foot. Issue the handout on turning strategy.
	Encourage patients to minimize the turning arc when approaching a chair. Instead of making a 180° turn, they can make a 90° turn by approaching from the side.
	To facilitate foot placement, use floor discs to create visual cues.
Improper footwear: feet catching, causing imbalance	Encourage patients to wear shoes with low-friction soles and no ridges. Shoe resurfacing is an option for current shoes.
Ambulatory assist devices	Assess for the safest and most practical ambulatory assist device. Canes can be detrimental because of problems with dual tasking. Walker velocity control is critical for safety. Patient education should focus on the potential to improve endurance and mobility by using the device and as well as improving walking capability.
	Review use of walker brakes 1. before the patient sits on the seat of the walker, 2. for general velocity control on level surfaces and ramps, and 3. to prepare for freezing episodes or onset of gait festination. Use stop-and-go drills with emphasis on squeezing the brakes first and stopping the feet second (observing this sequence prevents the walker from rolling away if the patients freezes). "If you freeze, you squeeze—immediately."
	Depending on the patient's mobility, cognition, and environmental barriers, review going up and down curbs with the walker or cane.
	Have the patient practice turns with the walker. The patient needs to stay within the walker boundaries and turn as a unit with the walker for greatest stability.
Instability on slopes	The patient should walk up and down slopes with each foot passing the other foot, stepping through for increased stability and avoiding a step-to gait.

From M. Boelen, 2009, *Health Professionals' Guide to Physical Management of Parkinson's Disease* (Champaign, IL: Human Kinetics).

(continued)

Gait *(continued)*

Table D.3 Gait Training Strategies When Using a Walker

Problem	Treatment suggestions
The patient walks too far behind the walker because the elbows are fully extended.	The patient should relax the elbows to allow a greater bend. By doing this the patient automatically has to step closer to the walker. Instead of repeatedly telling the person to step into the walker more, gently tap the volar surface of the elbow as needed for a reminder.
During turns the patient tends to turn the walker more quickly than the feet.	Make an analogy between turning in a car and turning with the walker. Passengers turn as a unit with the car, always facing the front of the car. When turning, the patient should try to turn as a unit with the walker.
The patient steps outside the walker during turns.	During turns the patient needs to stand more inside the walker so that the patient and the walker have the same turning circumference.
The patient starts to freeze as the walker keeps rolling forward. The patient then starts to lose balance.	Practice drills for sudden stops. On the cue of "stop," the patient first squeezes the brakes and then stops with the feet. Advise patients to "squeeze when you freeze."
The patient has difficulty with balance control when backing up with the walker.	Have the patient practice backward stepping with the walker. The patient should step back with the brakes on and then roll the walker back without moving the feet.

Floor Transfers

Treatment Interventions

Have the patient practice getting down to and up from the floor with or without the use of a chair for support. Encourage use of the least difficult method. Floor transfers should be reviewed with anyone who is at risk of falls.

Involve the caregiver with transfers to ensure understanding if help is needed. Issue a handout covering optimal methods of floor transfers.

May need to recommend a medical alert system if the patient or caregiver is unable to perform a floor transfer.

From M. Boelen, 2009, *Health Professionals' Guide to Physical Management of Parkinson's Disease* (Champaign, IL: Human Kinetics).

(continued)

Balance

Table D.4 Treatment Interventions

Impaired postural reflexes and stepping strategy	Discuss protective postural reflexes and the need for increased concentrated effort for an effective stepping response.
	Elicit induced stepping with progressive external perturbations to facilitate protective stepping responses. Fine-tune effectiveness with size, location, and speed of stepping. Issue a handout for a voluntary stepping home exercise program.
	Facilitate voluntary self-recovery stepping strategies by reducing base of support surfaces.
Instability with static standing	Instruct in staggered standing positions to increase base of support during static standing activities to increase stability. Issue a patient education handout.
	Review staggered standing positions to improve anterior stability for forward-reaching activities.
	Review staggered standing positions to improve posterior stability for higher-reaching activities.
Impaired balance because of deconditioning	Focus on power strengthening, weight shifting, and reaching activities. Target activities that were deficient in balance testing.

From M. Boelen, 2009, *Health Professionals' Guide to Physical Management of Parkinson's Disease* (Champaign, IL: Human Kinetics).

Glossary

Please note that the definitions of disability and functional limitation are from *Guide to Physical Therapist Practice, 2nd edition*, American Physical Therapy Association, 2001, *Physical Therapy, 81*(1), 9–746.

ablate—Destroy.

activities of daily living (ADLs)—Activities performed on a daily basis for self-care such as getting in or out of a bed or a chair, bathing, dressing, eating, and toileting (see instrumental activities of daily living).

akathisia—An often extremely unpleasant subjective sensation of "inner" restlessness that manifests itself with inability to sit still or remain motionless.

akinesia—The inability to initiate movement resulting from severe bradykinesia and hypokinesia. Akinesia is likely associated with the assumption of fixed postures and can last from seconds to hours.

ankle strategy—A balance strategy seen during quiet standing. The ankle muscles are activated to control anterior–posterior body sway so that the body remains within the limits of the base of support—no change in BOS is necessary to maintain or regain balance (feet-in-place strategy). The axis of motion occurs at the ankles.

anticipatory postural adjustments (APAs)—Activation of the postural muscles that occurs preceding volitional activities to prepare for any destabilizing forces that might upset balance.

arrhythmicity of gait—Inconsistent or variable step lengths.

athetosis—Involuntary slow sinusoidal writhing movements occurring primarily in the distal extremities.

autonomic failure hypotension—A fall in systolic BP below 20 mmHg and diastolic BP below 10 mmHg from baseline (from lying to standing) within 3 min of being in an upright position without a compensatory increase in heart rate.

basal ganglia—Subcortical nuclei in the brain consisting of the striatum (putamen and caudate nucleus), globus pallidus (internal and external segments), subthalamic nucleus, and substantia nigra (pars compacta and pars reticula). The basal ganglia are responsible for the automaticity of learned movements and sequential movements. The primary neurotransmitter is dopamine.

base of support (BOS)—The area of the object in contact with the support surface.

bradykinesia—Slowness of movement and difficulty initiating movement.

bradyphrenia—Slowness of thinking.

cadence—The number of steps per unit of time, typically steps per minute.

camptocormia—A posture characterized by marked anteroflexion of the trunk that increases on walking, disappears in the supine position, and has little or no response to L-dopa. The forward inclination of the trunk needs to be greater than 45° to be considered camptocormic.

catechol-O-methyltransferase (COMT) inhibitors—A class of drugs that inhibits catechol-O-methyltransferase, an enzyme that metabolizes levodopa, from breaking down exogenous levodopa to dopamine outside the CNS and allows higher concentrations to enter the brain.

center of gravity (COG)—The vertical projection of the COM. For example, with static standing the center of gravity falls between the feet.

center of mass (COM)—The point located in the center of the total body mass, established by finding the weighted average of each body segment. The center of mass in adults is at the L5–S1 level.

center of pressure (COP)—During quiet standing, vertical forces are projected from the COM. Each foot has its own COP. The net COP falls between the feet. These forces can be measured through force plates.

choreatic—A rapidly flowing movement that is unpredictable in direction or magnitude.

comorbidities—The combination of all other disease states that occur simultaneously but independently of the primary disease.

cues—Stimuli from the environment (auditory, tactile, or visual) to facilitate movements.

deep brain stimulation (DBS)—Involves the insertion of an electrode into a target site. For the control of Parkinson's symptoms, the target site is either the GPi or STN. The electrode is connected by a subcutaneous extension lead wire to a programmable pulse generator from which it receives the electrical stimulation.

destination hesitation—Freezing that occurs when approaching an object or intended destination.

disability—"The inability to perform or a limitation in the performance of actions, tasks, and activities usually expected in specific social roles that are customary for the individual or expected for the person's status or role in a specific sociocultural context and physical environment" (*Guide to Physical Therapist Practice, 2nd edition*, American Physical Therapy Association, 2001).

dopa—Produced from the amino acid tyrosine by the enzyme tyrosine hydroxylase. It is the precursor to the neurotransmitter dopamine.

dopamine—The neurotransmitter that is deficient in people with Parkinson's disease. This neurotransmitter is produced in the substantia nigra compacta and stored in its axonal terminals, which terminate in the striatum. Dopamine is responsible for normalization of sequential movements, automaticity of learned movements, and normalization of tone.

dopamine agonists—A class of drugs that stimulate the postsynaptic dopaminergic receptors.

dopaminergic—Pertaining to the nigrostriatal dopamine neurotransmitter system.

dyskinesia—An umbrella term used to describe involuntary movement disorders that include chorea, tics, tremors, athetosis, myoclonus, and dystonia. When referring to Parkinson's, the term *dyskinesia* is most commonly associated with choreiform type of movements that are rapidly flowing and unpredictable in direction or magnitude. These movements are drug induced in Parkinson's, resulting from disease progression in combination with L-dopa medications. Dyskinesias can occur at different times in the medication cycle.

dysphasia—Difficulty swallowing.

dystonia—A sustained muscle contraction that produces involuntary twisting and abnormal posturing.

entrainment—Means to be "attracted to" or "to lock into." This term is used in reference to rhythmic auditory stimulation and its application to cadence matching in which the patient is able to follow the auditory rhythm with a stepping rhythm.

essential tremor—A tremor that occurs with motion (also known as kinetic tremor) or while attempting to maintain a position in which any body part is not fully supported against gravity (also known as postural tremor).

extrinsic fall risk factors—Fall risk factors related to the environment such as poor lighting, loose throw rugs, lack of grab bars, and so on.

fading—Removing the auditory stimulus after gait training with rhythmic auditory stimulation. The patient attempts to replicate the beat of the music mentally to maintain optimal gait improvements without the stimulus.

fall—A sudden unintended change in position (displacement) that causes a person to land inadvertently at a lower level on an object, floor, or ground.

festination—A propulsive gait or involuntary speeding up of gait in a forward direction, resulting from a shortened stride length and the tendency to lean forward.

functional limitation—Restriction of the ability to perform a physical action, task, or activity in an efficient, typically expected, or competent manner at the level of the whole organism or person (*Guide to Physical Therapist Practice, 2nd edition.* American Physical Therapy Association, 2001).

freezing—Inability to take steps while walking or when attempting to start walking. Attempted movement is visible but nonproductive.

gait variability—A gait pattern of inconsistent step lengths and arrhythmic stepping.

gait velocity—A measure of gait speed, which is a function of distance covered per unit of time. Commonly used measures are m/s or m/min.

globus pallidus internus (GPi)—A subcortical nucleus in the brain that is part of the basal ganglia.

hip strategy—Occurs with a greater destabilizing force or if the BOS is limited, as when standing on a support surface smaller than the feet. No change in BOS is necessary to reestablish balance (feet-in-place strategy). The axis of motion is at the hips.

hypokinesia—Decreased amplitude of movement and progressive lessening of amplitude with each repetitive movement.

impairment—Abnormalities of anatomical, physiological, or psychological structures. Examples are limited ROM, muscle weakness, rigidity, or bradykinesia. Impairments can lead to functional limitations.

incidence—The number of new cases of a disease occurring in a population in a specified time interval. This number measures the risk of developing a disease and is usually reported as a percentage of a given number of a population. For example, the number of new cases of Parkinson's among those over the age of 50 in a 15 yr period is 49 per 100,000 people, or 0.05%. Hypothetically, the incidence of the flu (new cases) from December to March is 30% of the population, and the incidence of the flu from June to September is 2% (these fictitious numbers are used only as an example).

instrumental activities of daily living (IADLs)—Activities such as using the telephone, shopping, preparing meals, paying bills, light housework, and ability to manage medications correctly.

intrinsic fall risk factors—Fall risk factors related to the patient such as weakness, limited vision, reduced sensation, impaired cognitive status, and so on.

juvenile onset PD—When initial symptoms of PD are apparent before the age of 21.

kinetic tremor—A type of essential tremor that occurs with motion.

levodopa (L-dopa)—A dopamine replacement medication for the treatment of PD. It is the precursor to dopamine. After L-dopa has crossed the blood brain barrier, the enzyme aromatic amino acid dopa decarboxylase that converts L-dopa to dopamine.

limits of stability—The relative outermost point on the base of support where the forces of the COM can go before a stepping strategy is necessary.

loss of balance—Occurs when a change in the BOS is required to regain stability and prevent a fall.

micrographia—Small cramped handwriting.

monoamine oxidase B (MAO-B) inhibitors—A class of drug that interferes with the enzymatic action of monoamine oxidase, which is a major enzyme in the brain that breaks down dopamine. These drugs reduce the breakdown of dopamine at the synaptic cleft, resulting in higher levels of dopamine and improvement of PD symptoms.

motor fluctuation—A change in the ability to move in response to taking dopamine replacement medications. Motor fluctuations can be subtle or dramatic and are related to the dopamine levels in the brain. Low dopamine levels can result in increased bradykinesia, rigidity, dystonia, tremor, greater balance impairment, or worsening of gait including increased freezing. High dopamine levels can result primarily in choreatic dyskinesias.

multiple systems atrophy (MSA)—A category of movement disorders that generally has poor response to L-dopa medication but shares Parkinsonian symptoms. MSA includes the following diagnoses: Shy-Drager syndrome, striatonigral degeneration, and olivopontocerebellar degeneration.

myoclonus—A sudden brief, jerky, shocklike involuntary movement. Abrupt muscle contraction is called positive myoclonus. Abrupt cessation of muscle activity is called negative myoclonus.

neuroprotective—Slowing the progression of neurodegeneration. This term is often used when referring to the benefits of some PD drugs.

"off"—Relates to a general state of function that is below that of an "on" state. Dopamine levels are less than optimal. This response relates to people with Parkinson's who take L-dopa replacement medications.

"off" freezing—Freezing that occurs when the dopamine levels of the brain are low and diminishes with L-dopa replacement medications.

"on"—Relates to the general state of improved function when dopamine medications are working and dopamine levels are optimal. This response relates to people with Parkinson's who take L-dopa replacement medications.

"on" freezing—Freezing that occurs when dopamine levels are optimal with the use of dopamine replacement medications.

"on-off" phenomenon—The result of long-term L-dopa therapy and the progression of Parkinson's. There is typically an abrupt and unpredictable return of Parkinsonian symptoms that is unrelated to the medication cycle.

orthostatic hypotension (OH)—A fall in systolic BP below 20 mmHg and diastolic BP below 10 mmHg from baseline (from lying to standing) within 3 min of being in an upright position (also see autonomic failure hypotension and postprandial hypotension).

pallidotomy—Stereotactic surgical destruction of the neurons in the globus pallidus internus for the relief of PD symptoms.

period error—The difference between the duration of the step and the duration of the rhythmic interval.

phase error—The time difference from the sound of the beat and the step.

postprandial hypotension—Orthostatic hypotension that occurs after eating a meal.

postural tremor—A type of essential tremor that occurs while attempting to maintain a position in which any body part is not fully supported against gravity.

power strength—The ability to exert a force quickly. Power = force × velocity. Force is muscle strength.

prevalence—The number of existing cases of a disease for the total population at a given time. This number is a function of the longevity of the illness or disease. For example, the number of cases of the flu is higher in the winter and lower in the summer. The number of cases of Parkinson's will increase over time because after a person has it, it does not go away. The longevity of a disease coupled with the new cases diagnosed with increased age will increase the prevalence.

propulsion—Involuntary increased momentum, progressively smaller steps, and instability in the forward direction. This condition can be noted during a loss of balance forward with impaired ability to recover or during gait (see festination).

protective stepping strategies—Occur when balance can no longer be maintained unless a new base of support is established.

reliability—Degree of consistency or reproducibility of a test or rater measurement of a variable.

resting tremor—A tremor that presents itself when a body part is at rest and supported. This type of tremor is associated with PD.

retropulsion—Stepping backward with involuntarily increased momentum, progressively smaller steps, and instability.

rhythmic auditory stimulation (RAS)—Rhythmical sounds to facilitate motor movement.

rigidity—Increased resistance felt throughout the range of motion by an evaluator when passively moving a body part. It is not velocity dependent.

RPE (rating of perceived exertion)—A rating scale to establish a person's subjective feelings regarding the level of perceived exercise intensity.

sarcopenia—An involuntary loss of muscle mass, due to the aging process. Results in loss of strength and function.

sensitivity—A measure of validity of a test based on the probability that a person with a disease will test positive.

specificity—A measure of validity of a test based on the probability that someone who does not have a disease will test negative.

start hesitation—The difficulty with initiating the first step or "freezing" when attempting to start walking.

step length—The distance from the foot strike of one foot to the foot strike of the opposite foot when both feet are in contact with the ground.

stereotactic head frame—A frame attached to the skull to help with precise localization of the targeted areas in the brain.

stereotactic neurosurgery—A surgery that uses stereotactic techniques to map the structures of the brain, enabling precise localization of a targeted structure. A small hole is made in the skull, and a microelectrode is inserted into the brain through the hole. The microelectrode confirms target localization with visual and auditory feedback on an oscilloscope. The procedure is used for surgeries such as pallidotomy, thalamotomy, deep brain stimulation, and biopsies of brain tumors.

stereotactic—Pertains to precise localization of a specific target point based on three-dimensional coordinates.

strength—The ability of the muscle to exert a force.

stride length—The distance covered by one foot from one heel strike to the next heel strike of the same foot (which requires two steps).

subthalamic nucleus (STN)—A subcortical nucleus in the brain that is part of the basal ganglia.

syncope—A temporary interruption of cerebral perfusion with a sudden and transient loss of consciousness and spontaneous recovery.

tandem standing—A static standing position in which one foot is placed directly in front of the other, as when attempting to stand with both feet on a single straight line. This position can be used to evaluate lateral stability or for balance training in rehab.

TENS (transcutaneous electrical nerve stimulation)—An electrical modality used for pain control. Cutaneous electrodes are attached by lead wires to an electrical stimulator. Electrical intensity and waveforms can be adjusted.

thalamotomy—Stereotactic surgical destruction of neurons in the thalamus to control tremor.

tremor—A rhythmical, involuntary oscillation of a body part. Resting tremor is a characteristic symptom of Parkinson's. Essential tremor is a tremor that occurs with movement and is not associated with Parkinson's.

validity—The degree to which a test measures what it is intended to measure.

wearing off—The predictable return of Parkinsonian symptoms related to the medication cycle.

young onset Parkinson's disease (YOPD)—Constitutes approximately 10% of the PD population. Initial onset of symptoms occurs in the 21 through 39 age group.

References

Chapter 1

Clissold, B.G., McColl, C.D., Reardon, K.R., Shiff, M., & Kempster, P.A. (2006). Longitudinal study of the motor response to levodopa in Parkinson's disease. *Mov Disord*. Oct. 6.

Dewey, R.B. (2000). Clinical features of Parkinson's disease. In C.H. Adler & J.E. Ahlskog (Eds.), *Parkinson's disease and movement disorders: Diagnoses and treatment guidelines for the practicing physician* (pp. 71–84). Totowa, NJ: Humana Press.

Giladi, N., Kao, R., & Fahn, S. (1997). Freezing phenomenon in patients with Parkinsonian syndromes. *Mov Disord, 12*(3), 302–5.

Goetz, C.G., Poewe, W., Rascol, O., Sampaio, C., Stebbins, G.T., Counsell, C., et al. (2004). Movement disorder society task force report on the Hoehn and Yahr staging scale: Status and recommendations. *Mov Disord, 19*(9), 1020–28.

Goetz, C.G., Stebbins, G.T., & Blasucci, L.M. (2000). Differential progression of motor impairment in levodopa-treated Parkinson's disease. *Mov Disord, 15*(3), 479–84.

Goldman, S.M., & Tanner, C. (1998). Etiology of Parkinson's disease. In J. Jankovic & E. Tolosa (Eds.), *Parkinson's disease and movement disorders* (3rd ed., pp. 133–58). Baltimore: Lippincott Williams & Wilkins.

Hoehn, M.M., & Yahr, M.D. (1967). Parkinsonism: Onset, progression and mortality. *Neurology, 17*(5), 427–42.

McColl, C.D., Reardon, K.A., Shiff, M., & Kempster, P.A. (2002). Motor response to levodopa and the evolution of motor fluctuations in the first decade of treatment of Parkinson's disease. *Mov Disord, 17*(6), 1227–34.

Miller, N., Allcock, L., Jones, D., Noble, E., Hildreth, A.J., & Burn, D.J. (2007). Prevalence and pattern of perceived intelligibility changes in Parkinson's disease. *J Neurol Neurosurg Psychiatry, 78*(11), 1188–90.

Molho, E., & Factor, S. (2000). Secondary causes of Parkinsonism. In C.H. Adler & J.E. Ahlskog (Eds.), *Parkinson's disease and movement disorders: Diagnoses and treatment guidelines for the practicing physician* (pp. 211–28). Totowa, NJ: Humana Press.

Mori, K. (2001). Management of idiopathic normal-pressure hydrocephalus: A multi-institutional study conducted in Japan. *J Neurosurg, 95*(6), 970–73.

Nieuwboer, A., De Weerdt, W., Dom, R., Bogaerts, K., & Nuyens, G. (2000). Development of an activity scale for individuals with advanced Parkinson disease: Reliability and "on-off" variability. *Phys Ther, 80*(11), 1087–96.

Paulson, H., & Stern, M. (2004). Clinical manifestations of Parkinson's disease. In R. Watts & W. Koller (Eds.), *Movement disorders neurologic principles and practice* (2nd ed., pp. 233–245). New York: McGraw-Hill.

Potulska, A., Friedman, A., Krolicki, L., Jedrzejowski, M., & Spychala, A. (2002). [Swallowing disorders in Parkinson's disease]. *Neurol Neurochir Pol, 36*(3), 449–56.

Quinn, N., Critchley, P., & Marsden, C.D. (1987). Young onset Parkinson's disease. *Mov Disord, 2*(2), 73–91.

Sethi, K. (2003). Differential diagnosis of Parkinsonism. In R. Pahwa, K. Lyons, & W. Koller (Eds.), *Handbook of Parkinson's disease* (3rd ed., pp. 43–69). New York: Marcel Dekker.

Sibon, I., Fenelon, G., Quinn, N.P., & Tison, F. (2004). Vascular Parkinsonism. *J Neurol, 251*(5), 513–24.

Suchowersky, O., Reich, S., Perlmutter, J., Zesiewicz, T., Gronseth, G., & Weiner, W.J. (2006). Practice parameter: Diagnosis and prognosis of new onset Parkinson disease (an evidence-based review): Report of the quality standards subcommittee of the American Academy of Neurology. *Neurology, 66*(7), 968–75.

Volonte, M.A., Porta, M., & Comi, G. (2002). Clinical assessment of dysphagia in early phases of Parkinson's disease. *Neurol Sci, 23 Suppl 2,* S121–22.

Winikates, J., & Jankovic, J. (1999). Clinical correlates of vascular Parkinsonism. *Arch Neurol, 56*(1), 98–102.

Chapter 2

Ahlskog, J.E. (2000). Initial symptomatic treatment of Parkinson's disease. In C.H. Adler & J.E. Ahlskog (Eds.), *Parkinson's disease and movement disorders: Diagnoses and treatment guidelines for the practicing physician* (pp. 115–28). Totowa, NJ: Humana Press.

Ahsan Ejaz, A., Sekhon, I.S., & Munjal, S. (2006). Characteristic findings on 24-h ambulatory blood pressure monitoring in a series of patients with Parkinson's disease. *Eur J Intern Med, 17*(6), 417–20.

Alesch, F., Pinter, M. M., Helscher, R. J., Fertl, L., Benabid, A. L., & Koos, W. T. (1995). Stimulation of the ventral intermediate thalamic nucleus in tremor dominated parkinson's disease and essential tremor. *Acta Neurochir (Wien), 136*(1-2), 75-81.

Alves, G., Wentzel-Larsen, T., Aarsland, D., & Larsen, J.P. (2005). Progression of motor impairment and disability in Parkinson disease: A population-based study. *Neurology, 65*(9), 1436–41.

Bonuccelli, U., & Pavese, N. (2007). Role of dopamine agonists in Parkinson's disease: An update. *Expert Rev Neurother, 7*(10), 1391–99.

Bouhaddi, M., Vuillier, F., Fortrat, J.O., Cappelle, S., Henriet, M.T., Rumbach, L., et al. (2004). Impaired cardiovascular autonomic control in newly and long-term-treated patients with Parkinson's disease: Involvement of L-dopa therapy. *Auton Neurosci, 116*(1–2), 30–38.

Brooks, D. J., Agid, Y., Eggert, K., Widner, H., Ostergaard, K., & Holopainen, A. (2005). Treatment of end-of-dose wearing-off in parkinson's disease: Stalevo (levodopa/carbidopa/entacapone) and levodopa/ddci given in combination with comtess/comtan (entacapone) provide equivalent improvements in symptom control superior to that of traditional levodopa/ddci treatment. *Eur Neurol, 53*(4), 197-202.

Burleigh, A., Horak, F., Nutt, J., & Frank, J. (1995). Levodopa reduces muscle tone and lower extremity tremor in parkinson's disease. *Can J Neurol Sci, 22*(4), 280-285.

Chen, C.C., Lee, S.T., Wu, T., Chen, C.J., Chen, M.C., & Lu, C.S. (2003). Short-term effect of bilateral subthalamic stimulation for advanced Parkinson's disease. *Chang Gung Med J, 26*(5), 344–51.

Constantoyannis, C., Berk, C., Honey, C.R., Mendez, I., & Brownstone, R.M. (2005). Reducing hardware-related complications of deep brain stimulation. *Can J Neurol Sci, 32*(2), 194–200.

Davis, J. T., Lyons, K. E., & Pahwa, R. (2005). Freezing of gait after bilateral subthalamic nucleus stimulation for parkinson's disease. *Clin Neurol Neurosurg.*

Dewey, R.B. (2000). Clinical features of Parkinson's disease. In C.H. Adler & J.E. Ahlskog (Eds.), *Parkinson's disease and movement disorders: Diagnoses and treatment guidelines for the practicing physician* (pp. 71–84). Totowa, NJ: Humana Press.

Dodel, R.C., Berger, K., & Oertel, W.H. (2001). Health-related quality of life and health-care utilisation in patients with Parkinson's disease: Impact of motor fluctuations and dyskinesias. *Pharmacoeconomics, 19*(10), 1013–38.

Ejaz, A.A., Haley, W.E., Wasiluk, A., Meschia, J.F., & Fitzpatrick, P.M. (2004). Characteristics of 100 consecutive patients presenting with orthostatic hypotension. *Mayo Clin Proc, 79*(7), 890–94.

Goetz, C.G., Stebbins, G.T., Shale, H.M., Lang, A.E., Chernik, D.A., Chmura, T.A., et al. (1994). Utility of an objective dyskinesia rating scale for Parkinson's disease: Inter- and intrarater reliability assessment. *Mov Disord, 9*(4), 390–94.

Group, D.-B. S. f. P. s. D. S. (2001). Deep-brain stimulation of the subthalamic nucleus or the pars interna of the globus pallidus in parkinson's disease. *N Engl J Med, 345*(13), 956-963.

Hauser, R. A., McDermott, M. P., & Messing, S. (2006). Factors associated with the development of motor fluctuations and dyskinesias in parkinson's disease. *Arch Neurol, 63*(12), 1756-60.

Hauser, R., & Zesiewicz, T. (2000). *Parkinson's disease questions and answers* (3rd ed.). Coral Springs, FL: Merit Publishing International.

Hilz, M.J., Marthol, H., & Neundorfer, B. (2002). [Syncope—a systematic overview of classification, pathogenesis, diagnosis and management]. *Fortschr Neurol Psychiatr, 70*(2), 95–107.

Hoff, J.I., van Hilten, B.J., & Roos, R.A. (1999). A review of the assessment of dyskinesias. *Mov Disord, 14*(5), 737–43.

Horak, F. B., Frank, J., & Nutt, J. (1996). Effects of dopamine on postural control in parkinsonian subjects: Scaling, set, and tone. *J Neurophysiol, 75*(6), 2380-96.

Inzelberg, R., Bonuccelli, U., Schechtman, E., Miniowich, A., Strugatsky, R., Ceravolo, R., et al. (2006). Association between amantadine and the onset of dementia in Parkinson's disease. *Mov Disord, 21*(9), 1375–79.

Jankovic, J. (2001). Parkinson's disease therapy: Treatment of early and late disease. *Chin Med J (Engl), 114*(3), 227–34.

Jankovic, J. (2005). Motor fluctuations and dyskinesias in Parkinson's disease: Clinical manifestations. *Mov Disord, 20 Suppl 11*, S11–16.

Jankovic, J., & Stacy, M. (2007). Medical management of levodopa-associated motor complications in patients with Parkinson's disease. *CNS Drugs, 21*(8), 677–92.

Kaakkola, S. (2000). Clinical pharmacology, therapeutic use and potential of COMT inhibitors in Parkinson's disease. *Drugs, 59*(6), 1233–50.

Kompoliti K., G. C., Leurgans S., Morrissey M., Siegel I.M. (2000). "on" freezing in parkinson's disease: Resistance to visual cue walking devices. *Mov Disord, 15*(2), 309-12.

Krack, P., Batir, A., Van Blercom, N., Chabardes, S., Fraix, V., Ardouin, C., et al. (2003). Five-year follow-up of bilateral stimulation of the subthalamic nucleus in advanced parkinson's disease. *N Engl J Med, 349*(20), 1925-34.

Kujawa, K., Leurgans, S., Raman, R., Blasucci, L., & Goetz, C.G. (2000). Acute orthostatic hypotension when starting dopamine agonists in Parkinson's disease. *Arch Neurol, 57*(10), 1461–63.

Lahrmann, H., Cortelli, P., Hilz, M., Mathias, C.J., Struhal, W., & Tassinari, M. (2006). EFNS guidelines on the diagnosis and management of orthostatic hypotension. *Eur J Neurol, 13*(9), 930–36.

Lang, A.E., Houeto, J.L., Krack, P., Kubu, C., Lyons, K.E., Moro, E., et al. (2006). Deep brain stimulation: Preoperative issues. *Mov Disord, 21 Suppl 14*, S171–96.

Mathias, C.J., & Kimber, J.R. (1998). Treatment of postural hypotension. *J Neurol Neurosurg Psychiatry, 65*(3), 285–89.

Mathias, C.J., Mallipeddi, R., & Bleasdale-Barr, K. (1999). Symptoms associated with orthostatic hypotension in pure autonomic failure and multiple system atrophy. *J Neurol, 246*(10), 893–98.

Maurer, C., Mergner, T., Xie, J., Faist, M., Pollak, P., & Lucking, C. H. (2003). Effect of chronic bilateral subthalamic nucleus (stn) stimulation on postural control in parkinson's disease. *Brain, 126*(Pt 5), 1146-63.

Medtronic. Activa Parkinson's control therapy. From www.medtronic.com/physician/activa/parkinsons.html

Medtronic. (2005). *Compatibility guidelines for neurostimulation products.*

Melamed, E. (1992). Mechanism of action of levodopa. In W. Koller (Ed.), *Handbook of Parkinson's disease* (2nd ed., pp. 433–49). New York: Marcel Dekker.

Moro, E., Poon, Y.Y., Lozano, A.M., Saint-Cyr, J.A., & Lang, A.E. (2006). Subthalamic nucleus stimulation: Improvements in outcome with reprogramming. *Arch Neurol, 63*(9), 1266–72.

Pathak, A., & Senard, J.M. (2006). Blood pressure disorders during Parkinson's disease: Epidemiology, pathophysiology and management. *Expert Rev Neurother, 6*(8), 1173–80.

Pavese, N., Evans, A. H., Tai, Y. F., Hotton, G., Brooks, D. J., Lees, A. J., et al. (2006). Clinical correlates of levodopa-induced dopamine release in parkinson disease: A pet study. *Neurology, 67*(9), 1612-17.

Piboolnurak, P., Lang, A.E., Lozano, A.M., Miyasaki, J.M., Saint-Cyr, J.A., Poon, Y.Y., et al. (2007). Levodopa response in long-term bilateral subthalamic stimulation for Parkinson's disease. *Mov Disord, 22*(7), 990–97.

Pickering, T.G., Hall, J.E., Appel, L.J., Falkner, B.E., Graves, J., Hill, M.N., et al. (2005). Recommendations for blood pressure measurement in humans and experimental animals: Part 1: Blood pressure measurement in humans: A statement for professionals from the subcommittee of professional and public education of the American Heart Association Council on High Blood Pressure Research. *Circulation, 111*(5), 69–716.

Poluha, P. C., Teulings, H0. L., & Brookshire, R. H. (1998). Handwriting and speech changes across the levodopa cycle in parkinson's disease. *Acta Psychol (Amst), 100*(1-2), 71-84.

Pursiainen, V., Korpelainen, T.J., Haapaniemi, H.T., Sotaniemi, A.K., & Myllyla, V.V. (2007). Selegiline and blood pressure in patients with Parkinson's disease. *Acta Neurol Scand, 115*(2), 104–8.

Rezak, M., Marks, W., Cozzens, J., Bernstein, L., Novak, K., & Vergenz, S. (2004, May 22). *Deep brain stimulation: The role of deep brain stimulation for movement disorders*, Chicago.

Salarian, A., Russmann, H., Vingerhoets, F. J., Dehollain, C., Blanc, Y., Burkhard, P. R., et al. (2004). Gait assessment in parkinson's disease: Toward an ambulatory system for long-term monitoring. *IEEE Trans Biomed Eng, 51*(8), 1434-43.

Santiago, A., & Factor, S. (2003). Levodopa. In R. Pahwa, K. Lyons, & W. Koller (Eds.), *Handbook of Parkinson's disease* (3rd ed., pp. 381–405). New York: Marcel Dekker.

Schade, R., Andersohn, F., Suissa, S., Haverkamp, W., & Garbe, E. (2007). Dopamine agonists and the risk of cardiac-valve regurgitation. *N Engl J Med, 356*(1), 29–38.

Senard, J.M. (2003). [Blood pressure disorders during idiopathic Parkinson's disease]. *Presse Med, 32*(26), 1231–37.

Shaheda, N., Azher, S. N., & Jankovic, J. (2005). Camptocormia: Pathogenesis, classification, and response to therapy. *Neurology, 65*(3), 355-59.

Slawek, J. (2007). [Dopamine agonists in the treatment of motor complications in advanced Parkinson's disease]. *Neurol Neurochir Pol, 41*(2 Suppl 1), S29–33.

Stacy, M. (2003). Dopamine agonists. In R. Pahwa, K. Lyons & W. Koller (Eds.), *Handbook of parkinson's disease* (3rd ed., pp. 407-23). New York: Marcel Dekker, Inc.

Tir, M., Devos, D., Blond, S., Touzet, G., Reyns, N., Duhamel, A., et al. (2007). Exhaustive, one-year follow-up of subthalamic nucleus deep brain stimulation in a large, single-center cohort of Parkinsonian patients. *Neurosurgery, 61*(2), 297–305.

Tolosa, E., & Katzenschlager, R. (2007). Pharmacological management of Parkinson's disease. In J. Jankovic & E. Tolosa (Eds.), *Parkinson's disease & movement disorders* (5th ed., pp. 125–27). Philadelphia: Lippincott Williams & Wilkens.

Trepanier, L.L., Kumar, R., Lozano, A.M., Lang, A.E., & Saint-Cyr, J.A. (2000). Neuropsychological outcome of GPi pallidotomy and GPi or STN deep brain stimulation in Parkinson's disease. *Brain Cogn, 42*(3), 324–47.

Uitti, R. (2000). Advancing Parkinson's disease and treatment of motor complications. In C.H. Adler & J.E. Ahlskog (Eds.), *Parkinson's disease and movement disorders: Diagnoses and treatment guidelines for the practicing physician* (pp. 129–50). Totowa, NJ: Humana Press.

van Laar, T. (2003). Levodopa-induced response fluctuations in patients with Parkinson's disease: Strategies for management. *CNS Drugs, 17*(7), 475–89.

Victor, D., & Waters, C. (2003). Monoamine oxidase inhibitors in parkinson's disease. In R. Pahwa, K. Lyons & W. Koller (Eds.), *Handbook of parkinson's disease* (3rd ed., pp. 425-436). New York: Marcel Dekker, Inc.

Young, T.M., & Mathias, C.J. (2004). The effects of water ingestion on orthostatic hypotension in two groups of chronic autonomic failure: Multiple system atrophy and pure autonomic failure. *J Neurol Neurosurg Psychiatry, 75*(12), 1737–41.

Zibetti, M., Torre, E., Cinquepalmi, A., Rosso, M., Ducati, A., Bergamasco, B., et al. (2007). Motor and nonmotor symptom follow-up in parkinsonian patients after deep brain stimulation of the subthalamic nucleus. *Eur Neurol, 58*(4), 218-3.

Chapter 3

Brach J.S., Simonsick E.M., Kritchevsky S., Yaffe K., Newman A.B.; Health, Aging and Body Composition Study Research Group. (2004). The association between physical function and lifestyle activity and exercise in the health, aging and body composition study. *J Am Geriatr Soc, 52*(4), 502–9.

Bryant, C., Peterson, J., & Graves, J.E. (1998). Muscular strength and endurance. In E. Johnson (Ed.), *ACSM's resource manual for guidelines for exercise testing and prescription* (3rd ed., pp. 448–455). Baltimore: Williams & Wilkins.

Caglar, A.T., Gurses, H.N., Mutluay, F.K., & Kiziltan, G. (2005). Effects of home exercises on motor performance in patients with Parkinson's disease. *Clin Rehabil, 19*(8), 870–77.

Cipriani, D., Abel, B., & Pirrwitz, D. (2003). A comparison of two stretching protocols on hip range of motion: Implications for total daily stretch duration. *J Strength Cond Res, 17*(2), 274–78.

Coleman, K.J., Raynor, H.R., Mueller, D.M., Cerny, F.J., Dorn, J.M., & Epstein, L.H. (1999). Providing sedentary adults with choices for meeting their walking goals. *Prev Med, 28*(5), 510–19.

de Vos, N.J., Singh, N.A., Ross, D.A., Stavrinos, T.M., Orr, R., & Fiatarone Singh, M.A. (2005). Optimal load for increasing muscle power during explosive resistance training in older adults. *J Gerontol A Biol Sci Med Sci, 60*(5), 638–47.

Dimitrova, D., Horak, F.B., & Nutt, J.G. (2004). Postural muscle responses to multidirectional translations in patients with Parkinson's disease. *J Neurophysiol, 91*(1), 489–501.

Dodd, K., Taylor, N., & Bradley, S. (2004). Strength training for older people. In M. Morris & A. Schoo (Eds.), *Optimizing exercise and physical activity in older people* (pp. 125–57). Philadelphia: Butterworth-Heinemann.

Doherty, T.J. (2003). Invited review: Aging and sarcopenia. *J Appl Physiol, 95*(4), 1717–27.

Ekin, J.A., & Sinaki, M. (1993). Vertebral compression fractures sustained during golfing: Report of three cases. *Mayo Clin Proc, 68*(6), 566–70.

Exercise testing and prescription for children and elderly people. (2006). In M. Whaley, P. Brubaker, & M. Otto (Eds.), *ACSM's guidelines for exercise testing and prescription* (7th ed., pp. 237–51). Baltimore: Lippincott Williams & Wilkins.

Fatouros, I.G., Kambas, A., Katrabasas, I., Nikolaidis, K., Chatzinikolaou, A., Leontsini, D., et al. (2005). Strength training and detraining effects on muscular strength, anaerobic power, and mobility of inactive older men are intensity dependent. *Br J Sports Med, 39*(10), 776–80.

Feland, J.B., Myrer, J.W., Schulthies, S.S., Fellingham, G.W., & Measom, G.W. (2001). The effect of duration of stretching of the hamstring muscle group for increasing range of motion in people aged 65 years or older. *Phys Ther, 81*(5), 1110–17.

Fiatarone, M.A., Marks, E.C., Ryan, N.D., Meredith, C.N., Lipsitz, L.A., & Evans, W.J. (1990). High-intensity strength training in nonagenarians. Effects on skeletal muscle. *JAMA, 263*(22), 3029–34.

Fielding, R.A., LeBrasseur, N.K., Cuoco, A., Bean, J., Mizer, K., & Fiatarone Singh, M.A. (2002). High-velocity resistance training increases skeletal muscle peak power in older women. *J Am Geriatr Soc, 50*(4), 655–62.

Galvao, D.A., & Taaffe, D.R. (2005). Resistance exercise dosage in older adults: Single- versus multiset effects on physical performance and body composition. *J Am Geriatr Soc, 53*(12), 2090–97.

General principles of exercise prescription. (2006). In M. Whaley, P. Brubaker, & M. Otto (Eds.), *ACSM's guidelines for exercise testing and prescription* (7th ed., pp. 158–60). Baltimore: Lippincott Williams & Wilkins.

Jacobs, J.V., & Horak, F.B. (2006). Abnormal proprioceptive-motor integration contributes to hypometric postural responses of subjects with Parkinson's disease. *Neuroscience, 141*(2), 999–1009.

Lehman, D., Toole, T., Lofald, D., & Hirsch, M. (2005). Training with verbal instructional cues results in near-term improvement of gait in people with Parkinson disease. *Journal of Neurological Physical Therapy, 29*(1), 1–8.

Lewis, C., & Kellems, S. (2002). Musculoskeletal changes with age: Clinical implications. In C. Bernstein Lewis (Ed.), *Aging the health care challenge* (4th ed., pp. 104–26). Philadelphia: F.A. Davis.

Lun, V., Pullan, N., Labelle, N., Adams, C., & Suchowersky, O. (2005). Comparison of the effects of a self-supervised home exercise program with a physiotherapist-supervised exercise program on the motor symptoms of Parkinson's disease. *Mov Disord, 20*(8), 971–75.

Maurer, C., Mergner, T., Xie, J., Faist, M., Pollak, P., & Lucking, C.H. (2003). Effect of chronic bilateral subthalamic nucleus (STN) stimulation on postural control in Parkinson's disease. *Brain, 126*(Pt 5), 1146–63.

Miszko, T.A., Cress, M.E., Slade, J.M., Covey, C.J., Agrawal, S.K., & Doerr, C.E. (2003). Effect of strength and power training on physical function in community-dwelling older adults. *J Gerontol A Biol Sci Med Sci, 58*(2), 171–75.

Pal, P.K., Sathyaprabha, T.N., Tuhina, P., & Thennarasu, K. (2007). Pattern of subclinical pulmonary dysfunctions in Parkinson's disease and the effect of levodopa. *Mov Disord, 22*(3), 420–24.

Pavese, N., Evans, A.H., Tai, Y.F., Hotton, G., Brooks, D.J., Lees, A.J., et al. (2006). Clinical correlates of levodopa-induced dopamine release in Parkinson disease: A PET study. *Neurology, 67*(9), 1612–17.

Physical activity and health: A report of the surgeon general. (1996). Recommendations from the Centers for Disease Control and Prevention, the American College of Sports Medicine and the American Heart Association.

Roberts, J.M., & Wilson, K. (1999). Effect of stretching duration on active and passive range of motion in the lower extremity. *Br J Sports Med, 33*(4), 259–63.

Rogers, M.W., & Mille, M.L. (2003). Lateral stability and falls in older people. *Exerc Sport Sci Rev, 31*(4), 182–87.

Sabate, M., Gonzalez, I., Ruperez, F., & Rodriguez, M. (1996). Obstructive and restrictive pulmonary dysfunctions in Parkinson's disease. *J Neurol Sci, 138*(1–2), 114–19.

Scandalis, T.A., Bosak, A., Berliner, J.C., Helman, L.L., & Wells, M.R. (2001). Resistance training and gait function in patients with Parkinson's disease. *Am J Phys Med Rehabil, 80*(1), 38–43; quiz 44–36.

Seynnes, O., Fiatarone Singh, M.A., Hue, O., Pras, P., Legros, P., & Bernard, P.L. (2004). Physiological and functional responses to low-moderate versus high-intensity progressive resistance training in frail elders. *J Gerontol A Biol Sci Med Sci, 59*(5), 503–9.

Silverman, E.P., Sapienza, C.M., Saleem, A., Carmichael, C., Davenport, P.W., Hoffman-Ruddy, B., et al. (2006). Tutorial on maximum inspiratory and expiratory mouth pressures in individuals with idiopathic Parkinson disease (IPD) and the preliminary results of an expiratory muscle strength training program. *NeuroRehabilitation, 21*(1), 71–79.

Sinaki, M., & Mikkelsen, B.A. (1984). Postmenopausal spinal osteoporosis: Flexion versus extension exercises. *Arch Phys Med Rehabil, 65*(10), 593–96.

Slade, J.M., Miszko, T.A., Laity, J.H., Agrawal, S.K., & Cress, M.E. (2002). Anaerobic power and physical function in strength-trained and non-strength-trained older adults. *J Gerontol A Biol Sci Med Sci, 57*(3), M168–72.

Starkey, D.B., Pollock, M.L., Ishida, Y., Welsch, M.A., Brechue, W.F., Graves, J.E., et al. (1996). Effect of resistance training volume on strength and muscle thickness. *Med Sci Sports Exerc, 28*(10), 1311–20.

Suteerawattananon, M., Morris, G.S., Etnyre, B.R., Jankovic, J., & Protas, E.J. (2004). Effects of visual and auditory cues on gait in individuals with Parkinson's disease. *J Neurol Sci, 219*(1–2), 63–69.

Volpi, E., Nazemi, R., & Fujita, S. (2004). Muscle tissue changes with aging. *Curr Opin Clin Nutr Metab Care, 7*(4), 405–10.

Chapter 4

Boelen, M., Crawford, S., & Meyer, T. (2006). *"Can therapy help me?"* Glenview, IL: NorthShore University HealthSystem.

Davey, C., Wiles, R., Ashburn, A., & Murphy, C. (2004). Falling in Parkinson's disease:

The impact on informal caregivers. *Disabil Rehabil, 26*(23), 1360–66.

Edwards, N.E., & Scheetz, P.S. (2002). Predictors of burden for caregivers of patients with Parkinson's disease. *J Neurosci Nurs, 34*(4), 184–90.

Happe, S., & Berger, K. (2002). The association between caregiver burden and sleep disturbances in partners of patients with Parkinson's disease. *Age Ageing, 31*(5), 349–54.

Martinez-Martin, P., Benito-Leon, J., Alonso, F., Catalan, M.J., Pondal, M., Zamarbide, I., et al. (2005). Quality of life of caregivers in Parkinson's disease. *Qual Life Res, 14*(2), 463–72.

Miller, N., Allcock, L., Jones, D., Noble, E., Hildreth, A.J., & Burn, D.J. (2007). Prevalence and pattern of perceived intelligibility changes in Parkinson's disease. *J Neurol Neurosurg Psychiatry, 78*(11), 1188–90.

Sadagopan, N., & Huber, J.E. (2007). Effects of loudness cues on respiration in individuals with Parkinson's disease. *Mov Disord, 22*(5), 651–59.

Sapir, S., Spielman, J.L., Ramig, L.O., Story, B.H., & Fox, C. (2007). Effects of intensive voice treatment (the Lee Silverman Voice Treatment [LSVT]) on vowel articulation in dysarthric individuals with idiopathic Parkinson disease: Acoustic and perceptual findings. *J Speech Lang Hear Res, 50*(4), 899–912.

Schrag, A., Hovris, A., Morley, D., Quinn, N., & Jahanshahi, M. (2006). Caregiver-burden in Parkinson's disease is closely associated with psychiatric symptoms, falls, and disability. *Parkinsonism Relat Disord, 12*(1), 35–41.

Schrag, A., Morley, D., Quinn, N., & Jahanshahi, M. (2004). Impact of Parkinson's disease on patients' adolescent and adult children. *Parkinsonism Relat Disord, 10*(7), 391–97.

Vaugoyeau, M., Viel, S., Assaiante, C., Amblard, B., & Azulay, J.P. (2007). Impaired vertical postural control and proprioceptive integration deficits in Parkinson's disease. *Neuroscience, 146*(2), 852–63.

Chapter 5

Abbruzzese, G., & Berardelli, A. (2006). Neurophysiological effects of botulinum toxin type A. *Neurotox Res, 9*(2–3), 109–14.

Askmark, H., Eeg-Olofsson, K., Johansson, A., Nilsson, P., Olsson, Y., & Aquilonius, S. (2001). Parkinsonism and neck extensor myopathy: A new syndrome or coincidental findings? *Arch Neurol, 58*(2), 232–37.

Bloch, F., Houeto, J.L., Tezenas du Montcel, S., Bonneville, F., Etchepare, F., Welter, M.L., et al. (2006). Parkinson's disease with camptocormia. *J Neurol Neurosurg Psychiatry*.

Boesch, S.M., Wenning, G.K., Ransmayr, G., & Poewe, W. (2002). Dystonia in multiple system atrophy. *J Neurol Neurosurg Psychiatry, 72*(3), 300–303.

Charpentier, P., Dauphin, A., Stojkovic, T., Cotten, A., Hurtevent, J.F., Maurage, C.A., et al. (2005). [Parkinson's disease, progressive lumbar kyphosis and focal paraspinal myositis]. *Rev Neurol (Paris), 161*(4), 459–63.

Currie, L.J., Harrison, M.B., Trugman, J.M., Bennett, J.P., Jr., & Wooten, G.F. (1998). Early morning dystonia in Parkinson's disease. *Neurology, 51*(1), 283–85.

Djaldetti, R., & Melamed, E. (2006). Camptocormia in Parkinson's disease: New insights. *J Neurol Neurosurg Psychiatry, 77*(11), 1205.

Djaldetti, R., Mosberg-Galili, R., Sroka, H., Merims, D., & Melamed, E. (1999). Camptocormia (bent spine) in patients with Parkinson's disease—characterization and possible pathogenesis of an unusual phenomenon. *Mov Disord, 14*(3), 443–47.

Feriha, O., Aytul, M., & Hasan, M. (2004). A case of camptocormia (bent spine) secondary to early motor neuron disease. *Behav Neurol, 15*(1–2), 51–54.

Fujimoto, K. (2006). Dropped head in Parkinson's disease. *J Neurol, 253 Suppl 7*, vii21–vii26.

Hellmann, M.A., Djaldetti, R., Israel, Z., & Melamed, E. (2006). Effect of deep brain subthalamic stimulation on camptocormia and postural abnormalities in idiopathic Parkinson's disease. *Mov Disord, 21*(11), 2008–10.

Huang, W., Foster, J.A., & Rogachefsky, A.S. (2000). Pharmacology of botulinum toxin. *J Am Acad Dermatol, 43*(2 Pt 1), 249–59.

Karbowski, K. (1999). The old and the new camptocormia. *Spine, 24*(14), 1494–98.

Krack, P., Pollak, P., Limousin, P., Benazzouz, A., Deuschl, G., & Benabid, A.L. (1999). From off-period dystonia to peak-dose chorea. The clinical spectrum of varying subthalamic nucleus activity. *Brain, 122 (Pt 6)*, 1133–46.

Melamed, E. (1992). Mechanism of action of levodopa. In W. Koller (Ed.), *Handbook of Parkinson's disease* (2nd ed., pp. 433–449). New York: Marcel Dekker.

Micheli, F., Cersosimo, M.G., & Piedimonte, F. (2005). Camptocormia in a patient with Parkinson disease: Beneficial effects of pallidal deep brain stimulation. Case report. *J Neurosurg, 103*(6), 1081–83.

Nutt, J.G. (1990). Levodopa-induced dyskinesia: Review, observations, and speculations. *Neurology, 40*(2), 340–45.

Ozer, F., Ozturk, O., Meral, H., Serdaroglu, P., & Yayla, V. (2007). Camptocormia in a patient with Parkinson disease and a myopathy with nemaline rods. *Am J Phys Med Rehabil, 86*(1), 3–6.

Pacchetti, C., Albani, G., Martignoni, E., Godi, L., Alfonsi, E., & Nappi, G. (1995). "Off" painful dystonia in Parkinson's disease treated with botulinum toxin. *Mov Disord, 10*(3), 333–36.

Rivest, J., Quinn, N., & Marsden, C.D. (1990). Dystonia in Parkinson's disease, multiple system atrophy, and progressive supranuclear palsy. *Neurology, 40*(10), 1571–78.

Schabitz, W.R., Glatz, K., Schuhan, C., Sommer, C., Berger, C., Schwaninger, M., et al. (2003). Severe forward flexion of the trunk in Parkinson's disease: Focal myopathy of the paraspinal muscles mimicking camptocormia. *Mov Disord, 18*(4), 408–14.

Shaheda, N., Azher, S.N., & Jankovic, J. (2005). Camptocormia: Pathogenesis, classification, and response to therapy. *Neurology, 65*(3), 355–59.

Slawek, J., Derejko, M., Lass, P., & Dubaniewicz, M. (2006). Camptocormia or pisa syndrome in multiple system atrophy. *Clin Neurol Neurosurg, 108*(7), 699–704.

Slawek, J., Madalinski, M.H., Maciag-Tymecka, I., & Duzynski, W. (2005). [Frequency of side effects after botulinum toxin A injections in neurology, rehabilitation and gastroenterology]. *Pol Merkur Lekarski, 18*(105), 298–302.

Song, I.U., Kim, J.S., & Lee, K.S. (2007). Dopa-responsive camptocormia in a patient with multiple system atrophy. *Parkinsonism Relat Disord.*

Steiger, M., & Quinn, N. (1992). Levodopa-based therapy. In W. Koller (Ed.), *Handbook of Parkinson's disease* (2nd ed., pp. 391–410). New York: Marcel Dekker.

Tarsey, D. (2000). Dystonia. In C.H. Adler & J.E. Ahlskog (Eds.), *Parkinson's disease and movement disorders: Diagnoses and treatment guidelines for the practicing physician* (pp. 297–312). Totowa, NJ: Humana Press.

Tarsy, D., & Simon, D.K. (2006). Dystonia. *N Engl J Med, 355*(8), 818–29.

Tolosa, E., & Compta, Y. (2006). Dystonia in Parkinson's disease. *J Neurol, 253 Suppl 7*, vii7–vii13.

Uitti, R. (2000). Advancing Parkinson's disease and treatment of motor complications. In C.H. Adler & J.E. Ahlskog (Eds.), *Parkinson's disease and movement disorders: Diagnoses and treatment guidelines for the practicing physician* (pp. 129–50). Totowa, NJ: Humana Press.

Wenzel, R.G. (2004). Pharmacology of botulinum neurotoxin serotype A. *Am J Health Syst Pharm, 61*(22 Suppl 6), S5–10.

Yamada, K., Goto, S., Matsuzaki, K., Tamura, T., Murase, N., Shimazu, H., et al. (2006). Alleviation of camptocormia by bilateral subthalamic nucleus stimulation in a patient with Parkinson's disease. *Parkinsonism Relat Disord, 12*(6), 372–75.

Yoshiyama, Y., Takama, J., & Hattori, T. (1999). The dropped head sign in Parkinsonism. *J Neurol Sci, 167*(1), 22–25.

Chapter 6

Alesch, F., Pinter, M.M., Helscher, R.J., Fertl, L., Benabid, A.L., & Koos, W.T. (1995). Stimulation of the ventral intermediate thalamic nucleus in tremor dominated Parkinson's disease and essential tremor. *Acta Neurochir (Wien)*, *136*(1–2), 75–81.

Deuschl, G., Bain, P., & Brin, M. (1998). Consensus statement of the Movement Disorder Society on Tremor. Ad hoc scientific committee. *Mov Disord*, *13 Suppl 3*, 2–23.

Deuschl, G., Volkmann, J., & Raethjen, J. (2007). Tremors: Differential diagnosis, pathophysiology, and therapy. In J. Jankovic & E. Tolosa (Eds.), *Parkinson's disease & movement disorders* (5th ed., pp. 298–309). Philadelphia: Lippincott Williams and Wilkins.

Essential tremor. (2004). *The Harvard Medical School family health guide*, www.health.harvard.edu/fhg/updates/update1204c.shtml.

Giladi, N., McDermott, M.P., Fahn, S., Przedborski, S., Jankovic, J., Stern, M., et al. (2001). Freezing of gait in PD: Prospective assessment in the datatop cohort. *Neurology*, *56*(12), 1712–21.

Habib ur, R. (2000). Diagnosis and management of tremor. *Arch Intern Med*, *160*(16), 2438–44.

Hubble, J. (2000). Essential tremor: Diagnosis and treatment. In C.H. Adler & J.E. Ahlskog (Eds.), *Parkinson's disease and movement disorders: Diagnoses and treatment guidelines for the practicing physician* (pp. 283–96). Totowa, NJ: Humana Press.

Lyons, K.E., Pahwa, R., Comella, C.L., Eisa, M.S., Elble, R.J., Fahn, S., et al. (2003). Benefits and risks of pharmacological treatments for essential tremor. *Drug Saf*, *26*(7), 461–81.

Matsumoto, J. (2000). Tremor disorders: Overview. In C.H. Adler & J.E. Ahlskog (Eds.), *Parkinson's disease and movement disorders: Diagnoses and treatment guidelines for the practicing physician* (pp. 273–82). Totowa, NJ: Humana Press.

Pahwa, R., & Lyons, K.E. (2003). Essential tremor: Differential diagnosis and current therapy. *Am J Med*, *115*(2), 134–42.

Raethjen, J., & Deuschl, G. (2007). [Tremor]. *Ther Umsch*, *64*(1), 35–40.

Whitney, C.M. (2006). Essential tremor. *Neurologist*, *12*(6), 331–32.

Chapter 7

Bazalgette, D., Zattara, M., Bathien, N., Bouisset, S., & Rondot, P. (1987). Postural adjustments associated with rapid voluntary arm movements in patients with Parkinson's disease. *Adv Neurol*, *45*, 371–74.

Beckley, D.J., Bloem, B.R., & Remler, M.P. (1993). Impaired scaling of long latency postural reflexes in patients with Parkinson's disease. *Electroencephalogr Clin Neurophysiol*, *89*(1), 22–28.

Behrman, A.L., Teitelbaum, P., & Cauraugh, J.H. (1998). Verbal instructional sets to normalise the temporal and spatial gait variables in Parkinson's disease. *J Neurol Neurosurg Psychiatry*, *65*(4), 580–82.

Bloem, B.R. (1992). Postural instability in Parkinson's disease. *Clin Neurol Neurosurg*, *94 Suppl*, S41–45.

Dimitrova, D., Horak, F.B., & Nutt, J.G. (2004). Postural muscle responses to multidirectional translations in patients with Parkinson's disease. *J Neurophysiol*, *91*(1), 489–501.

Farley, B.G., & Koshland, G.F. (2005). Training big to move faster: The application of the speed-amplitude relation as a rehabilitation strategy for people with Parkinson's disease. *Exp Brain Res*, *167*(3), 462–67.

Frank, J.S., Horak, F.B., & Nutt, J. (2000). Centrally initiated postural adjustments in Parkinsonian patients on and off levodopa. *J Neurophysiol*, *84*(5), 2440–48.

Horak, F.B., Frank, J., & Nutt, J. (1996). Effects of dopamine on postural control in Parkinsonian subjects: Scaling, set, and tone. *J Neurophysiol*, *75*(6), 2380–96.

Horak, F.B., & Nashner, L.M. (1986). Central programming of postural movements: Adaptation to altered support-surface configurations. *J Neurophysiol*, *55*(6), 1369–81.

Jacobs, J.V., & Horak, F.B. (2006). Abnormal proprioceptive-motor integration contributes to hypometric postural responses of subjects with Parkinson's disease. *Neuroscience*, *141*(2), 999–1009.

Jacobs, J.V., Horak, F.B., Van Tran, K., & Nutt, J.G. (2006). An alternative clinical postural stability test for patients with Parkinson's disease. *J Neurol*, *253*(11), 1404–13.

Jobges, M., Heuschkel, G., Pretzel, C., Illhardt, C., Renner, C., & Hummelsheim, H. (2004). Repetitive training of compensatory steps: A therapeutic approach for postural instability in Parkinson's disease. *J Neurol Neurosurg Psychiatry, 75*(12), 1682–87.

Kaneoke, Y., Koike, Y., Sakurai, N., Takahashi, A., & Watanabe, S. (1989). Reaction times of movement preparation in patients with Parkinson's disease. *Neurology, 39*(12), 1615–18.

Keijsers, N.L., Admiraal, M.A., Cools, A.R., Bloem, B.R., & Gielen, C.C. (2005). Differential progression of proprioceptive and visual information processing deficits in Parkinson's disease. *Eur J Neurosci, 21*(1), 239–48.

King, L.A., & Horak, F.B. (2008). Lateral stepping for postural correction in Parkinson's disease. *Arch Phys Med Rehabil, 89*(3), 492–99.

Kirby, R.L., Price, N.A., & MacLeod, D.A. (1987). The influence of foot position on standing balance. *J Biomech, 20*(4), 423–27.

Mille, M.L., Rogers, M.W., Martinez, K., Hedman, L.D., Johnson, M.E., Lord, S.R., et al. (2003). Thresholds for inducing protective stepping responses to external perturbations of human standing. *J Neurophysiol, 90*(2), 666–74.

Munhoz, R.P., Li, J.Y., Kurtinecz, M., Piboolnurak, P., Constantino, A., Fahn, S., et al. (2004). Evaluation of the pull test technique in assessing postural instability in Parkinson's disease. *Neurology, 62*(1), 125–27.

Pai, Y.C. (2003). Movement termination and stability in standing. *Exerc Sport Sci Rev, 31*(1), 19–25.

Pai, Y.C., Maki, B.E., Iqbal, K., McIlroy, W.E., & Perry, S.D. (2000). Thresholds for step initiation induced by support-surface translation: A dynamic center-of-mass model provides much better prediction than a static model. *J Biomech, 33*(3), 387–92.

Rogers, M.W., Hain, T.C., Hanke, T.A., & Janssen, I. (1996). Stimulus parameters and inertial load: Effects on the incidence of protective stepping responses in healthy human subjects. *Arch Phys Med Rehabil, 77*(4), 363–68.

Rogers, M.W., Johnson, M.E., Martinez, K.M., Mille, M.L., & Hedman, L.D. (2003). Step training improves the speed of voluntary step initiation in aging. *J Gerontol A Biol Sci Med Sci, 58*(1), 46–51.

Rogers, M.W., Kukulka, C.G., & Soderberg, G.L. (1987). Postural adjustments preceding rapid arm movements in Parkinsonian subjects. *Neurosci Lett, 75*(2), 246–51.

Shumway-Cook, A., & Woollacott, M. (2001). *Motor control: Theory and practical applications* (2nd ed.). Baltimore: Lippincott Williams & Wilkins.

Visser, M., Marinus, J., Bloem, B.R., Kisjes, H., van den Berg, B.M., & van Hilten, J.J. (2003). Clinical tests for the evaluation of postural instability in patients with Parkinson's disease. *Arch Phys Med Rehabil, 84*(11), 1669–74.

Chapter 8

Aarsland, D., Zaccai, J., & Brayne, C. (2005). A systematic review of prevalence studies of dementia in Parkinson's disease. *Mov Disord, 20*(10), 1255–63.

Ashburn, A. (2001). Screening people with Parkinson's disease to identify those at risk of falling. *The Research Findings Register*.

Ashburn, A., Stack, E., Pickering, R.M., & Ward, C.D. (2001). A community-dwelling sample of people with Parkinson's disease: Characteristics of fallers and non-fallers. *Age Ageing, 30*(1), 47–52.

Balash, Y., Peretz, C., Leibovich, G., Herman, T., Hausdorff, J.M., & Giladi, N. (2005). Falls in outpatients with Parkinson's disease frequency, impact and identifying factors. *J Neurol*.

Behrman, A., Light, K., Flynn, S., & Thigpen, M. (2002). Is the functional reach test useful for identifying falls risk among individuals with Parkinson's disease? *Arch Phys Med Rehabil, 83*(4), 538–42.

Bloem B.R., Grimbergen Y.A., Cramer, M., et al. (2000). "Stops walking when talking" does not predict falls in Parkinson's disease. *Ann Neurol, 48*(2), 268.

Bloem, B.R., Grimbergen, Y.A., Cramer, M., Willemsen, M., & Zwinderman, A.H. (2001a). Prospective assessment of falls in Parkinson's disease. *J Neurol, 248*(11), 950–58.

Bloem, B.R., Hausdorff, J.M., Visser, J.E., & Giladi, N. (2004). Falls and freezing of gait in Parkinson's disease: A review of two interconnected, episodic phenomena. *Mov Disord, 19*(8), 871–84.

Bloem, B.R., van Vugt, J.P., & Beckley, D.J. (2001b). Postural instability and falls in Parkinson's disease. *Adv Neurol, 87,* 209–23.

Bond J.M., & Morris, M. (2000). Goal-directed secondary motor tasks: Their effects on gait in subjects with Parkinson disease. *Arch Phys Med Rehabil, 81*(1), 110–16.

Brusse, K.J., Zimdars, S., Zalewski, K.R., & Steffen, T.M. (2005). Testing functional performance in people with Parkinson disease. *Phys Ther, 85*(2), 134–41.

Canning, C.G. (2005). The effect of directing attention during walking under dual-task conditions in Parkinson's disease. *Parkinsonism Relat Disord, 11*(2), 95–99.

Duncan, P.W., Weiner, D.K., Chandler, J., & Studenski, S. (1990). Functional reach: A new clinical measure of balance. *J Gerontol, 45*(6), M192–97.

Frank, J.S., Horak, F.B., & Nutt, J. (2000). Centrally initiated postural adjustments in Parkinsonian patients on and off levodopa. *J Neurophysiol, 84*(5), 2440–48.

Giladi, N., Kao, R., & Fahn, S. (1997). Freezing phenomenon in patients with Parkinsonian syndromes. *Mov Disord, 12*(3), 302–5.

Hausdorff, J.M., Balash, J., & Giladi, N. (2003a). Effects of cognitive challenge on gait variability in patients with Parkinson's disease. *J Geriatr Psychiatry Neurol, 16*(1), 53–58.

Hausdorff, J.M., Schaafsma, J.D., Balash, Y., Bartels, A.L., Gurevich, T., & Giladi, N. (2003b). Impaired regulation of stride variability in Parkinson's disease subjects with freezing of gait. *Exp Brain Res, 149*(2), 187–94.

Jacobs, J.V., & Horak, F.B. (2006). Abnormal proprioceptive-motor integration contributes to hypometric postural responses of subjects with Parkinson's disease. *Neuroscience, 141*(2), 999–1009.

Kirby, R.L., Price, N.A., & MacLeod, D.A. (1987). The influence of foot position on standing balance. *J Biomech, 20*(4), 423–27.

Lim, I., van Wegen, E., de Goede, C., Deutekom, M., Nieuwboer, A., Willems, A., et al. (2005). Effects of external rhythmical cueing on gait in patients with Parkinson's disease: A systematic review. *Clin Rehabil, 19*(7), 695–713.

Lundin-Olsson, L., Nyberg, L., & Gustafson, Y. (1997). "Stops walking when talking" as a predictor of falls in elderly people. *Lancet, 1*(349:617).

Marchese, R., Bove, M., & Abbruzzese, G. (2003). Effect of cognitive and motor tasks on postural stability in Parkinson's disease: A posturographic study. *Mov Disord, 18*(6), 652–58.

Morris, M.E., Matyas, T.A., Iansek, R., & Summers, J.J. (1996). Temporal stability of gait in Parkinson's disease. *Physical Therapy, 76*(7), 763–77; discussion 778–80.

Morris, S., Morris, M.E., & Iansek, R. (2001). Reliability of measurements obtained with the timed "up and go" test in people with Parkinson disease. *Physical Therapy (United States), 81,* 810–18.

Nova, I., Perracini, M., & Ferraz, H. (2004). Levodopa effect upon functional balance of Parkinson's disease patients. *Parkinsonism Relat Disord, October* (10(7)), 411–15.

O'Shea, S., Morris, M.E., & Iansek, R. (Sep 2002). Dual task interference during gait in people with Parkinson disease: Effects of motor versus cognitive secondary tasks. *Physical Therapy (United States), 82,* 888–97.

Pickering, R.M., Grimbergen, Y.A., Rigney, U., Ashburn, A., Mazibrada, G., Wood, B., et al. (2007). A meta-analysis of six prospective studies of falling in Parkinson's disease. *Mov Disord, 22*(13), 1892–1900.

Qutubuddin, A.A., Pegg, P.O., Cifu, D.X., Brown, R., McNamee, S., & Carne, W. (2005). Validating the berg balance scale for patients with Parkinson's disease: A key to rehabilitation evaluation. *Arch Phys Med Rehabil, 86*(4), 789–92.

Rochester, L., Hetherington, V., Jones, D., Nieuwboer, A., Willems, A.M., Kwakkel, G., et al. (2005). The effect of external rhythmic cues (auditory and visual) on walking during a functional task in homes of people with Parkinson's disease. *Arch Phys Med Rehabil, 86*(5), 999–1006.

Rudzinska, M. (2007). Causes of falls in retrospective and prospective study in Parkinson's disease patients. *Parkinsonism Relat Disord, 13*, S175.

Scandalis, T.A., Bosak, A., Berliner, J.C., Helman, L.L., & Wells, M.R. (2001). Resistance training and gait function in patients with Parkinson's disease. *Am J Phys Med Rehabil, 80*(1), 38–43; quiz 44–36.

Schaafsma, J., Giladi, N., Balash, Y., Bartels, A.L., Gurevich, T., & Hausdorff, J.M. (2003). Gait dynamics in Parkinson's disease: Relationship to Parkinsonian features, falls and response to levodopa. *J Neurol Sci, 212*(1–2), 47–53.

Seynnes, O., Fiatarone Singh, M.A., Hue, O., Pras, P., Legros, P., & Bernard, P.L. (2004). Physiological and functional responses to low-moderate versus high-intensity progressive resistance training in frail elders. *J Gerontol A Biol Sci Med Sci, 59*(5), 503–9.

Sgadari, A., Lapane, K.L., Mor, V., Landi, F., Bernabei, R., & Gambassi, G. (2000). Oxidative and nonoxidative benzodiazepines and the risk of femur fracture. The systematic assessment of geriatric drug use via epidemiology study group. *J Clin Psychopharmacol, 20*(2), 234–39.

Smithson, F., Morris, M.E., & Iansek, R. (1998). Performance on clinical tests of balance in Parkinson's disease. *Physical Therapy (United States), 78*(6), 577–92.

Stack, E., Ashburn, A., & Jupp, K. (2006). Strategies used by people with Parkinson's disease who report difficulty turning. *Parkinsonism Relat Disord, 12*(2), 87–92.

Weiner, D.K., Bongiorni, D.R., Studenski, S.A., Duncan, P.W., & Kochersberger, G.G. (1993). Does functional reach improve with rehabilitation? *Arch Phys Med Rehabil, 74*(8), 796–800.

Willems, A.M., Nieuwboer, A., Chavret, F., Desloovere, K., Dom, R., Rochester, L., et al. (2007). Turning in Parkinson's disease patients and controls: The effect of auditory cues. *Mov Disord, 22*(13), 1871–78.

Willemsen, M.D., Grimbergen, Y.A.M., Slabbekoorn, M., Bloem, B.R. (2000). [Falling in Parkinson disease: More often due to postural instability than to environmental factors]. *Ned Tijdschr Geneeskd, 144*(48), 2309–14.

Chapter 9

Huxham, F., Baker, R., Morris, M.E., & Iansek, R. (2008). Footstep adjustments used to turn during walking in Parkinson's disease. *Mov Disord.*

Inkster, L.M., & Eng, J.J. (2004). Postural control during a sit-to-stand task in individuals with mild Parkinson's disease. *Exp Brain Res, 154*(1), 33–38.

Janssen, W.G., Bussmann, H.B., & Stam, H.J. (2002). Determinants of the sit-to-stand movement: A review. *Phys Ther, 82*(9), 866–79.

Kamsma, Y., Brouwer, W., & Lakke, J. (1995). Training of compensatory strategies for impaired gross motor skills in Parkinsons disease. *Physiother Theory Pract*(11), 209–29.

Kirby, R.L., Price, N.A., & MacLeod, D.A. (1987). The influence of foot position on standing balance. *J Biomech, 20*(4), 423–27.

Lord, S.R., Murray, S.M., Chapman, K., Munro, B., & Tiedemann, A. (2002). Sit-to-stand performance depends on sensation, speed, balance, and psychological status in addition to strength in older people. *J Gerontol A Biol Sci Med Sci, 57*(8), M539–43.

Mak, M.K., & Hui-Chan, C.W. (2002). Switching of movement direction is central to Parkinsonian bradykinesia in sit-to-stand. *Mov Disord, 17*(6), 1188–95.

Mak, M.K., & Hui-Chan, C.W. (2005). The speed of sit-to-stand can be modulated in Parkinson's disease. *Clin Neurophysiol, 116*(4), 780–89.

Mak, M.K., Levin, O., Mizrahi, J., & Hui-Chan, C.W. (2003). Joint torques during sit-to-stand in healthy subjects and people with Parkinson's disease. *Clin Biomech (Bristol, Avon), 18*(3), 197–206.

Mourey, F., Grishin, A., d'Athis, P., Pozzo, T., & Stapley, P. (2000). Standing up from a chair as a dynamic equilibrium task: A comparison between young and elderly subjects. *J Gerontol A Biol Sci Med Sci, 55*(9), B425–31.

Pai, Y.C., & Lee, W.A. (1994). Effect of a terminal constraint on control of balance during sit-to-stand. *J Mot Behav, 26*(3), 247–56.

Pai, Y.C., & Rogers, M.W. (1991). Segmental contributions to total body momentum in sit-to-stand. *Med Sci Sports Exerc, 23*(2), 225–30.

Rickli, R., & Jones, J. (2001). *Senior fitness test manual.* Champaign, IL: Human Kinetics.

Schaafsma, J., Balash, Y., Gurevich, T., Bartels, A., Hausdorff, J., & Giladi, N. (2003). Characterization of freezing of gait subtypes and the response of each to levodopa in Parkinson's disease. *Eur J Neurol, 10*(4), 341–48.

Stack, E., Ashburn, A., & Jupp, K. (2006). Strategies used by people with Parkinson's disease who report difficulty turning. *Parkinsonism Relat Disord, 12*(2), 87–92.

Chapter 10

Adamovich, S.V., Berkinblit, M.B., Hening, W., Sage, J., & Poizner, H. (2001). The interaction of visual and proprioceptive inputs in pointing to actual and remembered targets in Parkinson's disease. *Neuroscience, 104*(4), 1027–41.

Bergonzi, P., Chiurulla, C., & Cianchetti, C. (1974). Clinical pharmacology as an approach to the study of biochemical sleep mechanisms: The action of L-dopa. *Confin Neurol,* (36), 5–22.

Bergonzi, P., Chiurulla, C., & Gambi, D. (1975). L-dopa plus dopa-decarboxylase inhibitor. Sleep organization in Parkinson's syndrome before and after treatment. *Acta Neurol Belg,* (75), 5–10.

Jansen, E.N., & Meerwaldt, J.D. (1988). Madopar HBS in Parkinson patients with nocturnal akinesia. *Clin Neurol Neurosurg, 90*(1), 35–39.

Keijsers, N.L., Admiraal, M.A., Cools, A.R., Bloem, B.R., & Gielen, C.C. (2005). Differential progression of proprioceptive and visual information processing deficits in Parkinson's disease. *Eur J Neurosci, 21*(1), 239–48.

Mathias, C.J., & Kimber, J.R. (1998). Treatment of postural hypotension. *J Neurol Neurosurg Psychiatry, 65*(3), 285–89.

Morecraft, R.J., & Hoesen, G.W.V. (1996). Cortical motor systems. In C.M. Fredericks & L.K. Saladin (Eds.), *Pathophysiology of the motor systems: Principles and clinical presentations* (pp. 158–180). Philadelphia: FA Davis.

Praamstra, P., Stegeman, D.F., Cools, A.R., & Horstink, M.W. (1998). Reliance on external cues for movement initiation in Parkinson's disease. Evidence from movement-related potentials. *Brain, 121 (Pt 1),* 167–77.

Rye, D., & Bliwise, D. (2004). Movement disorders specific to sleep and nocturnal manifestations of waking movement disorders. In R. Watts & W.C. Koller (Eds.), *Movement disorders neurologic principles and practice* (2nd ed., pp. 855–90). New York: McGraw-Hill.

Seitz, R., & Roland, P. (1992). Learning of sequential finger movements in man: A combinated kinematic and positron emission tomography (PET) study. *Eur J Neurosci* (4), 154.

Steiger, M.J., Thompson, P.D., & Marsden, C.D. (1996). Disordered axial movement in Parkinson's disease. *J Neurol Neurosurg Psychiatry, 61*(6), 645–48.

Turner, R.S., Grafton, S.T., McIntosh, A.R., DeLong, M.R., & Hoffman, J.M. (2003). The functional anatomy of Parkinsonian bradykinesia. *Neuroimage, 19*(1), 163–79.

Chapter 11

Davey, C., Wiles, R., Ashburn, A., & Murphy, C. (2004). Falling in Parkinson's disease: The impact on informal caregivers. *Disabil Rehabil, 26*(23), 1360–66.

Grimbergen, Y.A., Munneke, M., & Bloem, B.R. (2004). Falls in Parkinson's disease. *Curr Opin Neurol, 17*(4), 405–15.

Sethi, K. (2003). Differential diagnosis of Parkinsonism. In R. Pahwa, K. Lyons, & W. Koller (Eds.), *Handbook of Parkinson's disease* (3rd ed., pp. 43–69). New York: Marcel Dekker.

Williams, D.R., Watt, H.C., & Lees, A.J. (2006). Predictors of falls and fractures in bradykinetic rigid syndromes: A retrospective study. *J Neurol Neurosurg Psychiatry, 77*(4), 468–73.

Chapter 12

Behrman, A.L., Teitelbaum, P., & Cauraugh, J.H. (1998). Verbal instructional sets to normalise the temporal and spatial gait variables in Parkinson's disease. *J Neurol Neurosurg Psychiatry*, 65(4), 580–82.

Blin, O., Ferrandez, A.M., Pailhous, J., & Serratrice, G. (1991). Dopa-sensitive and dopa-resistant gait parameters in Parkinson's disease. *J Neurol Sci*, 103(1), 51–54.

Bloem, B.R., Grimbergen, Y.A., van Dijk, J.G., & Munneke, M. (2006). The "posture second" strategy: A review of wrong priorities in Parkinson's disease. *J Neurol Sci*, 248(1–2), 196–204.

Bohannon, R.W. (1997). Comfortable and maximum walking speed of adults aged 20–79 years: Reference values and determinants. *Age Ageing*, 26(1), 15–19.

Bond, J.M., & Morris, M. (2000). Goal-directed secondary motor tasks: Their effects on gait in subjects with Parkinson disease. *Arch Phys Med Rehabil*, 81(1), 110–16.

Canning, C.G. (2005). The effect of directing attention during walking under dual-task conditions in Parkinson's disease. *Parkinsonism Relat Disord*, 11(2), 95–99.

Dewey, R.B. (2000). Clinical features of Parkinson's disease. In C.H. Adler & J.E. Ahlskog (Eds.), *Parkinson's disease and movement disorders: Diagnosis and treatment guidelines for the practicing physician* (pp. 75). Totowa, NJ: Humana Press.

Hausdorff, J.M., Balash, J., & Giladi, N. (2003a). Effects of cognitive challenge on gait variability in patients with Parkinson's disease. *J Geriatr Psychiatry Neurol*, 16(1), 53–58.

Hausdorff, J.M., Schaafsma, J.D., Balash, Y., Bartels, A.L., Gurevich, T., & Giladi, N. (2003b). Impaired regulation of stride variability in Parkinson's disease subjects with freezing of gait. *Exp Brain Res*, 149(2), 187–94.

Kemoun, G., & Defebvre, L. (2001). Gait disorders in Parkinson disease. Gait freezing and falls: Therapeutic management. *Presse Med*, 30(9), 460–68.

Kimmeskamp, S., & Hennig, E.M. (2001). Heel to toe motion characteristics in Parkinson patients during free walking. *Clin Biomech (Bristol, Avon)*, 16(9), 806–12.

Lim, I., van Wegen, E., de Goede, C., Deutekom, M., Nieuwboer, A., Willems, A., et al. (2005). Effects of external rhythmical cueing on gait in patients with Parkinson's disease: A systematic review. *Clin Rehabil*, 19(7), 695–713.

Morris, M.E., Huxham, F., McGinley, J., Dodd, K., & Iansek, R. (2001). The biomechanics and motor control of gait in Parkinson disease. *Clin Biomech*, 16(Jul), 459–70.

Morris, M.E., Iansek, R., Matyas, T.A., & Summers, J.J. (1996). Stride length regulation in Parkinson's disease. Normalization strategies and underlying mechanisms. *Brain*, 119, 551–68.

Nieuwboer, A., Dom, R., De Weerdt, W., Desloovere, K., Fieuws, S., & Broens-Kaucsik, E. (2001). Abnormalities of the spatiotemporal characteristics of gait at the onset of freezing in Parkinson's disease. *Mov Disord*, 16(6), 1066–75.

Nieuwboer, A., Kwakkel G., Rochester, L., Jones, D., van Wegen, E., Willems, A.M., Chavret, F., Hetherington, V., Baker, K., & Lim, I. (2007). Cueing training in the home improves gait-related mobility in Parkinson's disease: The rescue trial. *J Neurol Neurosurg Psychiatry*, 78(2),111.

Oberg, T., Karsznia, A., & Oberg, K. (1993). Basic gait parameters: Reference data for normal subjects, 10–79 years of age. *J Rehabil Res Dev*, 30(2), 210–23.

O'Shea, S., Morris, M.E., & Iansek, R. (Sep 2002). Dual task interference during gait in people with Parkinson disease: Effects of motor versus cognitive secondary tasks. *Physical Therapy (United States)*, 82, 888–97.

Perry, J. (1992). *Gait analysis normal and pathological function*. Thorofare, NJ: SLACK.

Perry, J., Garrett, M., Gronley, J.K., & Mulroy, S.J. (1995). Classification of walking handicap in the stroke population. *Stroke*, 26(6), 982–89.

Rikli, R., & Jones, C. (2001). *Senior fitness test manual*: Champaign, IL: Human Kinetics.

Rochester, L., Hetherington, V., Jones, D., Nieuwboer, A., Willems, A.M., Kwakkel, G., et al. (2004). Attending to the task: Interference effects of functional tasks on walking in Parkinson's disease and the roles of cognition, depression, fatigue, and balance. *Arch Phys Med Rehabil, 85*(10), 1578–85.

Rochester, L., Hetherington, V., Jones, D., Nieuwboer, A., Willems, A.M., Kwakkel, G., et al. (2005). The effect of external rhythmic cues (auditory and visual) on walking during a functional task in homes of people with Parkinson's disease. *Arch Phys Med Rehabil, 86*(5), 999–1006.

Sofuwa, O., Nieuwboer, A., Desloovere, K., Willems, A.M., Chavret, F., & Jonkers, I. (2005). Quantitative gait analysis in Parkinson's disease: Comparison with a healthy control group. *Arch Phys Med Rehabil, 86*(5), 1007–13.

Steffen, T.M., Hacker, T.A., & Mollinger, L. (2002). Age- and gender-related test performance in community-dwelling elderly people: Six-minute walk test, berg balance scale, timed up & go test, and gait speeds. *Phys Ther, 82*(2), 128–37.

Warshaw, G. (1999). Rehabilitation and the aged. In J.J. Gallo, J. Busby-Whitehead, P.V. Rabins, R.A. Silliman, J.B. Murphy, & W. Reichel (Eds.), *Reichel's care of the elderly: Clinical aspects of aging* (5th ed.). Philadelphia: Lippincott Williams & Wilkins.

Willemsen, M.D., Grimbergen, Y.A.M., Slabbekoorn, M., Bloem, B.R. (2000). [Falling in Parkinson disease: More often due to postural instability than to environmental factors]. *Ned Tijdschr Geneeskd, 144*(48), 2309–14.

Yogev, G., Giladi, N., Peretz, C., Springer, S., Simon, E.S., & Hausdorff, J.M. (2005). Dual tasking, gait rhythmicity, and Parkinson's disease: Which aspects of gait are attention demanding? *Eur J Neurosci, 22*(5), 1248–56.

Chapter 13

Azulay, J.P., Mesure, S., Amblard, B., Blin, O., Sangla, I., & Pouget, J. (1999). Visual control of locomotion in Parkinson's disease. *Brain, 122 (Pt 1)*, 111–20.

Behrman, A.L., Teitelbaum, P., & Cauraugh, J.H. (1998). Verbal instructional sets to normalise the temporal and spatial gait variables in Parkinson's disease. *J Neurol Neurosurg Psychiatry, 65*(4), 580–82.

Coleman, K.J., Raynor, H.R., Mueller, D.M., Cerny, F.J., Dorn, J.M., Epstein, L.H. (1999). Providing sedentary adults with choices for meeting their walking goals. *Prev Med, 28*(5), 510–19.

Hausdorff, J.M., Schaafsma, J.D., Balash, Y., Bartels, A.L., Gurevich, T., & Giladi, N. (2003). Impaired regulation of stride variability in Parkinson's disease subjects with freezing of gait. *Exp Brain Res, 149*(2), 187–94.

Jiang, Y., & Norman, K.E. (2006). Effects of visual and auditory cues on gait initiation in people with Parkinson's disease. *Clin Rehabil, 20*(1), 36–45.

Kemoun, G., & Defebvre, L. (2001). Gait disorders in Parkinson disease. Gait freezing and falls: Therapeutic management. *Presse Med, 30*(9), 460–68.

Kompoliti, K., Goetz, C.G., Leurgans, S., Morrissey, M., Siegel, I.M. (2000). "On" freezing in Parkinson's disease: Resistance to visual cue walking devices. *Mov Disord, 15*(2), 309–12.

Lehman, D., Took, T., Lofald, D., & Hirsch, M. (2005). Training with verbal instructional cues results in near-term improvement of gait in people with Parkinson's disease. *Journal of Neurological Physical Therapy, 29*(1), 1-8.

Lim, I., van Wegen, E., de Goede, C., Deutekom, M., Nieuwboer, A., Willems, A., et al. (2005). Effects of external rhythmical cueing on gait in patients with Parkinson's disease: A systematic review. *Clin Rehabil, 19*(7), 695–713.

McIntosh, G.C., Brown, S.H., Rice, R.R., & Thaut, M.H. (1997). Rhythmic auditory-motor facilitation of gait patterns in patients with Parkinson's disease. *J Neurol Neurosurg Psychiatry, 62*(1), 22–26.

McIntosh, G.C., Rice, R.R., Hurt, C.P., & Thaut, M.H. (1998). Long-term training effects of rhythmic auditory stimulation on gait in patients with Parkinson's disease. *Movement Disorders, 13 (suppl 2)*.

Miller, R.A., Thaut, M.H., McIntosh, G.C., & Rice, R.R. (1996). Components of EMG symmetry and variability in Parkinsonian and healthy elderly gait. *Electroencephalogr Clin Neurophysiol, 101*(1), 1–7.

Nieuwboer, A., Dom, R., De Weerdt, W., Desloovere, K., Janssens, L., & Stijn, V. (2004a). Electromyographic profiles of gait prior to onset of freezing episodes in patients with Parkinson's disease. *Brain, 127*(Pt 7), 1650–60.

Nieuwboer, A., Kwakkel G., Rochester, L., Jones, D., van Wegen, E., Willems, A.M., Chavret, F., Hetherington, V., Baker, K., & Lim, I. (2007). Cueing training in the home improves gait-related mobility in Parkinson's disease: The rescue trial. *J Neurol Neurosurg Psychiatry, 78*(2), 111.

Nieuwboer, A., Williams, A., Chavret, F., Kwakkel G, Jones, D., & Dom, R. (2004b). Synchronising walking to various auditory cueing frequencies: Differences between freezers and nonfreezers with Parkinson's disease, *Movement Disorders Conference*. Rome: The Rescue Project/Consortium, copyright 10 Sept 2004.

Perry, J. (1992). *Gait analysis normal and pathological function*. Thorofare, NJ: SLACK.

Physical activity and health: A report of the surgeon general. (1996). Recommendations from the Centers for Disease Control and Prevention, the American College of Sports Medicine and the American Heart Association.

Rochester, L., Hetherington, V., Jones, D., Nieuwboer, A., Willems, A.M., Kwakkel, G., et al. (2005). The effect of external rhythmic cues (auditory and visual) on walking during a functional task in homes of people with Parkinson's disease. *Arch Phys Med Rehabil, 86*(5), 999–1006.

Sabate, M., Gonzalez, I., Ruperez, F., & Rodriguez, M. (1996). Obstructive and restrictive pulmonary dysfunctions in Parkinson's disease. *J Neurol Sci, 138*(1–2), 114–19.

Skinner, R.D., Homma, Y., & Garcia-Rill, E. (2004). Arousal mechanisms related to posture and locomotion: 2. Ascending modulation. *Prog Brain Res, 143*, 291–98.

Suteerawattananon, M., Morris, G.S., Etnyre, B.R., Jankovic, J., & Protas, E.J. (2004). Effects of visual and auditory cues on gait in individuals with Parkinson's disease. *J Neurol Sci, 219*(1–2), 63–69.

Thaut, M.H. (2005). *Rhythm, music, and the brain: Scientific foundations and clinical applications*. New York: Taylor & Francis Group.

Thaut, M.H., Kenyon, G.P., Schauer, M.L., & McIntosh, G.C. (1999). The connection between rhythmicity and brain function. *IEEE Engineering in Medicine and Biology, 0739–5175* (March/April), 101–8.

Thaut, M.H., McIntosh, G.C., Rice, R.R., Miller, R.A., Rathbun, J., & Brault, J.M. (1996). Rhythmic auditory stimulation in gait training for Parkinson's disease patients. *Mov Disord, 11*(2), 193–200.

Thaut, M.H., Rathbun, J.A., & Miller, R.A. (1997). Music versus metronome timekeeper in a rhythmic motor task. *International Journal of Arts Medicine, 5*(1), 4–12.

Willems, A.M., Nieuwboer, A., Chavret, F., Desloovere, K., Dom, R., Rochester, L., et al. (2006). The use of rhythmic auditory cues to influence gait in patients with Parkinson's disease, the differential effect for freezers and non-freezers, an explorative study. *Disabil Rehabil, 28*(11), 721–28.

Chapter 14

Albani, G., Sandrini, G., Kunig, G., Martin-Soelch, C., Mauro, A., Pignatti, R., et al. (2003). Differences in the EMG pattern of leg muscle activation during locomotion in Parkinson's disease. *Funct Neurol, 18*(3), 165–70.

Atchison, P.R., Thompson, P.D., Frackowiak, R.S., & Marsden, C.D. (1993). The syndrome of gait ignition failure: A report of six cases. *Mov Disord, 8*(3), 285–92.

Burleigh-Jacobs, A., Horak, F.B., Nutt, J.G., & Obeso, J.A. (1997). Step initiation in Parkinson's disease: Influence of levodopa and external sensory triggers. *Mov Disord, 12*(2), 206–15.

Davis, J.T., Lyons, K.E., & Pahwa, R. (2005). Freezing of gait after bilateral subthalamic nucleus stimulation for Parkinson's disease. *Clin Neurol Neurosurg*.

del Olmo, M.F., & Cudeiro, J. (2005). Temporal variability of gait in Parkinson disease: Effects of a rehabilitation programme based on rhythmic sound cues. *Parkinsonism Relat Disord, 11*(1), 25–33.

Dietz, M.A., Goetz, C.G., & Stebbins, G.T. (1990). Evaluation of a modified inverted walking stick as a treatment for Parkinsonian freezing episodes. *Mov Disord, 5*(3), 243–47.

Fahn, S. (1995). The freezing phenomenon in Parkinsonism. *Adv Neurol*(67), 53–63.

Gantchev, N., Viallet, F., Aurenty, R., & Massion, J. (1996). Impairment of posturokinetic co-ordination during initiation of forward oriented stepping movements in Parkinsonian patients. *Electroencephalogr Clin Neurophysiol, 101*(2), 110–20.

Giladi, N., Kao, R., & Fahn, S. (1997). Freezing phenomenon in patients with Parkinsonian syndromes. *Mov Disord, 12*(3), 302–5.

Giladi, N., McDermott, M.P., Fahn, S., Przedborski, S., Jankovic, J., Stern, M., et al. (2001). Freezing of gait in PD: Prospective assessment in the datatop cohort. *Neurology, 56*(12), 1712–21.

Giladi, N., McMahon, D., Przedborski, S., Flaster, E., Guillory, S., Kostic, V., et al. (1992). Motor blocks in Parkinson's disease. *Neurology, 42*(2), 333–39.

Giladi, N., Shabtai, H., Simon, E.S., Biran, S., Tal, J., & Korczyn, A.D. (2000). Construction of freezing of gait questionnaire for patients with Parkinsonism. *Parkinsonism Relat Disord, 6*(3), 165–70.

Halliday, S.E., Winter, D.A., Frank, J.S., Patla, A.E., & Prince, F. (1998). The initiation of gait in young, elderly, and Parkinson's disease subjects. *Gait Posture, 8*(1), 8–14.

Hass, C.J., Waddell, D.E., Fleming, R.P., Juncos, J.L., & Gregor, R.J. (2005). Gait initiation and dynamic balance control in Parkinson's disease. *Arch Phys Med Rehabil, 86*(11), 2172–76.

Hausdorff, J.M., Schaafsma, J.D., Balash, Y., Bartels, A.L., Gurevich, T., & Giladi, N. (2003). Impaired regulation of stride variability in Parkinson's disease subjects with freezing of gait. *Exp Brain Res, 149*(2), 187–94.

Jiang, Y., & Norman, K.E. (2006). Effects of visual and auditory cues on gait initiation in people with Parkinson's disease. *Clin Rehabil, 20*(1), 36–45.

Kompoliti, K., Goetz, C.G., Leurgans, S., Morrissey, M., Siegel, I.M. (2000). "On" freezing in Parkinson's disease: Resistance to visual cue walking devices. *Mov Disord, 15*(2), 309–12.

McIntosh, G.C., Brown, S.H., Rice, R.R., & Thaut, M.H. (1997). Rhythmic auditory-motor facilitation of gait patterns in patients with Parkinson's disease. *J Neurol Neurosurg Psychiatry, 62*(1), 22–26.

McIntosh, G.C., Rice, R.R., Hurt, C.P., & Thaut, M.H. (1998). Long-term training effects of rhythmic auditory stimulation on gait in patients with Parkinson's disease. *Movement Disorders, 13 (suppl 2)*.

Michalowska, M., Fiszer, U., Krygowska-Wajs, A., & Owczarek, K. (2005). Falls in Parkinson's disease. Causes and impact on patients' quality of life. *Funct Neurol, 20*(4), 163–68.

Nieuwboer, A., De Weerdt, W., Dom, R., & Lesaffre, E. (1998). A frequency and correlation analysis of motor deficits in Parkinson patients. *Disabil Rehabil, 20*(4), 142–50.

Nieuwboer, A., Dom, R., De Weerdt, W., Desloovere, K., Fieuws, S., & Broens-Kaucsik, E. (2001). Abnormalities of the spatiotemporal characteristics of gait at the onset of freezing in Parkinson's disease. *Mov Disord, 16*(6), 1066–75.

Nieuwboer, A., Dom, R., De Weerdt, W., Desloovere, K., Janssens, L., & Stijn, V. (2004). Electromyographic profiles of gait prior to onset of freezing episodes in patients with Parkinson's disease. *Brain, 127*(Pt 7), 1650–60.

Nieuwboer, A., Kwakkel G., Rochester, L., Jones, D., van Wegen, E., Willems, A.M., Chavret, F., Hetherington, V., Baker, K., & Lim, I. (2007). Cueing training in the home improves gait-related mobility in Parkinson's disease: The rescue trial. *J Neurol Neurosurg Psychiatry, 78*(2), 111.

Plotnik, M., Giladi, N., Balash, Y., Peretz, C., & Hausdorff, J.M. (2005). Is freezing of gait in Parkinson's disease related to asymmetric motor function? *Ann Neurol, 57*(5), 656–63.

Schaafsma, J., Balash, Y., Gurevich, T., Bartels, A., Hausdorff, J., & Giladi, N. (2003). Characterization of freezing of gait subtypes and the response of each to levodopa in Parkinson's disease. *Eur J Neurol, 10*(4), 341–48.

Shumway-Cook, A., & Woollacott, M. (2001). *Motor control: Theory and practical applications* (2nd ed.). Baltimore: Lippincott Williams & Wilkins.

Sibon, I., & Tison, F. (2004). Vascular Parkinsonism. *Curr Opin Neurol, 17*(1), 49–54.

Thaut, M.H., Kenyon, G.P., Schauer, M.L., & McIntosh, G.C. (1999). The connection between rhythmicity and brain function. *IEEE Engineering in Medicine and Biology, 0739–5175* (March/April), 101–8.

Chapter 15

Bloem, B.R., Hausdorff, J.M., Visser, J.E., & Giladi, N. (2004). Falls and freezing of gait in Parkinson's disease: A review of two interconnected, episodic phenomena. *Mov Disord, 19*(8), 871–84.

Crenna, P., Carpinella, I., Rabuffetti, M., Calabrese, E., Mazzoleni, P., Nemni, R., et al. (2007). The association between impaired turning and normal straight walking in Parkinson's disease. *Gait Posture, 26*(2), 172–78.

Dimitrova, D., Horak, F.B., & Nutt, J.G. (2004). Postural muscle responses to multidirectional translations in patients with Parkinson's disease. *J Neurophysiol, 91*(1), 489–501.

Ferrarin, M., Carpinella, I., Rabuffetti, M., Calabrese, E., Mazzoleni, P., & Nemni, R. (2006). Locomotor disorders in patients at early stages of Parkinson's disease: A quantitative analysis. *Conf Proc IEEE Eng Med Biol Soc, 1*, 1224–27.

Huxham, F., Baker, R., Morris, M.E., & Iansek, R. (2008). Footstep adjustments used to turn during walking in Parkinson's disease. *Mov Disord.*

Morris, M.E., Huxham, F., McGinley, J., Dodd, K., & Iansek, R. (2001). The biomechanics and motor control of gait in Parkinson disease. *Clin Biomech, 16*(Jul), 459–70.

Pai, Y.C., Maki, B.E., Iqbal, K., McIlroy, W.E., & Perry, S.D. (2000). Thresholds for step initiation induced by support-surface translation: A dynamic center-of-mass model provides much better prediction than a static model. *J Biomech, 33*(3), 387–92.

Rogers, M.W., & Mille, M.L. (2003). Lateral stability and falls in older people. *Exerc Sport Sci Rev, 31*(4), 182–87.

Schaafsma, J., Balash, Y., Gurevich, T., Bartels, A., Hausdorff, J., & Giladi, N. (2003). Characterization of freezing of gait subtypes and the response of each to levodopa in Parkinson's disease. *Eur J Neurol, 10*(4), 341–48.

Stack, E., Ashburn, A., & Jupp, K. (2006). Strategies used by people with Parkinson's disease who report difficulty turning. *Parkinsonism Relat Disord, 12*(2), 87–92.

Willems, A.M., Nieuwboer, A., Chavret, F., Desloovere, K., Dom, R., Rochester, L., et al. (2007). Turning in Parkinson's disease patients and controls: The effect of auditory cues. *Mov Disord, 22*(13), 1871–78.

Willemsen, M.D., Grimbergen, Y.A.M., Slabbekoorn, M., Bloem, B.R. (2000). [Falling in Parkinson disease: More often due to postural instability than to environmental factors]. *Ned Tijdschr Geneeskd, 144*(48), 2309–14.

Chapter 16

Bateni, H., Zecevic, A., McIlroy, W.E., & Maki, B.E. (2004). Resolving conflicts in task demands during balance recovery: Does holding an object inhibit compensatory grasping? *Exp Brain Res, 157*(1), 49–58.

Dunne, R.G., Bergman, A.B., Rogers, L.W., Inglin, B., & Rivara, F.P. (1993). Elderly persons' attitudes towards footwear—a factor in preventing falls. *Public Health Rep, 108*(2), 245–48.

Kimmeskamp, S., & Hennig, E.M. (2001). Heel to toe motion characteristics in Parkinson patients during free walking. *Clin Biomech (Bristol, Avon), 16*(9), 806–12.

Tencer, A.F., Koepsell, T.D., Wolf, M.E., Frankenfeld, C.L., Buchner, D.M., Kukull, W.A., et al. (2004). Biomechanical properties of shoes and risk of falls in older adults. *J Am Geriatr Soc, 52*(11), 1840–46.

Warshaw, G. (1999). Rehabilitation and the aged. In J.J. Gallo, J. Busby-Whitehead, P.V. Rabins, R.A. Silliman, J.B. Murphy, & W. Reichel (Eds.), *Reichel's care of the elderly: Clinical aspects of aging* (5th ed.). Philadelphia: Lippincott Williams & Wilkins.

Appendix A

Fahn, S., Elton, R.L., & UPDRS Development Committee. (1987). Unified Parkinson's Disease Rating Scale. In S. Fahn, C. Marsden, D. Calne, & M. Goldstein (Eds.), *Recent developments in Parkinson's disease* (Vol. 2, pp. 153–64). Florham Park, NJ: Macmillan Health Care Information.

Giladi, N., Shabtai, H., Simon, E.S., Biran, S., Tal, J., & Korczyn, A.D. (2000). Construction of freezing of gait questionnaire for patients with Parkinsonism. *Parkinsonism Relat Disord, 6*(3), 165–70.

Hoehn, M.M, & Yahr, M.D. (1967). Parkinsonism: Onset, progression and mortality. *Neurology, 17*(5),427–42.

Jenkinson, C., Fitzpatrick, R., Peto, V., Greenhall, R., & Hyman, N. (1997). The Parkinson's Disease Questionnaire (PDQ-39): Development and validation of a Parkinson's disease summary index score. *Age Ageing, 26*(5), 353–57.

Schwab, R.S., & England, A.C. (1969). Projection technique for evaluating surgery in Parkinson's disease. In F.J. Gillingham & I.M.L. Donaldson (Eds.), *Third symposium on Parkinson's disease* (pp. 152–157). Edinburgh: Livingstone.

Appendix B

Berg, K.O., Maki, B.E., Williams, J.I., Holliday, P.J., & Wood Dauphinee, S.L. (1992a). Clinical and laboratory measures of postural balance in an elderly population. *Arch Phys Med Rehabil, 73*(11), 1073–80.

Berg, K., Wood-Dauphinee, S., & Williams, J.I. (1995). The balance scale: Reliability assessment with elderly residents and patients with an acute stroke. *Scand J Rehabil Med, 27*(1), 27–36.

Berg, K.O., Wood-Dauphinee, S.L., Williams, J.I., & Maki, B. (1992b). Measuring balance in the elderly: Validation of an instrument. *Can J Public Health, 83 Suppl 2*, S7–11.

Duncan, P.W., Weiner, D.K., Chandler, J., & Studenski, S. (1990). Functional reach: A new clinical measure of balance. *J Gerontol, 45*(6), M192–97.

Podsiadlo, D., & Richardson, S. (1991). The timed "up & go": A test of basic functional mobility for frail elderly persons. *J Am Geriatr Soc, 39*(2), 142–48.

Rickli, R., & Jones, J. (2001). *Senior fitness test manual*. Champaign, IL: Human Kinetics.

Index

Note: The italicized *f* and *t* following page numbers refer to figures and tables, respectively.

About the Author

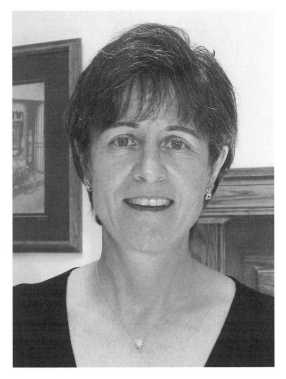

Miriam P. Boelen, PT, has been a licensed physical therapist for 31 years and currently is senior staff physical therapist at NorthShore University HealthSystem/Glenbrook Hospital in Glenview, Illinois. As a movement disorder specialist since 1990, she has worked with patients in all stages of Parkinson's disease and those with implanted deep brain stimulators. Boelen has lectured extensively on issues related to the physical management of Parkinson's disease, including exercise, walking aids, caregiver instruction, and education. She has also taught patients how to regain a sense of control over their physical capabilities while clearing up misconceptions and allowing for renewed hope.

Boelen is a member of the American Physical Therapy Association and the American College of Sports Medicine. She wrote an article on the role of rehabilitative modalities and exercise in Parkinson's disease that was published in *Disease-a-Month*. She earned a B.S. in physical therapy from the University of Health Sciences at the Chicago Medical School and is certified by the American College of Sports Medicine as a health fitness specialist.